*Savage*

*1991.*

# Principles of Hand Surgery

# Principles of Hand Surgery

**F. D. Burke** MBBS FRCS
Consultant Orthopaedic and Hand Surgeon,
Derbyshire Royal Infirmary,
Derby, UK

**D. A. McGrouther** MSc MD (Hons) FRCS
Professor of Plastic and Reconstructive Surgery,
University College Hospital,
London, UK

**P. J. Smith** MB BS FRCS
Consultant Plastic and Hand Surgeon,
Mount Vernon Hospital,
Middlesex;
The Hospital for Sick Children,
Great Ormond Street,
London, UK

Foreword by
**H. E. Kleinert**

CHURCHILL LIVINGSTONE
EDINBURGH LONDON MELBOURNE AND NEW YORK 1990

CHURCHILL LIVINGSTONE
Medical Division of Longman Group UK Limited

Distributed in the United States of America by
Churchill Livingstone Inc., 1560 Broadway, New York,
N.Y. 10036, and by associated companies, branches
and representatives throughout the world.

First published 1990

ISBN 0–443–03466–4

**British Library Cataloguing in Publication Data**
Burke, F. D.
    Principles of hand surgery
    1. Man. Hands: Surgery
    I. Title   II. McGrouther, D. A. (Duncan
Angus)   III. Smith, P. J.
    617′.575059

**Library of Congress Cataloging in Publication Data**
Burke, F. D.
    Principles of hand surgery.
    1. Hand—Surgery.   I. McGrouther, D. A.   II. Smith,
P. J. (Paul John) III. Title.   [DNLM: 1. Hand—surgery.
WE 830 B959p]
RD559.B86      1990      617′.575059      88–35268

Produced by Longman Singapore Publishers (Pte) Ltd.
Printed in Singapore.

# Foreword

Hand surgery as a specialty in America, developed during and immediately after World War II under the guidance and stimulation of Sterling Bunnell.

The basic principles he established and recorded were accepted by all hand surgeons and served as a guide for at least 20 years. With the introduction of magnification, as stated in this book, the eye provided the brain with a more precise, detailed image which, in turn, directed the surgeon's hand to a new and more precise, detailed correction of our most magnificent tool, the hand, in both injury and disease.

The authors, representing a new generation of hand surgeons trained with the established hand surgery principles as well as surgery under magnification, have, after years of personal experience provided us with an overview of present-day hand surgery.

The practising hand surgeon must be familiar with all this information and be able to combine it with a knowledge of anatomy and biomechanics unheard of 20 years ago and then be able to apply it to the treatment of patients. A look at recent hand surgery reveals an expanding library of research, diagnoses and techniques all important in the improved treatment of patients. The plethora of detailed technical information available today permits us to correct and restore function in previously hopeless situations.

Drs Burke, McGrouther and Smith have drawn on years of practical clinical experience and personal research to enable them to present us an overview of not just the 'how' of hand surgery, but more importantly the 'when' and 'why'.

With the understanding of the principles of hand and microsurgery they have emphasised the importance of proper assessment, the application of up-to-date technical knowledge for diagnosis and treatment and the necessary rehabilitation to obtain maximum function and cosmesis.

It was a pleasure for me to read, to write a foreword, and to recommend this excellent book to the trainee and the experienced surgeon.

Louisville, Kentucky          Harold E. Kleinert, MD

# Preface

In this book, we have attempted to fuse the philosophical approaches of three different surgeons. *Principles of Hand Surgery* has been born out of a desire to produce a book for surgeons in training, which explains the concepts underlying the management of hand injuries or abnormalities. It attempts to cover the 'why' rather than the 'how', although it is inevitable that a certain amount of the latter is included. We hope that we are helping trainees to think about the principles of hand surgery rather than the practicalities of how to operate. Techniques are often transient, but principles rarely change. We have chosen to leave the chapters unreferenced, believing that principles are derived from many sources and cannot readily be attributed to a single publication. The contents should serve as an introduction to hand surgery and must be supplemented by wider reading of text books and journals. Theoretical knowledge must always be complemented by sound clinical and operative experience under the guidance of a knowledgeable surgeon.

The book is aimed principally at the surgeon who wishes to learn surgery of the hand and is concise enough to be read in a few evenings. We hope, however, that it will also be considered on other levels, being stimulating or provocative to the experienced hand surgeon, and also valuable to hand therapists, who play such an important role in our speciality. Surgery is but one small episode in the total care of the patient. The importance of rehabilitation is underlined by its position in Chapter 2 rather than being relegated (as is more usual) to the final pages.

The text is a mixture of the strengths and frailties of the three authors. The principal author of each chapter has submitted his draft to simultaneous cross-examination and discussion by his co-authors. The process has been repeated at frequent meetings and some chapters have required 12 or 13 revisions. Each chapter was debated, to arrive at a set of principles acceptable to all three authors. There has been no predominance of one philosophy, intellect or effort and the final result is a true amalgam of the three authors' attitudes. Alphabetical order of authorship has been used for this reason.

Many practices are based more on tradition than well researched literature. We have been obliged during our discussions to justify our attitudes, and this has often resulted in the development of a fresh approach. The writing of this book has been an educational experience for us and we hope it will prove as informative and stimulating for the reader.

Derby, Glasgow, London 1990        F.D.B.
D.A.M.
P.J.S.

# ACKNOWLEDGEMENTS

## F.D.B.

My thanks to David Brown for his teaching skills and enthusiasm which developed my interest in orthopaedics. For his surgical skill in the repair of a ruptured profundus tendon, with the subsequent brutal realisation that finger mobility, once lost, is only regained by personal commitment, and in this case, by the very special expertise of a physiotherapist, Mrs Biddy Sherwin.

To George Brewis for career advice ('when in doubt aim high'), and to Brian O'Connor for permitting a somewhat unbalanced orthopaedic training programme to favour hand surgery, and for his continuing support of the Derby Hand Unit.

To Harold Kleinert for an understanding of the management of the injured hand and Adrian Flatt for an appreciation of the very specialised requirements of the rheumatoid patient.

To John Varian for his guidance during my early years in Derby and to my colleague Peter Lunn, our residents, therapists and secretaries for making work a pleasure. Particular thanks to my wife, Linda, for all her efforts related to the book, hosting visits and tolerating absences.

## D.A.M.

I am grateful to the many teachers who have encouraged my interest in surgery of the hand, especially Maurice Kinmonth, Ian Jackson, Graham Lister and Ian McGregor. They have each set high standards in technical surgery, in judgement and philosophy.

Many of my own trainees have contributed to the management of cases illustrated and their enthusiasm has continued to be a source of inspiration.

My wife Sandy and my children, Jill and Gordon, have waited patiently during the many wanderings necessitated by the debates over *Principles of Hand Surgery*.

## P.J.S.

To my father, for stimulating my interest in medicine. To Harry Jones in the Sunderland Royal Infirmary for directing me towards surgery and to Athol Parkes for showing me the sphere of hand surgery. To David Hamblen for being interested in my career and providing guidance and to Campbell Semple in the same department, for teaching me how to suture tendons and showing me how to organise a hand surgery service. To Ian McGregor for his enthusiasm and analytical comments and for pointing me in the direction of plastic surgery. To Ian Jackson for his timely intervention and career guidance and to Stewart Harrison for taking me under his wing. To Harold Kleinert, who then took over, along with all of his colleagues in Louisville, and who confirmed and stimulated my interest in hand surgery. To Graham Lister for his great example that we all try to copy. For his support during the whole of my career and his guidance, and in particular for his teaching. To my wife Anne and to my children Mark, Jaime, Victoria and Francesca, who have perhaps made the greatest sacrifices in the writing of this book. Without their support, it would never have been completed.

Our grateful thanks to our secretaries who have been involved in the preparation of the drafts—Moira Warren, Jean Leiper, Jackie Olive, Gill Lock and Elsa Gordon; our respective hospital photographers—Barry Wilkes, Margaret Murray and Ron Blake. Thanks also to Alan Poole for proof reading the final drafts. We are particularly grateful to Patrick Elliott for his excellent illustrations to the book.

# Contents

# 1. Introduction

*Principal author: P. J. Smith*

The hand is a unique mobile sensor and effector mechanism — its integrated function being ideally suited to exploring a hostile environment. In appreciation and control the hand has a dual relationship with the brain. As sensor it is the brain's master. As effector, its obedient servant, responding instantaneously to commands. This mechanism stretches from cortex to fingertip, from the conceptual to the practical. Such functional sophistication is reflected in the anatomical density which renders it particularly vulnerable to the insults and abuses of everyday life. It is a curious paradox of nature that evolution has provided our species with hands whose motor skills exceed the performance of the human eye. The hand is capable of such fine precision of movement that the eye can neither see nor control it unaided. Magnification may be necessary for us to exert such control, and fully utilise such precision skills, which can permit surgery at a cellular level.

The dynamic integration between sensor and effector actions is so complete that sensation cannot properly be interpreted by stiff and immobile fingers. Rapid movements, which are quite subconscious, are necessary to appreciate texture and contour change. Such movements provide alternating sensory data allowing the central appreciation of three-dimensional relationships. The fingertips are capable of 'feeling all' and 'knowing all'. Such conceptual appreciation of sensation is tactile gnosis: it produces an *instantaneous* appropriate motor response.

The sensory perception of the hand may be heightened when called upon to substitute for deficient special senses. The blind may read braille using their fingertips, which contain a dense network of peripheral receptors monitored by a large area of sensory cortex. The posture and movement of the human hand convey a wealth of information in a subtle and silent fashion and may be used to substitute for speech, or to emphasise it by gestures which transcend language difficulties.

The hand surgeon, contemplating interfering with so complex a mechanism, must make a logical assessment based on the history and physical findings to localise the site of the lesion. A profound knowledge of anatomy is essential. The patient's psychological status and determination to overcome his disability are as important as the assessment of the more distal mechanical problem.

Following such careful assessment, operative intervention must be precise. The delicate mechanisms of the hand are easily disturbed and surgery must therefore be gentle. Poor technique will manifest itself in prolonged morbidity or failure of the procedure. By contrast, purposeful intervention, performed with care, will lead to a rapid resolution of symptoms and a shorter rehabilitation period.

Operative treatment is only part of the overall care of a patient with a hand problem. It must be preceded by a sound judgement and followed by appropriate rehabilitation to return the hand to its normal automatic functions. There are thus three elements in hand surgery:

1. Assessment.
2. Surgical technique.
3. Rehabilitation.

The quality of the patient's recovery will reflect the surgeon's attention to all three areas. Perhaps in no other sphere of surgery is the final result more dependent upon the degree of skill that the surgeon imparts to the treatment of his patient. The hand is an area of unique surgical challenge.

## INITIAL ASSESSMENT

It is always preferable for the initial assessment to be undertaken by an experienced hand surgeon, particularly in the management of complex and difficult problems. This inspires confidence and establishes rapport with the patient. The general health of the patient, his motivation and personal circumstances must be considered before formulating a treatment plan. The surgeon's recommendations must be balanced against the patient's requirements. Limitation of locally available facilities may necessitate secondary referral in order to obtain the best results for the patient.

A careful history should always be taken specifically to elicit the details that are likely to influence treatment. The patient's age, sex, occupation, hand dominance, hobbies and interests should be noted. An assessment of general health and ability to co-operate with rehabilitation should be undertaken. The dramatic mechanism of presentation of many hand injuries can serve to distract the examiner from important associated injuries. It is necessary to exclude concomitant serious injury before proceeding to detailed examination or treatment of the hand. Detailed information about the precise mechanism of injury is essential. This will indicate whether the tissues have been incised, crushed, avulsed, degloved or burned.

The patient with an injured hand is apprehensive and in pain. The examination should be thorough, but expeditious, and cause no additional discomfort. If wound exploration is indicated, it should always be undertaken in theatre under tourniquet control, with adequate lighting and fine instrumentation. Blunt probing in the casualty department serves only to add to the patient's anxiety, contributes little to the surgeon's knowledge and may inflict further injury. Troublesome haemorrhage may be controlled by elevation and the use of a padded pressure dressing. An artery clamp must never be blindly applied in such circumstances. Attempts to clamp a bleeding ulnar artery in this way may result in damage to the ulnar nerve.

The examination of the injured hand should answer five questions:

1. Is the viability of the hand or digit in doubt?
2. Is the skeleton stable?
3. Is there an associated nerve injury?
4. Is there evidence of tendon damage?
5. Is there actual or impending skin loss?

These questions can be answered briefly by inspection of the skin colour, the use of high-quality radiographs in two planes, the plastic pen test and the tenodesis test. A rapid examination will indicate the sort of complexity of procedure that is going to be necessary in theatre. It should be emphasised that in such cases the definitive examination is surgical exploration. Examination of the non-traumatised patient is quite different and a detailed examination should be undertaken as described in Chapter 20.

## SURGICAL TECHNIQUE

Surgical exploration requires organised supporting facilities. Fine instruments appropriate to the size of the structures which are being operated upon are necessary (Fig. 1.1). An adequate hand table with a stable base is essential, as many procedures now require microsurgical reconstruction. Magnifying loupes should be used and an operating microscope should be available if there is any question of revascularisation or nerve repair. In centres where replantation is undertaken, a theatre should be permanently available for the immediate exploration of amputated digits or re-exploration of previously revascularised digits. Rapid surgical assessment should be possible and replantation commenced without delay. Support from the anaesthetic department in the provision of general anaesthesia and regional nerve block anaesthesia is essential. The trauma patient is an unknown quantity and deserves the supervision of his vital functions when nerve block anaesthesia is undertaken. In supraclavicular blocks, an inadvertent high spinal anaesthetic may be given, resulting in cessation of respiration. A skilled anaesthetist should always be available. In general, intravenous Bier's blocks do not provide a satisfactory operative field and are potentially hazardous if the

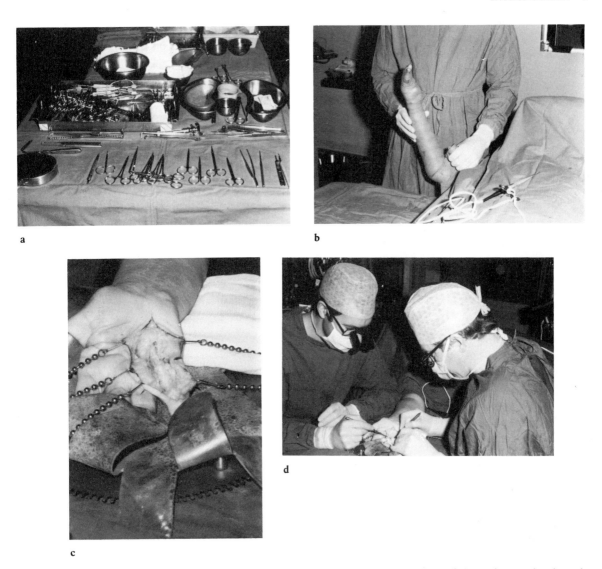

**Fig. 1.1** **a** Refined instruments are essential in atraumatic hand surgery. **b** An adequately applied tourniquet and eschmarch bandage is used to exsanguinate the limb to allow a bloodless field. **c** The use of the lead hand and special retractors allows adequate exposure and enables the assistant to assist the surgeon rather than simply retract. **d** Adequate illumination and magnification are essential

tourniquet should deflate. If the tourniquet requires release prior to wound closure, such a technique cannot be applied. The majority of hand operations may be undertaken under brachial or axillary blocks. The use of an adequate tourniquet is essential. The tourniquet should, by choice, be attached to an air cylinder to allow steady pressure control. It should be standardised at least once every week. Excessive and prolonged pressure may lead to nerve palsies. After the limb has undergone normal surgical preparation prior to surgery, it is advisable for the wound to be subjected to pulsatile lavage (Fig. 1.2). This mechanically irrigates the tissues, removing dirt and contaminants and thereby reducing the quantitative bacteriological count. Three to five minutes should be spent using this technique at the beginning of surgery on every traumatic case.

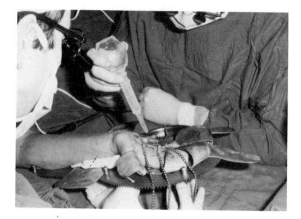

**Fig. 1.2** Pulsatile lavage is used to cleanse debris from contaminated wounds prior to the commencement of surgical treatment, or to remove blood clots following haemostasis at the end of a routine operative procedure

At the same time all blood clots should be removed from the wound with the gloved finger. Upon completion of this procedure, wound débridement may be required if indicated by the nature of the injury.

### Incisions and extension of existing wounds

In planning incisions or extensions of wounds in the hand, care must be taken to ensure that the resulting scars do not produce contractures. Particular attention should be paid to designing the scars so that they do not cross flexion creases at right angles and are placed in areas of the hand where skin movement is at its mimimum. In general the zig-zag approach of Bruner or midlateral incisions satisfy these requirements (see Ch. 3). The Bruner incision allows adequate exposure of the tendon sheath and the neurovascular bundles, which lie protected in their subcutaneous fat, at the base of the reflected flaps. In long, thin fingers however, such incisions tend to become straight with advancing time and a mini Bruner may then be used to avoid this situation. When performing a midlateral incision, the neurovascular bundle may either be elevated along with the flap, or be left on the digit and not incorporated into the flap. Both techniques inevitably produce a certain amount of local denervation. Skin flaps and skin grafts should comply with the neutral lines when applied to digits and should not

parallel a web space, or cross flexion creases. To do so will invite a flexion contracture or web space constriction at a later date.

### The timing of repair

There are widely differing philosophical approaches in the management of upper limb injuries. At one end of the spectrum lies the 'Everest' philosophy, in which everything is repaired primarily 'because it is there'. At the other end of the spectrum there is the philosophy of masterly inactivity in which nothing is primarily repaired, wound closure may or may not be achieved, and the hand is simply elevated and observed. The state of the wound may force such decisions. An experienced surgeon will form a balanced judgement between these extreme policies. The more complex the injury the more important is this judgement. Historically there have been three philosophical approaches in the development of hand surgery:

1. Secondary repair of nerves and tendons.
2. Primary repair of all structures.
3. A balanced view where the role of primary and secondary reconstruction is recognised. The surgeon must visualise the functional outcome. He may aim to achieve this in one stage or in a number of stages, depending upon a plan which is conceived at the initial assessment and modified from time to time thereafter, according to the patient's progress and needs.

The surgeon must see the far horizon of his endeavours, but he will not necessarily reach this in one stride. How far he can step depends upon his ability and experience.

Wounds may be classified as tidy or untidy (Fig. 1.3). Tidy wounds are clean-cut lacerations, such as those sustained by a knife. The damage to the tissues is well localised and primary repair can usually be undertaken. It should be performed by an experienced surgeon. The wound should be clean and there should be no swelling. If underlying joints, tendons or fractures are exposed, primary repair and immediate wound closure is highly desirable. Delayed primary repair may be undertaken in less favourable circumstances. Untidy wounds are caused by crushing, avulsion or bursting injuries. Damage tends to involve

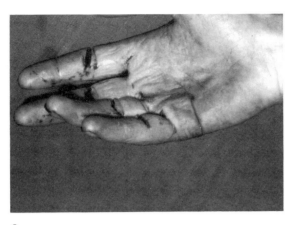

a

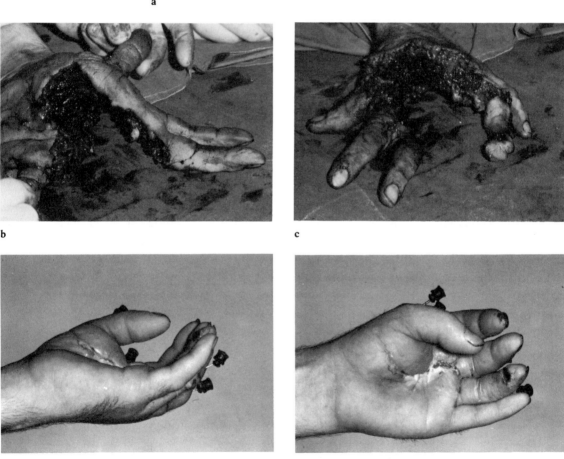

b

c

d

e

**Fig. 1.3** **a** An example of a tidy wound caused by a laceration by a sharp object dividing flexor tendons. **b, c** An example of an untidy wound caused by a rotating circular saw devascularising the fingers. **d, e** The result of surgical revascularisation in the untidy wound

skin, blood vessels and bones, but may involve other structures as well. Such wounds are rarely capable of being treated by primary repair. Untidy or contaminated wounds, the presence of gross swelling, or extensive injury all favour the delayed approach.

The terms 'primary', 'delayed primary' and 'secondary repair', are confusing. From the moment of injury a biological clock of tissue response is activated. This clock ticks at different rates for different tissues, so that while 80% of dermal tensile strength returns within the first 2 weeks, tendons require 5–7 weeks to regain adequate strength. Thus, there is one wound in which healing is proceeding in a multilayered fashion. A therapeutic window exists between the time of injury and the height of the inflammatory response (Fig. 1.4). Another window exists between the decline of the inflammatory response and the commencement of the repair processes. During both these periods it is possible to operate on structures which are relatively unaltered. Once the repair processes have commenced, there is an irreversible alteration in the quality of the tissues, which dictates the type of repair possible. The first therapeutic window corresponds to primary repair. The second to delayed primary repair. As the repair processes proceed, the repaired tissues

undergo changes which result in the acquisition of tensile strength. The terms 'primary' and 'secondary' were developed in an era when fear of infection governed the approach to surgical management. It is still important to consider the possibility of wound contamination and clearly, if this seems likely, early repair would not be advisable. It is now more relevant to assess the biological state of the wound in terms of the inflammatory response and repair processes. Nevertheless, to operate at the height of the inflammatory response would produce a summation of tissue responses leading to induration and immobility and perhaps the potentiation of an incipient post-traumatic sympathetic dystrophy.

Thus it can be seen that the timing of surgical intervention depends on numerous factors. Delay in referring the patient is crucial to the initial decision. Surgical management may also be influenced by the organization and workload of the hand unit. The actual state of the tissues at the time of injury and the pace of change within the tissues following injury will determine a decision about early or later surgical intervention.

Where primary repair is indicated, but the surgeon is unfamiliar with the techniques required, simple wound closure may be performed and the patient referred immediately to a centre

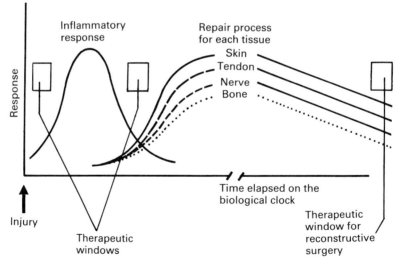

**Fig. 1.4**  The inflammatory response of the tissues to injury, followed by the rate of progress of healing in the various tissues. It can be seen that there are therapeutic windows during which surgical intervention will not significantly potentiate the normal physiological responses, adding insult to injury. The timing of such intervention is crucial

where a delayed primary repair of the underlying structures may be undertaken. Following wound closure in such circumstances, the hand should be elevated and the patient placed on a course of antibiotics. Re-exploration should be undertaken as soon as possible, but certainly within the first 5 days, to permit delayed primary repair. After 5 days, granulation tissue is developing and the nature of the tissues has been altered irreversibly. Primary repair is thus no longer feasible. Meticulous wound care is required to minimise the risk of superficial infection complicating delayed primary repair.

The most fundamental aim in primary treatment must be to ensure the viability of the hand. The next most important factor must be maintenance of a soft and supple hand by avoiding joint stiffness. A viable, supple, soft, mobile hand is suitable for secondary surgery, but the presence of stiffness and joint contractures would so prejudice any reconstructive procedures that in many cases they would be fruitless (Fig. 1.5). If the nature of the wound permits, it would seem rational to undertake primary repair of any damaged structures, provided this repair and postoperative care would be unlikely to compromise

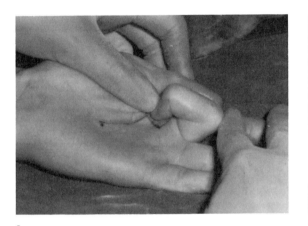

a

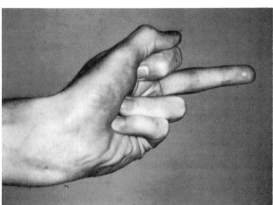

b

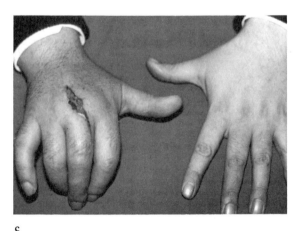

c

**Fig. 1.5  a, b** This patient illustrates a soft and supple hand. He has already undergone surgery involving a primary tendon repair, which failed. Following this, intensive physiotherapy and determination on the patient's part has produced a situation in which he has a full passive range of motion and the tissues are soft. This often takes up to 6 months or more following the last surgical event. He was then ready for secondary surgery and went on to have a successful tendon graft. **c** This patient illustrates an exaggerated physiological response to injury. He suffered a human bite and developed an infected wound which healed following adequate surgical treatment. However, 8 weeks after injury, he has obvious signs of reflex sympathetic dystrophy with swelling, stiffness and discoloration of his right hand. This will take many months to settle

joint function. In practice, this means that early active or passive mobilisation, using accepted techniques, should be chosen to permit maximum mobilisation. Where practical, uninvolved joints should be left free. If immobilisation is essential, care must be taken to ensure that the hand is held in the correct position. Electively this may be needed after tendon transfers to prevent tension on the tenorrhaphy site or in trauma, following the treatment of certain fractures. In the (grossly) swollen hand, the position of immobilisation is crucial if subsequent contractures are to be avoided. The metacarpophalangeal joints should be flexed and the interphalangeal joints extended with the thumb held in abduction (Fig. 1.6). In severe complex injuries, it may only be possible to stabilise the skeleton and revascularise the limb, achieving early skin cover by the simplest means. The hand is then subjected to early active or passive mobilisation with the aim of achieving a soft, supple and mobile hand. Once this has been achieved, secondary reconstruction of the skin may be necessary prior to later work on tendons and nerves. It is important to realise that the presence of an open wound in no way contraindicates the use of active or passive motion as can be seen in the McCash open palm technique (p. 306) used after release of Dupuytren's contracture. Mobilisation enhances collagen orientation, producing a soft and supple scar irrespective of whether a wound is open or closed.

## Dressings

Dressings are required for specific purposes. They are best avoided after replantation and skin flaps which should always be free for visual inspection. The principles underlying the application of dressings to the hand are:

1. To clean or débride wounds.
2. To prevent dead space between skin and underlying structures.
3. To assist in the application of a skin graft to its bed.
4. To protect suture lines until they are physiologically sealed.

It should be noted that a dressing should not be used to achieve haemostasis. To acquire perfect haemostasis a dressing would be so tight as to produce skin necrosis. Haemostasis should be achieved intra-operatively (Fig. 1.7). As incisions are made, obvious vessels should be coagulated with bipolar diathermy. At the end of the surgical procedure the tourniquet may be released and haemostasis achieved. The surgeon should be confident that haemostasis is adequate prior to

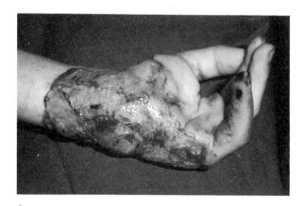
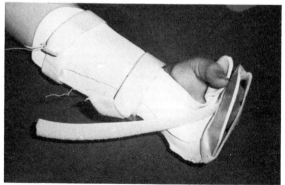

a                                                    b

Fig. 1.6  a, b This patient sustained a bomb blast injury to his hand which became grossly swollen. It was treated by initial surgical débridement followed by a secondary débridement and grafting. The hand was immobilised with metacarpophalangeal joint flexion and interphalangeal joint extension. Once his skin grafts had fully taken, he was capable of a full range of joint movement. It is imperative to immobilise swollen hands in this position, to prevent shortening of the collateral ligaments of the metacarpophalangeal joints

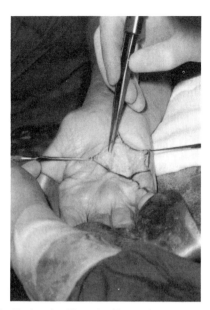

**Fig. 1.7** Drains should rarely, if ever, be necessary in elective hand surgery as haemostasis should be as perfect as possible. This is best achieved by using a bipolar coagulator as the tissues are exposed, and then once more upon release of the tourniquet

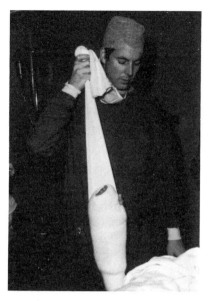

**Fig. 1.8** Elevation of the hand must be maintained from the time of surgery, until any tendency towards swelling has passed. Dependency produces pain, swelling and bleeding deep to skin grafts. Elevation should be maintained for some 4 or 5 days following hand surgical procedures

closing the wound. The use of a drain does not justify poor haemostasis.

Dressings may also act as splints:

a. To rest the hand.
b. To protect repaired structures, e.g. nerves and tendons transfers.
c. To prevent joint contractures.

## Postoperative care of the patient

Upon completion of the surgical procedure and the application of the dressing, the hand should be immediately elevated — a position that should be maintained for the next 4 or 5 days. Dependency produces pain and discomfort as well as the possibility of bleeding into the tissues. Simple elevation reduces the need for narcotic analgesics in hand surgery. There are many different ways of elevating the hand. A method should be chosen which guarantees that elevation occurs without constriction, such as the use of a roller towel, or foam support. Tube gauze may be used, provided it is not too tight. No circumferential attachment

of tape should be necessary to secure any form of elevation (Fig. 1.8). In general, patients do not have a great deal of discomfort following hand surgery except when bony surgery has been undertaken. The presence of persistent pain requires immediate dressing removal and wound inspection. Pain which does not respond to mild analgesia is a serious sign, indicating haematoma, ischaemia or infection.

The circulation in all of the digits should be carefully monitored in the postoperative phase. Any evidence of circulatory impairment requires immediate release of the dressing. A tight dressing may produce localised pressure sores. It may contribute to venous stasis and, following microvascular surgical procedures, this may be enough to diminish flow across an anastomosis and produce thrombosis. If the circulation is in question, the dressing should be removed, and it may be necessary to remove stitches from the wound. In the absence of a rapid return to normal circulation, an urgent re-exploration of the anastomosis is required in theatre. The surgeon must be aware of the possibilities of internal swelling as well as external compression. Crush injuries to muscle cause a great deal of swelling. Such muscular swelling may produce an internal compartment syndrome, in which the swelling itself compresses the venous outflow and arterial input into a muscle compartment, resulting in muscle ischaemia and infarction. Urgent fasciotomy, associated with interosseous muscle release, may be required.

## REHABILITATION

From the moment of injury or surgery, a biological clock is set in motion which provokes a malignant physiological response, producing oedema and stiffness. The aim of rehabilitation is to counteract these processes, producing a soft and supple hand. This aim must be achieved before undertaking any further secondary reconstruction. It is important to realise that, during the first 3 or 4 months following surgical treatment, there is a therapeutic window, during which time appropriate rehabilitation will return the hand to a soft and supple state. Surgery generates scar tissue which will contract unless prevented from doing so. Static or dynamic splints are most beneficial at this stage and if the opportunity that the therapeutic window presents is lost, it may never be regained.

Initially, the rehabilitation process concentrates on the reduction of oedema and the acquisition of a full range of passive mobility. Later, the re-acquisition of co-ordination in the performance of manipulative tasks is encouraged. Following nerve regeneration, sensory re-education may be used to enhance perception. While the surgical treatment of injury may take a matter of hours, the rehabilitation process may last for months.

The organisation of the rehabilitation service is of paramount importance in the running of a hand surgery unit. The logistics involved in providing physiotherapy, with a particular expertise in the management of hands, orthotics and prosthetics, is such that special centres should be set up to serve the local population and their district hospitals.

In future, a 'hand therapist' may well provide all of these services, and already does so in certain countries. In trauma cases, the hand therapist should see the patient on the day following surgery and receive a comprehensive account of the injuries received and the rehabilitation programme required. The therapists should attend the outpatient department for both new and follow-up patients. Ideally, they should present sufficiently frequently at the time of elective surgery to become acquainted with the pathological processes. This team approach is useful postoperatively when any member of the team may be needed to provide encouragement. Those responsible for the manufacture of splints should be available in the clinics. Each patient requires purpose-built splints for specific needs and a discussion in the clinic can clarify such needs. The construction of these splints is highly skilled and requires special training. The occupational therapist encourages the re-acquisition of motor skills providing a sequence of activities, progressing from simple exercises to more complex manufacturing tasks in a workshop environment. A liaison between an industrial rehabilitation officer, the place of work, and the occupational therapy department is beneficial. An early return to an occupation, which is appropriate to the patient's stage of rehabilitation, may be possible. Progressive firms will have their own rehabilitation unit which liaises with those responsible for the care of the patient.

## THE ORGANISATION OF HAND SURGERY SERVICES

The hand surgery centre should be readily accessible. Local casualty departments should feel free to seek advice by telephone and refer patients, if only for assessment. It is through their willingness to provide opinions in casualty departments that hand surgeons may establish their speciality. Hand clinics should be held in the local hospitals which the centre serves, in order to identify those patients who require early treatment. In the centre itself there should be a daily dressing clinic, as many soft tissue injuries undergo rapid changes and require careful monitoring. One operating theatre needs to be permanently available for microsurgical procedures, as these need to be undertaken as soon as possible. This theatre should be serviced by dedicated staff with specific training in microsurgical expertise, and should be equipped with two microscopes so that simultaneous work can be undertaken on amputated parts and injured hands. Another theatre is necessary for elective cases and this can be used in the mornings to deal with emergency cases from the preceding night, so that all such cases are seen by the most experienced member of the team. In this way control over the management of all hand trauma can be exercised. It is often necessary to balance the enthusiasm of youth with the wisdom of experience.

One-third of all patients who present to casualty departments have hand injuries. The work loss each year through hand trauma means that the provision of an expert hand service would have profound financial benefits for any country. The availability of such expertise would guarantee a more rapid return to work and, in some cases, would prevent patients from becoming permanently unemployed.

Hand surgery requires specific training in many aspects of surgical technique. The surgeon must be aware of orthopaedic, plastic and microvascular techniques and be able to apply them. A critical number of patients is necessary upon which to base such a service. The ability to adapt rapidly to changes in surgical practice is greater in a service driven by patient demand. The institutional inertia of government-led health care systems renders them less flexible. The aim for the patient should be the highest standard of care rather than the most convenient, or the least expensive.

The hand, which is such a unique sensor and effector mechanism, deserves professional assessment, surgical technique and rehabilitation.

# 2. Rehabilitation

*Principal author: D. A. McGrouther*

Rehabilitation is the process by which the patient's hand is returned to automatic and integrated use without conscious effort and with restoration of as much of the original function as possible. The aim of rehabilitation is to enable the patient to re-assume his previous occupation and social activities. Both physical and psychological support may be necessary to achieve this objective.

The organisation of the rehabilitation service must allow the surgeon and therapist together to monitor the postoperative progress of all patients. Those in need of treatment can be identified early and selectively instructed and treated. The resources of a rehabilitation service are a scarce commodity and must not be dispensed in a gratuitous fashion, but carefully applied to those in need.

## AUTOMATIC USE OF THE HAND

In normal use, the hand automatically performs everyday functions and the subject is unaware of the individual components that comprise such activities. Changes in loading and position of joints, tendons and skin provide a mass of information which is normally transmitted to the central nervous system but not consciously appreciated. The range of motion required at particular joints does not rise to consciousness. However, should there be a pathological process affecting a joint producing pain or stiffness, the patient will become aware of the resulting limitation of movement. Use of the hand will be modified to achieve the desired position, perhaps by altering the arc of motion of adjacent joints, or by an overall change in the positioning and posture of the hand. This requires a conscious effort, which makes activity slow and clumsy, heightening patients' awareness of their limitations. Visual control may even prove necessary.

Hand motion commences *in utero*. Grip is seen in the newborn, but individual digital motion is unco-ordinated. The patterns of automatic usage of the hand develop in infancy, but the learning of particular forms of dexterity continues throughout life. The brain and the hand can be regarded as a computer and its robotic terminal respectively. This hardware may be damaged by injury or disease, necessitating software modification. Rehabilitation is this reprogramming process. Well-motivated patients may achieve this on their own; others require help.

After an injury, sudden and obvious adaptation is required. A pathological process of slower onset promotes a gradual adaptive response which may result in progressive exclusion of the affected part of the hand. Thereafter restoration of automatic function of the part requires considerable effort by the hand therapist, as the patient must be re-educated in the use of the whole hand. This may explain why the correction of longstanding deformity may produce a disappointing improvement in function.

## FACTORS INFLUENCING RECOVERY

Rehabilitation is one of the major influences on the outcome of hand surgery, but its role must be considered in relation to other factors which are summarised in Table 2.1.

**Table 2.1** Factors influencing rehabilitation

| Patient factors | Physical |
|---|---|
| | The type and severity of the injury |
| | The variation in the normal healing response |
| | Post-traumatic sympathetic dystrophy |
| | Psychological |
| | Premorbid personality |
| | Postinjury; motivation, pain, litigation |
| Treatment factors | Surgical |
| | Additional tissue trauma due to surgery |
| | Rehabilitation |
| | Physiotherapy |
| | Occupational therapy |
| | Splintage |

## Physical factors

### The type and severity of the injury

The magnitude of tissue trauma sustained at injury has a profound effect on the outcome. A classification of injuries into tidy or untidy wounds reflects this level of tissue damage:

*Types of injury*
Contusions
Abrasions
Open wounds
   Tidy       — sharp laceration
   wound
   Untidy    — crush ⎫
   wound     — avulsion ⎬ or in combination
               — compound fracture
               — burns

A sharp laceration will traumatise only a few cells, whereas bursting lacerations or avulsion and tearing injuries will inflict cellular damage some considerable distance from the wound edge. Vascular damage and occlusion, with resulting exudation and ischaemia, will aggravate the direct cellular injury.

It must be appreciated that when a fracture occurs, major forces have been applied to hard and soft tissues alike and there is always associated soft tissue trauma. The skeletal disturbance apparent on the initial radiograph bears little relationship to the maximal displacement which occurred at the time of injury, and it is the latter which dictates the amount of soft tissue damage.

The greater the initial tissue damage, the greater the need for subsequent rehabilitation.

### The variation in healing response

From the moment of injury a biological clock starts to tick as a series of pathophysiological responses commence in the wound and adjacent tissues. From this point on, surgery and rehabilitation must be timed with precision, as there are favourable and unfavourable intervals for each.

Rehabilitation must be timed against this biological clock. Movement must commence before stiffness is established and the encouragement to exercise must continue until there is no further risk of deterioration.

The oedematous hand tends to stiffen into a standard posture, with extension of the metacarphophalangeal joints and flexion of the interphalangeal joints (Fig. 2.1). Several factors contribute to this position. As the finger swells, the accumulation of fluid exudate expands the skin envelope in the manner of an inflatable splint. The skin of the hand has little elasticity, especially on the palmar aspect. As the redundant wrinkled skin over the dorsum of the proximal interphalangeal joint is 'blown up', this joint will flex. Dilatation of the soft distal palm will tend to extend the metacarpophalangeal joints.

Additional factors contribute to this pattern. The ability of the skin of the digit to adapt to flexion and extension is a complex process which relies on the integrity of the 'skin joints'. The skin is anchored in a fixed relation to the underlying skeleton by ligamentous attachments. Cleland's ligaments are the oblique anchors which maintain the relationship between the lateral digital skin and the underlying joints. As the finger swells, the oblique Cleland's ligaments become taut and perpendicular to the joints. As a result, the flexed position of the proximal interphalangeal joint becomes fixed. When these processes have taken place, the finger becomes resistant to extension or further flexion.

The abnormal joint postures are potentiated by the fact that, as the proximal interphalangeal joints flex, the metacarpophalangeal joints will extend by a tenodesis action of the long flexors and extensors which maintain their resting

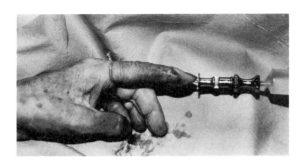

a

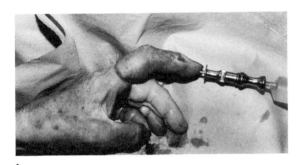

b

**Fig. 2.1** The posture of the oedematous hand, demonstrated by a cadaveric experiment. **a** A needle is inserted into the pulp of the straight digit. **b** When the digit is distended with fluid the proximal interphalangeal joint flexes (see also Fig. 12.3)

lengths. The extensor apparatus has a weak action at the proximal interphalangeal joint and does not have the power to overcome a tendency towards proximal interphalangeal flexion. Secondary changes include shortening of the collateral ligaments of the metacarpophalangeal and interphalangeal joints and adhesions of the volar plates of the proximal interphalangeal joints to the proximal phalanges. These changes together ensure that the hand stiffens in the well-recognised position (Fig. 2.1).

The severity of the inflammatory wound healing response and associated oedema depends on the degree of trauma, but there is considerable variation in the individual response. The obese hand, or workman's thickened hand, is predisposed to stiffness. There are racial differences in addition and the stiff Northern European hand is also at risk. It is difficult to quantify precisely these factors, but the wise surgeon will include them in the overall equation. Infection also aggravates the response to injury.

Mobilisation will mould and stretch adhesions to allow a return of normal excursion between tissue planes. The repaired structures, however, re-establish tensile strengths at different rates and the rehabilitation programme must be modified accordingly.

***Reactions in the wound.*** A wound is a breach in continuity of the tissues within which a fibrin clot forms filling all the dead space. This clot has a specific fibre orientation, rather like the grain in timber, and its direction is determined by early stresses. The surgeon should take steps to minimise wound dead space and avoid haematoma which augments it. Myofibroblasts (immature fibroblasts with contractile properties) grow into the fibrin clot and deposit collagen. This immature cell and collagen mix can be considered as internal granulation tissue. Its quantity in the closed wound is controlled by the wound dimensions, but in the open wound its generation is constrained only by infection, desiccation and marginal epithelialisation.

The orientation of collagen fibre deposition within the fibrin clot depends on the fibrin grain and the subsequent stresses and strains to which it is applied. Wound healing has been described as the introduction of slow setting fibrous cement to the dead space, causing adherence between layers which normally glide. *En bloc* healing of all layers must be avoided.

With the passage of time the wound is said to mature; the tissue becomes less cellular and more fibrous. The fibrous elements develop an orientation in response to the local tension and compression forces.

There is a 'window' during the healing phase within which specific dynamic stress loading can, with benefit, determine collagen orientation. Treatment at this stage can manipulate the orientation of collagen and the length of adhesions so as to permit movements.

***Pathophysiological events around the wound.*** Metabolites and humoral mediators control a sequence of events in the tissues adjacent to the wound, which depend on the amount of cellular and vascular damage in the area. These factors generate a 'whole hand problem' where oedema leads to abnormal posture. Serous exudation leads to a stiffening tendency of all structures; tendons, ligaments and joints. Oedema will be aggravated by dependency of the limbs or by loss of normal motion due to pain.

In the crushed hand, it is the invisible injury of cellular damage which leads to oedema and stiffness.

### Post-traumatic sympathetic dystrophy

The aetiology of this syndrome is uncertain, but it is considered to be a prolonged and exaggerated sympathetic response to injury. The condition may be regarded as having three phases which merge into one another.

The acute phase is heralded by disproportionate pain and a failure of the patient to make progress through the normal milestones of recovery. Clinical signs are of a swollen hyperaemic hand which perspires freely. The tissues are congested and there is increased hair growth. In this oedematous phase, acute carpal tunnel syndrome may arise. The subacute (and more prolonged phase) follows with continuing swelling and soft tissue hyperaemia associated with a dry skin. Radiographs reveal bone demineralisation. In the third (chronic) phase the swelling subsides to leave a dry skin with diffuse fibrosis and a frozen hand. A thickening of the palm, rather like early Dupuytren's, may be seen as a sequel to the condition. The surgeon and therapist must be constantly mindful of the possible development of post-traumatic sympathetic dystrophy. The patient is often of a particular personality type, with features of anxiety and a low pain threshold, and there may be a tendency to protect the hand. These features are not invariable, however.

There is a spectrum of severity. Probably many minor degrees are self limiting. Treatment is by active mobilisation, under the close supervision of a hand therapist, to prevent hand stiffness. There is an armamentarium of other treatments which may enable the physiotherapist to increase the range of motion. There may be benefit from guanethidine blocks, particularly if performed in the earliest stages of the acute phase, but it must be emphasised that these procedures require frequent repetition and they form only a part of the treatment programme, which must include appropriate physiotherapy. There may be a lag before guanethidine blocks effect an improvement. Stellate ganglion blocks are an alternative means of therapy; these again require repeated administration.

## Psychological factors

### The patient's pre-injury personality

The variation in outcome of injury and the need for rehabilitation will depend more on the patient's personality than any other factor. This can be difficult to quantify, but some form of assessment is valuable. The patient with an extrovert personality prior to surgery may subsequently be difficult to restrain from the use of the injured part. He may require little physiotherapy and may actually have to be cautioned from overuse of the hand for fear of rupture of repaired structures. By contrast, the anxious or depressed patient may be most reluctant to actively participate in treatment and may attempt to leave rehabilitation entirely to the therapist.

The patient may complain disproportionately about minor symptoms. It may be difficult to distinguish a low pain threshold from conscious exaggeration of symptoms or malingering. Symptoms may have an entirely psychological basis (hysteria). Even clinical signs may have a psychological origin; bizarre postures such as flexion or extension contractures are not uncommon. Apparent anaesthesia or motor weakness may require careful neurological examination and electrophysiological investigation to separate organic from functional disease. Patients may present with self-inflicted injuries, from the application of a tourniquet, self-inflicted burns or other wounds. Chronic percussion to the dorsum of the hand may cause peritendinous fibrosis (Secretan's disease), with local pain and swelling. Constant awareness is necessary to distinguish these unusual presentations.

### Post-injury factors

The patient's motivation is difficult to quantify and is not synonymous with intelligence or predictable from socio-economic grouping. It is a measure of the willingness of the patient to work towards recovery and his ability to adapt. Many factors may affect this, such as pain, the attitude to the appearance of the injury and a desire to return to work or to seek litigation. Some patients' interest in litigation exceeds their interest in a return to useful function. The highly motivated patient, with little assistance from rehabilitation, will achieve a good final result. At the opposite end of the spectrum lies the patient with poor motivation who, despite a massive rehabilitation effort, is unlikely to achieve a satisfactory outcome. Most patients lie between these two extremes. Their motivation fluctuates and requires constant prompting. The encouragement provided by rehabilitation will raise the level of ultimate function.

## Surgery

Any therapeutic intervention must inevitably increase the local tissue trauma. Even the application of a tourniquet may subsequently augment oedema due to reactive hyperaemia and tissue anoxia. By contrast, judicious surgical intervention (as in the treatment of infection) may achieve a reduction of inflammation. Surgery approximates divided structures thus reducing the volume of wound dead space and thereby diminishing the magnitude of the healing response. The timing and choice of procedure must be considered in relation to the underlying pathophysiological processes and the overall rehabilitation programme. Although the general rule of management for hand injuries is primary repair, there are exceptions to this principle. If a hand is at risk from stiffness due to major injury, secondary reconstruction of nerves and tendons may be chosen as a wise course, as it is more important to avoid joint stiffness. The hand which is viable and passively mobile can potentially be restored to active function by later reconstruction. The principle must be to choose a co-ordinated plan of surgery and rehabilitation which is most likely to give the best ultimate hand function. The quality and availability of both surgery and rehabilitation may modify judgements in this area.

## Rehabilitation

Rehabilitation aims to maintain joint mobility throughout the healing phase but, at the same time, to avoid wound dehiscence, rupture of repaired tendons and delayed union of fractures. Rehabilitation is therefore searching for a compromise between the integrity of repaired structures and the restoration of motion.

The principles of mobilisation are:

1. Mobilise early, if possible.
2. A safe range of motion should be decided upon.
3. Do not fear the open wound: wounds heal despite motion.

If a policy of immobilisation is chosen after repair of skin, tendon, nerve or bone, particular attention must be paid to joint positioning. *Although it is possible to immobilise the normal hand for a limited period of time without detriment, the oedematous hand is at risk and will rapidly become stiff.*

There is confusion about the terminology of the positions in which the hand may be immobilised. The terms 'functional position' and 'resting position' are best avoided. The *optimal position for immobilisation* is that in which the hand is least likely to become permanently stiff. The natural position in which the hand rests is that seen in the relaxed anaesthetised hand, when all of the digital joints are partially flexed, so that the position of the digits forms a cascade, with the fingers progressively more flexed towards the ulnar side of the hand. This position is due to the balance of forces between extrinsic flexors and extensors, modified by the action of the interossei and lumbricals. (The term 'intrinsic' is best avoided as the interossei and lumbricals have different actions.) The interossei act to flex the metacarpophalangeal joints and extend the interphalangeal joints. The action of the lumbricals is less certain; they may simply set the length of the flexor digitorum profundus, relative to the extensor apparatus, in all positions of the flexion arc. The lumbrical has been described as the 'mobile moderator band', and during roll-up these muscles maintain the maximum possible reach of the fingertips. The position of the hand in which the interphalangeal joints are extended and the metacarpophalangeal joints flexed is said to be 'intrinsic plus', and with the metacarpophalangeal joints extended and the interphalangeal joints flexed 'intrinsic minus'. It must be emphasised, however, that there are many explanations for the adoption of these postures and these descriptive terms do not necessarily imply an aetiological role by the muscles intrinsic to the hand. Therefore they are best not used.

The *ideal position for immobilisation* of the hand is with the metacarpophalangeal joints flexed and interphalangeal joints extended (see Figs 1.6 and 6.14). The thumb should be in full palmar abduction. Considerable difficulty is experienced in achieving this position by external fixation. However, the surgeon must compromise only to a very limited extent on acceptance of an unsatisfactory position. When the metacarpophalangeal joints flex, the collateral ligaments are taut due to the cam action of the metacarpal head. In extension, these ligaments become slack. At the interphalangeal joints, adhesion of the proximal portion of the volar plate is the principle cause of joint stiffness. Such adhesions develop most readily in the flexed position and this is avoided by maintaining the joint in extension. In addition to this classical description, it must be appreciated that the extensor tendons have a much weaker action at the proximal interphalangeal joints than the flexors, and it is therefore easier to regain flexion, rather than extension, at the interphalangeal joints.

*Physiotherapy*

Physiotherapy is a treatment regimen by which exercises and other physical means are used to restore normal muscle, tendon and joint function. The term 'therapist' mistakenly implies a passive role for the patient; physiotherapy is performed by a patient guided and instructed by the physiotherapist. Time spent in the department is principally teaching and it is vitally important that the patient should continue the prescribed exercises in the intervals between attendances. The patient must be instructed in active use of the hand and in passive manipulation by using the contralateral normal hand. Specific hand therapy should be administered on an individual basis, preferably by a therapist exclusively engaged in hand therapy. Each hand problem requires a specific treatment programme. The hand is such

a complex structure that there is no scope for group treatment, such as is used in quadriceps exercises. There is no place for using rehabilitation services as a general placebo when no other course is open to the surgeon. Not all hands will require physiotherapy, but it is crucially important to identify those that do and to commence therapy without delay and in an intensive manner. Waiting for therapy will cause progressive deterioration in the condition of the hand. To undertake intensive treatment, the patient must either be an inpatient, or attend sufficiently frequently to ensure that progress is being made. Stiffness often increases between therapy sessions. In practice, daily attendance is often necessary.

Certain specific surgical treatments require a short period of upper limb immobilisation. Elected positions may be chosen following specific procedures. Elbow and shoulder movements can be commenced at this time to prevent stiffness and to build up a relationship with the therapist. If only a part of the hand requires immobilisation, passive or active mobilisation of other parts of the hand may be continued at this time.

Communications between therapist and surgeon should be good so that the therapist understands the surgery performed and the surgeon's expectations for every patient. On occasion this will necessitate the therapist's presence in theatre. The relationship forged between patient and therapist in the rehabilitation phase completes the triangular relationship, with the therapist becoming the surgeon's eyes, ears and tongue!

Progress should be supervised until the patient's voluntary efforts are sufficient to overcome any stiffness arising from the healing process. This supervision may be required for several months.

Passive exercises consist of the gentle manipulation of joints by the physiotherapist, with resultant excursion of tendons and movement of subcutaneous tissue planes. Active exercises require voluntary muscle contraction by the patient. In performing active exercises without added resistance, the patient simply tries to move the joint through an arc of motion. In active, resisted (isometric) exercises, the joint is held still by the therapist, by the use of antagonistic muscle action or by working against external devices. The classical exercise of squeezing a ball in the hand is an isometric muscle exercise which aims to build up muscle power in the flexor muscles, but this form of exercise is not useful in increasing joint range or tendon excursion and has a very small role in hand rehabilitation. Active exercises may also be performed against graduated resistance, such as by squeezing a spring. Such exercises serve to increase both power and range of joint motion.

Tendons will, preferentially, move mobile joints and when they act on a chain of joints, those with the least stiffness will move through a full range of motion before there is any motion in the stiff joints. For this reason, if one joint in an intercalated chain (a linked digital system) is stiff, active exercises may only move the normal joints through the full range and have little effect in increasing the range of the pathological joint. To exercise a joint in such a situation, it is necessary for the normal joints to be restrained (Fig. 2.2) to direct the tendon forces towards the stiff joint. This can be guided by the physiotherapist, teaching the patient to use the uninvolved hand, during exercise periods (Fig. 2.3). For example, when the proximal interphalangeal joint is stiff, the normal metacarpophalangeal joint must be restrained in extension if an increase in the flexion range is being sought. This has the added advantage of increasing the mechanical benefit of the motor involved. Between exercise periods, motion at a particular joint may be encouraged by the use of splints, which block motion of the other joints.

In addition to exercise programmes, other forms of physical treatment may be of value. Heat treatment is generally administered by wax baths and is particularly useful in rheumatoid arthritis. However, care must be exercised in the application of heat to the denervated hand. Ultrasound may be used to diminish oedema and reduce

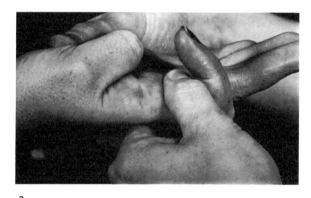

a

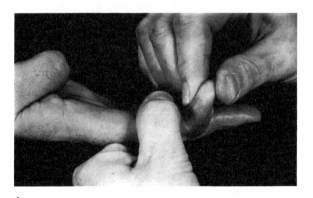

b

**Fig. 2.2 a** The therapist restrains the index metacarpophalangeal joint to encourage flexion of the proximal interphalangeal joint. **b** Restraint of the proximal interphalangeal joint to encourage flexion of the distal interphalangeal joint

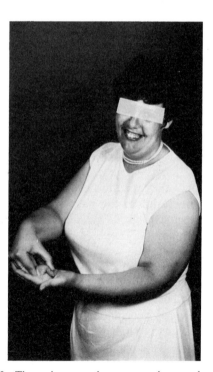

**Fig. 2.3** The patient must be encouraged to use the uninjured hand to assist in physiotherapy, either undertaking passive exercises as shown, or restraining uninjured joints as in Figure 2.2

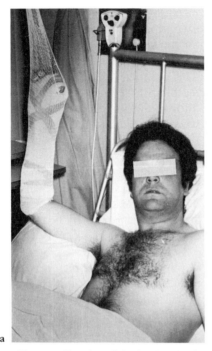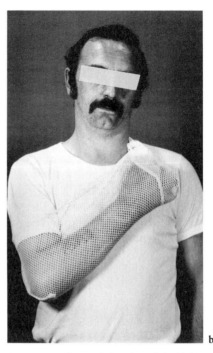

a                                                                                           b

Fig. 2.4   Elevation of the hand. **a** In the early postoperative period and at night high
elevation from a drip stand is best. **b** During ambulation a high sling is the most
practical method

adhesions. Pulsed electrical stimulation has been
reported to facilitate wound healing, but further
objective scientific evaluation is necessary and it
does not supercede other elements of rehabilitation.

The patient and therapist must not fear an open
hand wound, as no group of patients is more in
need of therapy. When dressings are applied to a
raw wound, they tend to become firm and inhibit
motion. In addition, the pain due to traction on
the wound edge by a coagulated dressing will
inhibit movement. Exercises may be undertaken,
free of dressing, in a water or silicon oil bath,
which facilitates the separation of crust and debris
and prevents desiccation of the raw surface. A
small whirlpool bath may be used.

The exercise programme must be co-ordinated
with measures to relieve oedema; in the early
stages after a severe injury, elevation will be
necessary between exercise periods (Fig. 2.4).
Further measures to control oedema are the application of pressure using elasticated gloves (Fig.
2.5) and pneumatic sleeves.

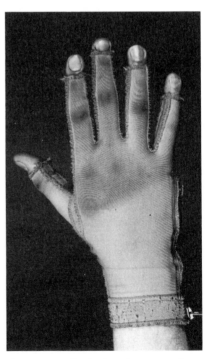

Fig. 2.5   A custom-made elasticated pressure glove may help
to control oedema and to promote scar maturation

*Occupational therapy*

The occupational therapist has a number of roles in relation to the hand patient.

**Assessment.** Before operation, the needs and functional deficiencies of the patient can be assessed in a domestic or workshop environment. Specific problems are identified which dictate the direction of the surgeon's reconstructive plans, particularly in post-traumatic or rheumatoid arthritis patients. Postoperatively, the occupational therapist can assess the value of the surgery in practical terms. The patient's further needs can be reviewed and a management plan formulated together with the surgeon.

**Preventive role.** The experience of the occupational therapist, in assessing the activities of daily living in a simulated domestic environment, provides a unique situation for advising rheumatoid patients on joint preservation and protection. This advice is designed to instruct the patients in the avoidance of powerful movements and shock loadings, which are considered to aggravate deformity. An example is the avoidance of unscrewing of jar-tops, which requires a large ulnar deviating force on the metacarpophalangeal joints of the right hand. Advice can be given on ways of limiting joint loading, for example, by using the left hand. Additionally, aids can be provided.

**Treatment role.** The varying role of the occupational therapist is exemplified by the different challenges of trauma and rheumatoid arthritis. The functional end-point in trauma is a return to pre-injury activities in relation to work and recreation. In rheumatoid arthritis, the end-point may be to achieve personal and domestic independence by concentration on cooking, housework, etc. together with personal hygiene.

The occupational therapist exercises her skills in easing the patient's transition towards normal activities. This therapy, therefore, has a role, not only in the promotion of physical rehabilitation, but also in providing psychological support. On the physical side motor skills can be improved and sensory re-education encouraged. This is achieved by the patient performing tasks in a workshop environment in the company of others. The aim is to assist the patient's return to automatic use of the hand, which in turn will mobilise tissue adhesions and increase joint range and muscle strength.

Grip may be strengthened by the use of tools in a workshop environment, to increase power and joint range. Different types of grip can be encouraged by adjusting tool handles. Pinch function and manipulation can also be facilitated. In addition to exercising, the manufacture of a product encourages a sense of achievement, and by providing an end-point may distract the patient from his pain or residual difficulty. This has a significant role in the restoration of the patient's confidence prior to return to gainful employment. The patient is once again made familiar with a daily routine and given confidence in undertaking everyday tasks.

Whereas physiotherapy often starts immediately after operation, occupational therapy generally commences rather later in the sequence of events, after sound wound healing is achieved. However, it usually continues longer than physiotherapy, until the patient has returned to his employment, and therefore forms part of the graduated return to normal activity.

Sensory re-education is the relearning of the appreciation of textures and shapes after nerve injury and repair. This can be encouraged by the identification of shapes and objects buried in lentils or similar light granular material. The exercise may be done initially under visual control, progressing to touch recognition alone. The patient can practise his ability to distinguish between materials of different textures. There is a feedback between sensation and motion, and sensory re-education and development of motor skills proceed together.

In addition to the problem of limited sensibility during the recovery phase after nerve injury, there is the additional problem of definite areas of neuroma pain. Much can be done to desensitise the neuroma or distract the patient's attention (see Ch. 8).

The ideal is to re-establish the patient's motor and sensory skills to a level where he can cope with his previous occupation. If this is not possible, job adjustment or retraining should be discussed with the patient's employers. The occupational therapist's role is only completed when

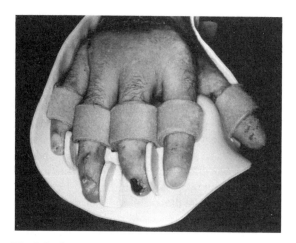

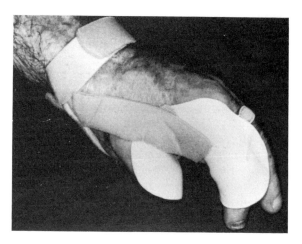

**Fig. 2.6**  A custom-made night resting splint made of thermoplastic material and incorporating Velcro loops to prevent proximal interphalangeal joint flexion contracture

**Fig. 2.7**  A web abduction splint

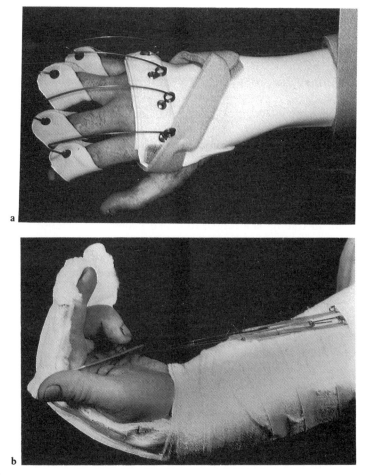

**Fig. 2.8**  Custom made splints. **a** An outrigger splint to encourage proximal interphalangeal joint extension. **b** Modified Kleinert splint using rubber bands to flex the digit after flexor tendon repair

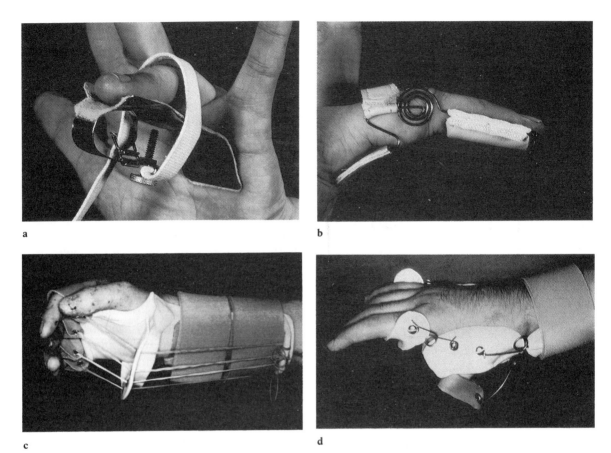

a                                                    b

c                                                    d

**Fig. 2.9** Proprietary splints. **a** The joint jack. **b** The Capener splint. **c** Outrigger splint using rubber bands to encourage metacarpophalangeal joint flexion. **d** Complex dynamic splint using springs to encourage wrist and metacarpophalangeal joint extension and thumb abduction

the patient has been returned to as active a role in society as his injury permits.

### Splintage

Splintage may be static to immobilise the hand, or dynamic, to apply force to the hand while allowing motion.

Indications for static splintage are:

1. Postoperative immobilisation, usually in the optimal position (Fig. 6.14).

2. Fracture immobilisation in a position of election.

3. Immobilisation to prevent tendon dehiscence.

4. Night splintage of the oedematous hand to maintain the ideal position.

5. To temporarily rest the acutely infected hand in the position of optimal function.

6. To maintain a gain in range of motion following surgical release. Incremental improvement in joint range can be achieved by serial static splintage. The stiff joint should be splinted at the extreme of current range of motion to allow a gradual 'loosening' and increase of range. (Retain the gain.) The joint jack is an extreme example of this where a three-point fixation splint is applied to a digit and tightened by means of a buckle.

Static splintage is usually achieved by a plaster of Paris slab. Complete circumferential plaster of Paris immobilisaton has virtually no role in hand fractures, nor does it have a value in the management of soft tissue injury. Volar slabs which are not circumferential should be used. They are removed during exercise periods and are less likely to be constrictive. Digits may be immobilised by aluminium splints covered with foam rubber (Zimmer). Great care must be taken in their application to prevent pressure sores. For more prolonged usage, thermoplastic materials allow individual manufacture of custom-made splints (Fig. 2.6). The fingers and thumb can be held in the ideal position. Other splints in common use are a web abduction splint (Fig. 2.7) or a slot-through splint to maintain abduction and flexion contracture release.

Dynamic splints aim to achieve a certain task, while allowing hand movements. Indications for dynamic splintage are:

1. To encourage movement at certain joints. To maximise this effect other joints should be restrained or blocked. An example of this is the use of an outrigger splint to increase proximal interphalangeal joint extension. The metacarpophalangeal joint should be prevented from hyperextension (Fig. 2.8a).

2. To apply a continuous force to overcome flexion contracture. An example of this is the use of a Capener splint to extend the proximal interphalangeal joint (Fig. 2.9b).

3. To protect a ligament reconstruction during mobilisation. An example of this is the use of a Capener splint to hold the proximal interphalangeal joint in extension when the hand is relaxed.

4. To protect a tendon repair during mobilisation. The Kleinert dynamic splintage system uses rubber bands to limit tensile loading on the digits during finger flexion. This may be used after surgical boutonnière correction.

5. To provide a force to exercise against. This is a secondary effect of 1 and 2 above.

6. To control the range of joint motion. An extension block splint prevents the proximal interphalangeal joint moving in to a chosen part of the extension range. This type of splint is used after injuries which disrupt the volar plate or its bony attachments.

The same splint may have different effects and may therefore be indicated for different problems. The Capener splint, for example, acts to produce many of the above effects. For example, when used to overcome a proximal interphalangeal flexion contracture (see 2 above) it also tends to hold the metacarpophalangeal joint in extension (1) and provides a force to exercise against (5).

The force of a dynamic splint may be provided by rubber bands (Kleinert splint, outrigger splint) or springs (Fig. 2.8b). The Capener splint uses watch springs, which should be located at the axis of joint motion. The 'joint spring' uses a leaf spring. Constant tension springs may also be used in place of rubber bands in the Kleinert system.

The splint made to fit every hand, fits none, and although there is a role for proprietary splints, they are not universally applicable. It is better to manufacture an individual splint for each hand. All splints require frequent adjustment and checking to ensure a satisfactory fit and action, for the hand may change its posture as contractures are overcome. The services of a professional orthotist or suitably trained hand therapist are required.

## REHABILITATION IN CONTEXT

The functional aim of hand surgery must not be merely wound healing or the achievement of a high points score in the academic pursuit of joint, tendon and nerve function. The patients should ideally be returned to their pre-injury lifestyles, encompassing all vocational, domestic and recreational pursuits, without physical or pyschological impairment.

# 3. Skin loss and scar contractures

*Principal author: P. J. Smith*

The provision of adequate skin cover is the basis of successful hand surgery. Without this ability, all other efforts by the hand surgeon are impaired. It is a rapidly evolving area which has dramatically changed in the past 10 years and will continue to do so as technical advances occur. Therefore it is essential for the hand surgeon to keep pace with these changes.

Skin loss initiates a sequence of wound healing processes, some of which are beneficial to the patient but many prove detrimental to subsequent hand function. If the loss exposes tissue which is well vascularised, granulation tissue will form and the wound will heal by secondary intention with resulting contraction. If the exposed tissue is non-vascularised, granulation tissue creeps centrally from the healthy wound margins and wound healing is a prolonged process generating much fibrous tissue.

Delayed or inadequate repair may lead to secondary damage to underlying structures. Delicate tissues vulnerable to desiccation, such as paratenon or periosteum, are lost rapidly upon exposure. Infection may become established destroying tendon or leading to sequestration of bone.

Skin cover will change the wound healing response, promoting healing by primary intention. This eliminates the granulation tissue and fibrosis associated with secondary healing at the periphery and deep surface of the newly applied skin. A well-vascularised wound bed is capable of sustaining a skin graft. Where the viability of the bed is less certain, a skin flap is indicated as it imports its own blood supply.

The provision of skin cover, whether in graft or flap form, will prevent many of the undesirable effects of the wound healing process. Following traumatic loss, skin replacement is required for a number of reasons; in the short term the immediate aims are:

1. To encourage primary healing.
2. To prevent infection.
3. To preserve the viability of exposed underlying structures.

The long-term benefits of adequate skin provision are:

4. To provide a durable envelope which will withstand everyday use.
5. To provide sensation at key points in the hand.
6. To permit mobility of underlying structures, particularly tendons.
7. To permit later reconstructive procedures upon the deeper structures should this prove necessary.
8. To prevent the development of contractures.

Skin loss may present as a congenital deficiency as in aplasia cutis congenita. It may be 'acquired' as a result of many types of trauma. Infections, such as synergistic gangrene, may produce skin loss, as may the surgical excision of neoplasms. A minimal injury to an area where the vascular supply to the skin is impaired may fail to heal. Vasculitis or changes following irradiation may lead to skin loss in this way. Relative shortening may occur as an adaptation to longstanding deformity.

Delicate surgical techniques must be used in even the simplest wound closure. Atraumatic handling of the skin using skin hooks, the elimination of dead space and careful haemostasis prior

31

to closure with appropriate suture material are all important details which affect the quality of the result. In particular, sutures should not be allowed to leave marks. These can be prominent on the dorsum of the hand and, where possible, subcuticular suturing techniques should be employed.

---

# METHODS OF OBTAINING SKIN COVER

---

Reconstructive surgical replacement of skin shortages may be grouped into two types: those where a large area of skin requires replacement and those where there are linear shortages or scar contractures which require release.

The two basic methods of obtaining skin closure when dealing with an area of skin loss are the application of skin graft or the use of a skin flap. Grafts are completely detached and have no intrinsic blood supply. Skin flaps contain full thickness dermis and subcutaneous tissue and are elevated retaining an attachment (the pedicle) to their donor sites. Through this attachment, the circulation and thus viability is maintained. The essential difference between a skin graft and a skin flap is that the former depends for its immediate viability upon nutrients from tissue fluids exuding from the recipient bed (plasmatic imbibition) whereas the latter has its viability maintained through its pedicle. Alternatively the vascular pedicle of skin flaps may be divided and re-attached to vessels in the recipient area by microvascular techniques. Such transfers of skin flaps are called 'free tissue transfers' or 'free flaps' because they do not remain attached to their donor sites. In all cases, neovascularisation (the ingrowth of new blood vessels) will occur from the surrounding tissues. New vessels link up with grafts within 5–7 days. In distant skin flaps, the pedicle may be safely divided once the area to which the flap is applied (the inset) is capable of maintaining flap viability by the ingrowth of new vessels. The length of time that this takes depends on the extent of the inset and varies from 10 days to 3 weeks. After free flap transfer, if further surgical treatment is required, more care should

be taken of the pedicle as this remains a dominant source of supply. In general, grafts are receptive to the ingress of new vessels because, for a small volume of tissue, they have a large contact area between themselves and the underlying bed. The intrinsic vascularity of the donor tissue may be of significance and determine the ease with which different grafts revascularise. Flaps are in general applied to avascular beds and revascularisation occurs slowly from the periphery as the contact area is small relative to the volume of tissue.

## SKIN GRAFTING TECHNIQUE

Skin grafts may be applied successfully to any defect which is capable of producing granulation tissue (which consists of new capillary buds and fibroblasts). Clinically such a bed is judged to be suitable for grafting if it produces punctate bleeding when abraded. Partial thickness skin grafts are shavings of the dermis and are usually harvested with any one of a variety of skin grafting knives or dermatomes. The thickness of the dermis and overlying epidermis within the graft is controlled by setting the blade angle. Their donor defects epithelialise spontaneously and they are thus the most commonly used type of graft. Split skin grafts have a major role in the initial management of traumatic defects because of their reliability and simplicity. They may also cover secondary defects produced by the elevation of flaps or may line their pedicles. However, they may be cosmetically unacceptable or incapable of withstanding trauma and the grafted recipient bed tends to contract.

Full thickness skin grafts are more durable, have a more natural texture and contract less. They have a certain inherent elasticity which allows them to stretch on movement. This may be important on dorsal digital defects. Extensive scarring on the volar surface of the digits may require excision leaving a large defect which should be covered by a full thickness skin graft. This is usually performed as an elective procedure because full thickness grafts take less well on recently traumatised beds. Ideally, donor sites should lie in an unobtrusive area and should be closed directly. The 'take' of such grafts is more difficult to achieve and is proportional to their thickness during the phase of plasmatic imbibition. It should be noted that large full thickness grafts may be used in degloving injuries, when the degloved skin is defatted and re-applied to the defect.

Any donor site or graft may alter in pigmentation following surgery. The site of these potential cosmetic blemishes should be chosen with care.

## Indications

Skin grafts are indicated:

1. In wounds which are too wide to close primarily.
2. In wounds which would spontaneously heal but where time would be saved by grafting.
3. To minimise the contraction resulting from secondary intention wound healing.
4. To preserve the viability of underlying structures on a temporary basis prior to the elective use of skin flaps.
5. Where there is no functional or cosmetic advantage to be obtained by using a skin flap to achieve skin closure.

## The recipient bed

When a skin graft is indicated it is necessary to assess the state of the recipient bed. The surgical excision of an area will leave a defect which is suitable for grafting provided there is no cartilage denuded of periochondrium, bone denuded of periosteum or tendon denuded of paratendon. The absence of these vascular lining tissues precludes the use of a skin graft except as a temporary biological dressing.

Traumatic wounds that have been left to granulate have a different appearance from the fresh wound. The bed of such a wound is suitable for the application of a split skin graft when it has a bright red granular appearance. The surface will bleed when scraped and it should be free of any membranous covering. Large pale flat pink granulations require treatment with hypotonic saline or Terra-Cortril prior to the application of a skin graft. When dealing with such unsuitable granulations time can be saved by shaving them and immediately applying the graft. The wound

should be clean with no evidence of existing infection. Streptococcal contamination is an absolute contraindication. *Pseudomonas* infection should also be eradicated prior to grafting.

One of the main difficulties may be in obtaining graft conformity to the contour of the defect. There should be no tenting of the graft across the defect and its dimensions should be enough to line the defect fully. It may be necessary to use special dressing techniques to maintain the application of the graft to a defect with a particularly irregular contour.

## Donor sites

### Partial or split skin grafts

Cosmetic considerations are of such importance that they govern the choice of donor site. For large areas of skin the commonly used donor sites are illustrated in Figure 3.1. The volar surface of

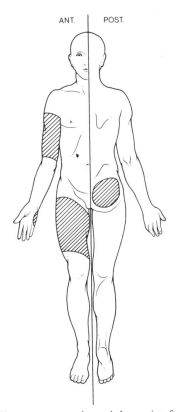

**Fig. 3.1** The most commonly used donor sites for split skin grafts are the thigh, buttock, hypothenar eminence and upper arm

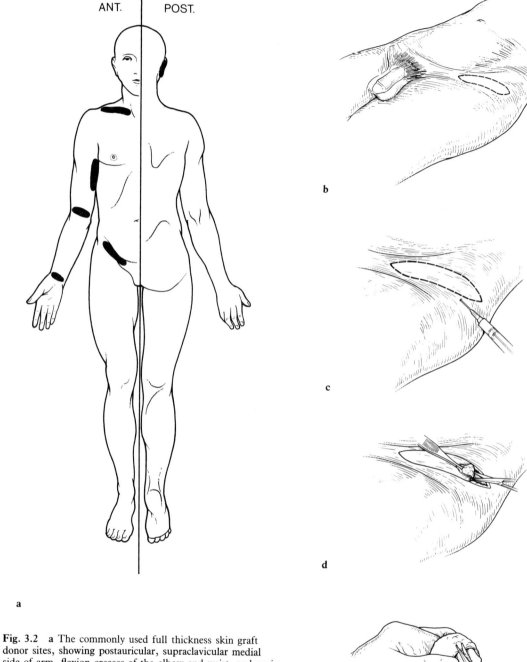

**Fig. 3.2** **a** The commonly used full thickness skin graft donor sites, showing postauricular, supraclavicular medial side of arm, flexion creases of the elbow and wrist, and groin donor sites. The flexion creases of the wrist and elbow are best avoided. **b** An outline of a proposed full thickness skin graft from the groin. **c** The area shown in **b** is injected with 0.5% lignocaine and 1:200 000 adrenaline. **d** After incising around the margin of the graft, the graft is elevated using either a knife or scissors. **e** The underside of the graft is then defatted until the dermis is visible

the forearm should only be used in the presence of severe burns where possible donor sites are restricted. It leaves an area of altered pigmentation and frequently produces hypertrophic scarring. It is an area that is exposed, particularly in women. Caution should be exercised in the use of the medial thigh in elderly patients; a full thickness skin graft may be inadvertently raised because of the progressive thinning of the dermis associated with advancing age. The upper aspects of the arm, both medially and laterally, present technical difficulties because of the use of tourniquets and both are areas that are frequently visible in female patients. *For larger sheets of skin the best donor site is the buttock.* If a smaller area of split skin graft is required to cover a fingertip a good source of graft is the hypothenar eminence.

## *Full thickness grafts* (Fig. 3.2)

Full thickness grafts are best taken from the groin (the flexor surfaces of the elbow and wrist are unsatisfactory donor sites as dehiscence may occur or a restricted range of movement result). Prior to removing the full thickness graft a template is made of the defect in the recipient site. The template is cut out of Jaconet or foam and is transferred to the donor site and an outline of the defect is made. This area is then excised and the secondary defect closed directly. The subcutaneous fat on the skin graft should be removed from the deep surface to permit more effective revascularisation. This may be done either when the graft is elevated using a knife or with scissors when the graft is free. The technique of using a template ensures that when the full thickness graft is sutured into the recipient defect the patency of the microcirculation of the graft is facilitated by the correct skin tension.

## Application of the graft

For a skin graft to survive it must receive a blood supply from the underlying bed. It is uncertain whether this process of neovascularisation involves end-to-end apposition of existing vessels or invasion of new blood vessels into the graft. The presence of haematoma or excessive exudate between the graft and its bed will interfere with

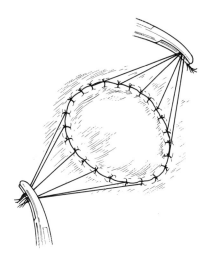

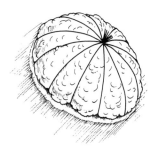

**Fig. 3.3** The full thickness graft is applied to the recipient defect and long sutures are left around the margin, which are then used to tie over a wool dressing. This helps to keep the skin graft applied. A further dressing above this is essential

this process. Prior to the application of any skin graft, haemostasis of the underlying bed must be achieved using bipolar coagulation. Shearing between the graft and its bed must be avoided during the first 5 days. Immobilisation of the grafted part is therefore essential and may be achieved by appropriate splintage and dressings (Fig. 3.3).

The application of a skin graft may be immediate (i.e. at the time of surgery) or delayed until later. In recent years, delayed exposed grafting has become the method of choice for the application of split skin graft in many situations (Fig. 3.4), but it does require expert nursing care. The defect to be grafted is dressed at the time of surgery with a non-adherent dressing. A skin graft

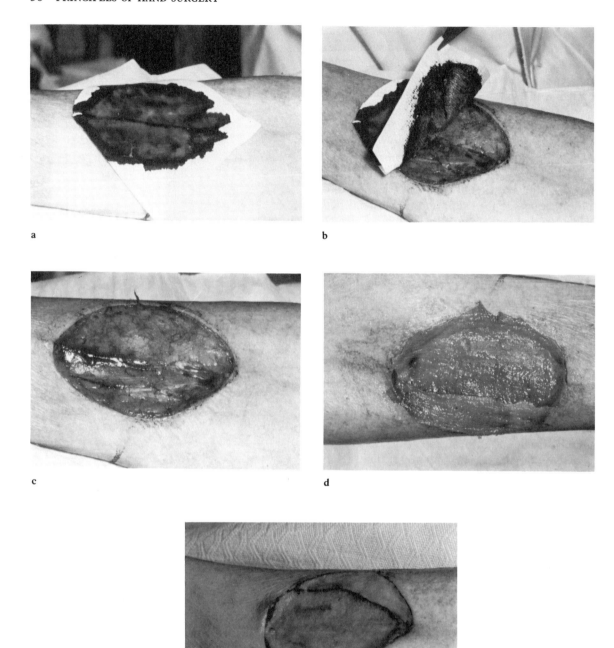

**Fig. 3.4** Delayed exposed grafting. **a** A non-adherent dressing has been applied to the recipient defect, which requires subsequent grafting. **b** The non-adherent dressing is removed after 24 hours. **c** The recipient bed shows no sign of residual haematoma. **d** A skin graft is immediately applied. **e** The appearance of the delayed exposed graft on day 7

is taken and stored. On the next day the dressing is removed and the graft applied to the defect. This technique may be performed in a ward dressing room using normal sterile dressing technique. The graft is left exposed. The nursing staff express any blood or serum collecting under the graft. Thus with careful postoperative care, haematoma can be avoided. The real advantage over other methods is that blood may be removed while still liquid and thus no graft should fail for this reason. The graft thickens and becomes pinker as revascularisation proceeds. However, there are certain situations where this technique cannot be used. For example, where the graft is applied to a cavity or to a mobile surface, a tie-over dressing is used to maintain graft contact with the bed. The dressing is secured by using long sutures around the periphery of the graft attachment, which are then tied over the top of the dressing. The aim of this dressing is to immobilise the graft rather than to apply pressure. A compressive dressing is applied over this. The whole dressing may be taken down after 48 hours if the site can be relatively easily re-dressed. At this time it is still possible to evacuate any liquid haematoma. If the site is more difficult to dress, the tie-over is left for 7 days.

The successful take of any skin graft is thus dependent upon the presence of a suitable bed, perfect haemostasis, and appropriate postoperative rest of the affected part. Such conditions are best achieved with the patient in hospital. When at home, patients are less likely to rest and elevate the grafted part.

## Meshed grafting

Skin meshing allows both expansion of the donor skin and drainage of the recipient bed. This technique is used where there is either a donor site shortage or suspected contamination of the recipient bed. A skin mesher is used which makes multiple longitudinal cuts allowing the skin graft to expand, assuming an appearance like a string vest (Fig. 3.5). The bare areas in the mesh are covered by epithelial migration from the grafted margins once the graft has taken. It is therefore important to use a dressing which maintains a moist environment on the surface of the wound to allow the migration of epithelial cells. If the wound is producing an exudate a meshed graft will allow the egress of the exudate and there will be a higher likelihood of skin graft take.

## Donor site dressings

Skin graft donor sites have traditionally been dressed by applying tulle gras to the raw areas, and a dressing of gauze, wool and crêpe bandages on top of this. It is important that when this technique is used the tulle gras should cover the whole area, otherwise the patient is subjected to severe

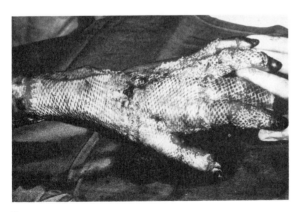 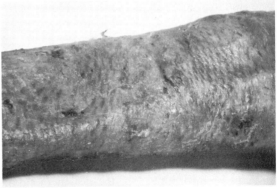

a                            b

**Fig. 3.5** Meshed grafting. **a** A meshed skin graft used to cover a burned hand. **b** Close-up view showing the resultant scarring following meshed grafting. This is less acceptable than conventional grafting, but meshed grafts are useful where there is a shortage of skin or possible contamination of the recipient site

discomfort. This type of dressing can be reduced at 10 days, but the tulle gras layer should not be removed until it detaches spontaneously. If it is pulled off, a more noticeable scar will result. This conventional dressing may be painful. Alternatively, the outer layers may be removed at 24 hours leaving the tulle gras; a hairdryer may be used to produce a dry eschar and the patient allowed home. However, this technique does not give as satisfactory a result in terms of appearance as the previously described method, since an additional layer of cellular death results from desiccation.

Studies of the methods of wound healing have shown that a slightly moist environment is ideal for optimal healing. Adhesive semipermeable membranes such as Opsite provide this environment, however they are difficult to apply and blood blisters may appear beneath them leading to leakage of fluid. More recently, solid gel dressings have been developed, which also relieve pain and produce cosmetically satisfactory donor sites.

## SKIN FLAPS

### Indications

The indications for flaps are of necessity situations in which a graft is not satisfactory. The use of a flap is therefore essential when the bed of a defect is such that an applied skin graft would fail to take because of poor vascularity. In addition, the long-term benefits of skin cover may be better served by a skin flap, for example, for later reconstructive procedures, the provision of more durable skin cover or sensation at key points in the hand.

A skin flap is a trap-door of dermis and subcutaneous tissue which has been elevated from its underlying bed, and whose vascularity is maintained through its base (pedicle). This pedicle consists of the full thickness of the dermis and subcutaneous tissues and contains the subdermal vascular plexus (Fig. 3.6). In certain flaps, large arteries and veins run in the subcutaneous tissue and can be incorporated in the design to supply the area of the skin flap (axial flap). The pedicle can be reduced to include only these vessels and all other structures may be divided; such a flap is called an island flap. The advantage of this tech-

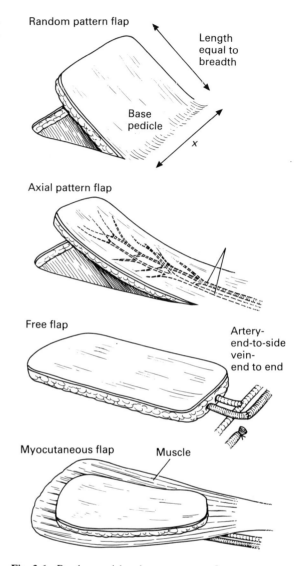

**Fig. 3.6** Random, axial and myocutaneous flaps

nique is that the mobility of the flap is less restricted than it would be with a thick and bulky pedicle. Where a flap includes fascia, the blood supply of the flap may be enhanced by vessels running on the surface of the fascia (fascial flap). Where muscle is included in the pedicle, the blood supply of the flap arises from the vascular pedicle of the muscle. Branches of these vessels then run throughout the substance of the muscles and supply perforating vessels to the overlying skin and subcutaneous tissues. It is possible to reduce

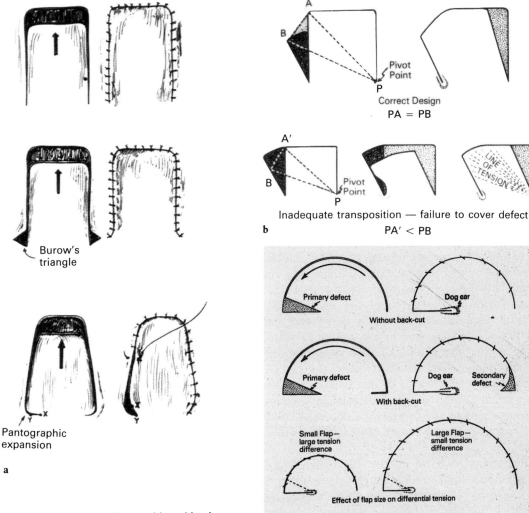

Burow's triangle

Pantographic expansion

**a**

A

B

Pivot Point

P

Correct Design

PA = PB

A′

B

Pivot Point

P

Inadequate transposition — failure to cover defect

**b**

PA′ < PB

LINE OF TENSION

Primary defect

Dog ear

**Without back-cut**

Primary defect

Dog ear

Secondary defect

**With back-cut**

Small Flap— large tension difference

Large Flap— small tension difference

**Effect of flap size on differential tension**

**c**

**Fig. 3.7** Local flaps are moved into position, either by **a** advancement, **b** transposition or **c** rotation

the pedicle to include only the muscle, and a paddle of skin may then be left overlying the muscle pedicle (myocutaneous flap).

Skin flaps elevated from tissues adjacent to defects are called local flaps. Such local flaps provide skin cover of a quality similar to the defect. Local flaps may not be possible, and a skin flap may have to be applied from a distance. To apply a distant flap, the defect and flap donor site must be approximated.

A *local flap* may be moved to its new site in three ways, *transposition*, *rotation* or *advancement*

(Fig. 3.7). When the flap is moved to its new position a line of tension develops between the point of the flap which moves most and the point which moves least (the pivot point). The significance of this line of tension is that it may impair the blood supply to the flap. The surgeon must check that the flap will have sufficient length to cover the defect after transposition. This is particularly important on the dorsum of the fingers. Rotation flaps involve the rotation of the flap into the defect and the secondary defect may often be closed directly. In both rotation and transposition flaps, triangulation of the defect is the initial step. Advancement flaps do not require triangulation of the defect but may require the removal of triangles of tissue from their bases.

Because *random skin flaps* are dependent for their blood supply on the subdermal plexus they can be raised at any site of the body or in any direction. They are, however, subject to certain dimension limitations and it is unwise to raise a flap whose length exceeds the width of its pedicle. Longer flaps may result in distal necrosis.

An *axial pattern flap* has specific cutaneous vessels in the design. The vessels are included in the pedicle and the flap comprises either part or the whole of their vascular territory. Such flaps are inherently safer because of their better blood supply. They have less tendency towards venous engorgement and in general are rather pale. An example is the groin flap based on the superficial iliac vessel. The blood supply of an axial flap remains predominantly from the donor end and the neovascularisation occurring around the inset must be encouraged to play a more significant role in maintaining flap viability should the pedicle subsequently be required in reconstruction. This requires a *delay* procedure effected by locating the arterial input and dividing it 2 or 3 weeks after the flap transfer and 1 week prior to pedicle division.

Flaps may be based on the underlying fascia. In the upper limb, the radial (or Chinese) flap is an example. The skin of the forearm may be elevated and its viability maintained by the blood supply arising from the deep fascia of the forearm, supplied through the radial artery via the intermuscular septum. The flap may be raised on a pedicle which may be proximally or distally based. A distally based flap may be used to reconstruct the thumb or provide cover for the palm or dorsum of the hand; proximally based, it may be used as a free tissue transfer.

A large skin flap may be safely elevated when mobilised on its underlying muscle. *Myocutaneous flaps* based on the latissimus dorsi or gracilis may be used to provide immediate skin cover and if the muscle is innervated they can simultaneously provide motor power in an otherwise damaged upper limb. Such transfers may be useful following Volkmann's ischaemic contractures or gunshot wounds to the forearm.

It is possible to design skin flaps so that they include other tissues such as tendons and bone. These compound flaps may provide vascularised living bone but have the disadvantage that planning must be performed with caution to ensure that the bone fragment coincides with the bone defect without compromising the overlying position of the skin flap. In this regard, the radial flap is more versatile than the deep circumflex iliac artery flap, which includes the iliac crest and its overlying skin. However, there is less flexibility in adapting skin and bone to fit the respective defects than if both were transferred separately.

## FREE FLAPS — THE ROLE OF MICROSURGERY IN SKIN COVER

Small vessel anastomosis using the operating microscope allows one-stage transfer of tissues with reliable success. A flap may be transferred by dividing its vascular pedicle and resuturing the pedicle to recipient vessels in a new site. By this technique, immediate transfer of tissue can be achieved in one stage. In the past, using a tube pedicle, the same result took on average 5 months and several stages to achieve. The advantages of immediate free flap transfers in the provision of skin cover for large areas in the upper limb make this the method of choice. The wound healing response is modified preventing healing by secondary intention with its resultant granulation tissue and fibrosis. There are no positional problems for the patient. There is an immediate reconstruction of the defect, permitting the early institution of intensive rehabilitation so that the ultimate return of function will be as complete as possible. The use of free skin flap and composite tissue transfers is associated with a higher success rate than conventional techniques and avoids the necessity for repeated operations. The value of these techniques as emergency procedures has been demonstrated by MarcoGodina. The recipient tissues are in the best state for surgical intervention at this early phase and there is a reduced incidence of infection. Free flaps suitable for upper limb reconstruction may be axial, myocutaneous or fascial in basis. All contain vascular systems suitable for small vessel microanastomosis. Many donor sites are available, but their selection depends on the area and thickness of skin required. Anatomical consistency and large vessel size increase flap reliability. A long vascular pedicle may avoid the use of a vein graft. The ease with which the flap can be elevated may also influence choice. The cosmetic appearance of the donor site is of importance. Innervated skin or muscle may be required in certain sites.

The groin flap provides the best cosmetic donor site but has a short, small and inconsistent pedicle which is difficult to raise. The scapular flap provides cover of similar thickness to the groin flap but with a long, large diameter pedicle. The dorsalis pedis flap provides very thin skin cover ideal for the hand, but the healing of the donor site can be troublesome. Toe-pulp may be raised in isolation or in conjunction with web space skin or the dorsalis pedis flap skin. The pulp is ideal for thumb-tip reconstruction. The radial flap can provide a large area of thin skin. It is reliable and easy to raise but leaves an ugly cosmetic blemish. However, this can be improved by raising a fascial flap alone without the overlying forearm skin; skin grafts are required to cover the fascia at the recipient site. The lateral arm flap may also be raised as a fascial flap alone or in conjunction with overlying skin. The pedicle is adequate in size and length for most applications in the hand leaving a straight-line donor scar. Latissimus dorsi is in general too bulky for use in the hand.

A specialised microvascular team is required. Members of the team must have experienced intensive laboratory training and be capable of performing microanastomoses with ease. A detailed anatomical knowledge of donor sites is necessary. Investigation of the recipient vascular tree may be required. A specialised anaesthetic service is necessary as prolonged anaesthesia may be required; peripheral vasodilatation must be encouraged and a temperature-controlled environment is necessary during both the operation and the postoperative period. Specialised instrumentation is required and its careful maintenance is essential. In the postoperative phase, flap monitoring in a warm room is required. There is a necessity for permanent theatre availability should re-exploration prove necessary as this must be performed expeditiously.

## THE TREATMENT OF SKIN LOSS ACCORDING TO SITE

### Dorsal digital defects

These defects are often the result of grinding or abrading injuries and are associated with exposure of underlying tendon, bone or joints, producing an unsatisfactory bed for graft take. The application of split skin grafts to the dorsum of the fingers will produce restriction of flexion if the area to be covered is extensive. Full thickness grafts will produce a better result. The majority of defects will need flap cover.

Such defects may be extensive or well localised, but even small defects must be reconstructed with care. If the bed is not satisfactory a flap must be provided to protect the extensor apparatus. Commonly, multiple adjacent digits are involved. Localised defects may lie on phalangeal or joint areas. Each area has its own particular problems and requirements and is treated by different techniques. In general local flaps provide an almost identical replacement for the tissue that has been lost. Their use can prove difficult as there is an absolute restriction on the amount of tissue available and its mobility. Laterally it is tethered by Cleland's ligament. The pronounced curvature of the dorsal digital area often leads to problems in the design of skin flaps. Flaps need to be considerably longer than they would have to be on a flat surface in order to reach and completely cover the defect. After rotation or transposition, the marginal scar lines must not extend anterior to the midlateral line or cross the dorsal wrinkled skin overlying the interphalangeal joints. Such transgressions will lead to either flexion or extension contractures respectively. The oblique pattern of the vascularity to the digits should be taken into account when designing skin flaps. A variable amount of the dorsal skin in the proximal phalangeal area is supplied by the termination of the dorsal metacarpal arteries. Distal to this the digit is usually supplied by the volar digital arteries and the oblique vessels arising from them. There is also an oblique dorsal nerve and care should be taken not to damage this, particularly in the index or little fingers as these are important contact areas in the hand.

### Nail-fold area

The aim of reconstruction in this region is to retain the eponychial fold, even in the absence of the germinal matrix, so that an artificial nail can be used by the patient. Transposition flaps from the area proximal to the defect are used to reconstruct loss in this region. These flaps must be large enough to transpose adequately. The secondary defect should be overlying a phalangeal area not over the interphalangeal joints. If the whole of the eponychial fold is lost then the deep surface of the transposed flap will require lining with a split skin graft. This can be kept in position by using a splint for the nail-bed. If the eponychial fold and

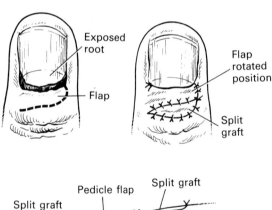

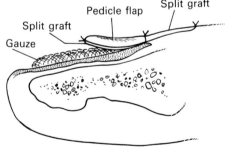

**Fig. 3.8** Reconstruction of the nail-fold area may require local flaps and skin grafts are used in combination, to reconstruct the eponychial fold

germinal matrix are missing both may be replaced by a split skin graft wrapped around a nail-bed splint and a transposed flap to recreate the eponychial fold. This will allow the patient to use an artificial nail at a later date. Where a large transposition flap is used the secondary defect lying on the dorsal phalangeal area is small (Fig. 3.8).

### The distal interphalangeal joint area

For small defects a flap of similar design to that used in the nail-bed area can be used. It is also possible to use a flag flap from the middle phalangeal area of adjacent digits, but flap viability is unreliable; it requires two procedures and a local transposition flap is preferable. If this is not possible then a proximally based cross-finger flap of reversed dermis from an adjacent digit should be considered (see below).

### The proximal interphalangeal joint area

Exposure of the underlying dorsal apparatus in this area can, if neglected, lead to a boutonnière deformity (Fig. 3.9a). If damage to the central slip has occurred and a tendon repair is undertaken provision of flap cover is essential to allow movement and promote healing of the underlying tendon. If the defect is small and tranversely orientated a conventional transposition flap may be taken from the dorsal skin over the proximal or middle phalangeal areas (Fig. 3.9b). Such flaps do however place a line of tension running from the pivot point of the flap to the contralateral apical corner of the defect, directly parallel to the desired direction of flexion. There is therefore an intrinsic conflict built into the design of these flaps. In the majority of patients the skin does slowly stretch and full flexion is retained, despite the theoretical design fault.

In obliquely sited or elliptical defects over the proximal interphalangeal joint, the sliding transposition flap is preferred. This has the advantage of providing a longitudinal redundancy of skin over the dorsum of the joint which allows rapid acquisition of the full range of flexion postoperatively.

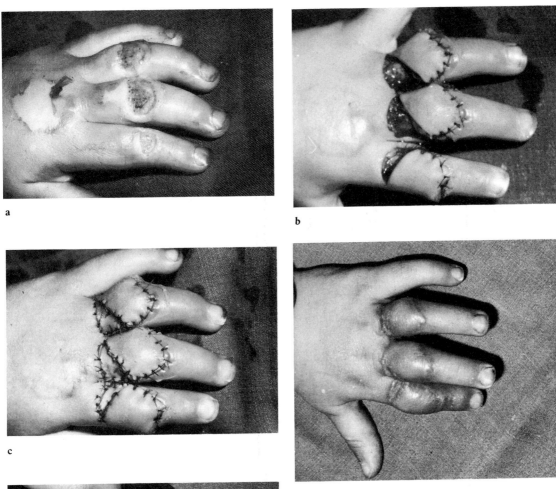

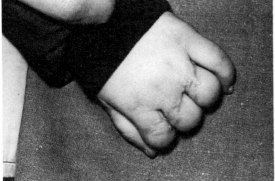

**Fig. 3.9** **a** Exposure of the proximal interphalangeal joints in a young child due to a burn. **b** The use of local transposition flaps to cover the exposed joints. **c** Full thickness grafts have been applied to the secondary defects left by the local flaps and one can see that it is possible now to fully flex the digits. **d** The result at 8 weeks, showing a well healed proximal interphalangeal joint area. **e** The range of flexion possible at the injured proximal interphalangeal joints

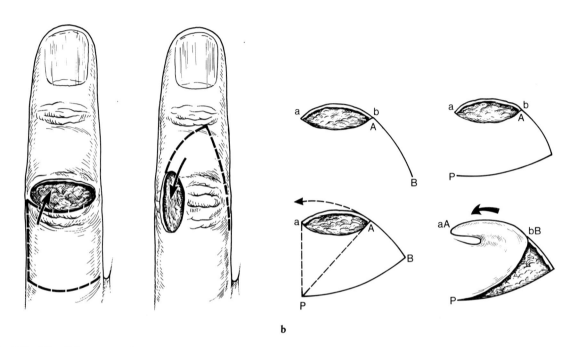

**Fig. 3.10** The sliding transposition flap. **a** It can be seen that more longitudinal or obliquely placed defects are suitable for the sliding transposition flap. Transverse defects are more suitable for the previously described transposition flap. **b** In designing the sliding transposition flap a line AB is projected in a smooth continuation of the contralateral edge of the defect ab. A line is then projected from B proximally to the pivot point P. This line is roughly parallel to aA, but does diverge more widely at the base. It can be seen that the pivot point line PA easily exceeds the distance aP. There is thus no tension on the flap in the transposed position and in fact a dog ear results, which is useful when placed over the proximal interphalangeal joint to allow full flexion of the digit. The secondary defect is grafted.

*The technique of the sliding transposition flap* (Fig. 3.10)

The defect should be oval and if it is not so, may be converted to the appropriate shape by minor adjustments. The flap is designed on the side of the defect which shows the maximum availability of local skin. Sliding the flap into its new position produces a dog ear or redundancy of skin. This is placed over the proximal interphalangeal joint and allows the patient to achieve a full range of joint flexion. The dog ear diminishes in time to acceptable cosmetic levels without losing its functional advantage. A full thickness graft is applied to the secondary defect. The secondary defect does not transgress the midaxial line of the finger and is placed on the dorsal phalangeal region.

Alternatively the reverse dermis flap may be

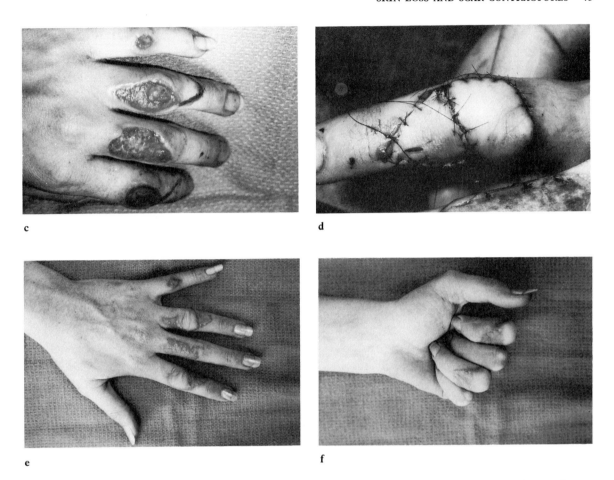

**Fig. 3.10** **c** A burn injury exposing the proximal interphalangeal joints of the index and ring fingers. The other two fingers did not expose underlying tendon or joints, and were treated by grafting. **d** Sliding transposition flaps were designed and then slid into position. The dog ear can be seen proximally and the secondary defect has been grafted. **e** Result at 4 weeks showing full extension. **f** Result at 4 weeks showing full flexion of the proximal interphalangeal joint

used (Fig. 3.11). The skin over a dorsal phalangeal area of an adjacent digit is de-epithelialised and then elevated as if it were a conventional cross-finger flap, but is turned over upon itself 180° and inset into the defect with the de-epithelialised dermis lying on the wound bed. A skin graft is placed on the turned-over flap and on the donor defect. Reverse dermis flaps do not provide the subcutaneous tissue which is so necessary for tendon gliding and they should not be used in an area where tendon movement is important. They are acceptable over the dorsum of the hand and over the bare area just distal to the proximal interphalangeal joint and perhaps, more particularly, in reconstruction of the nail-fold.

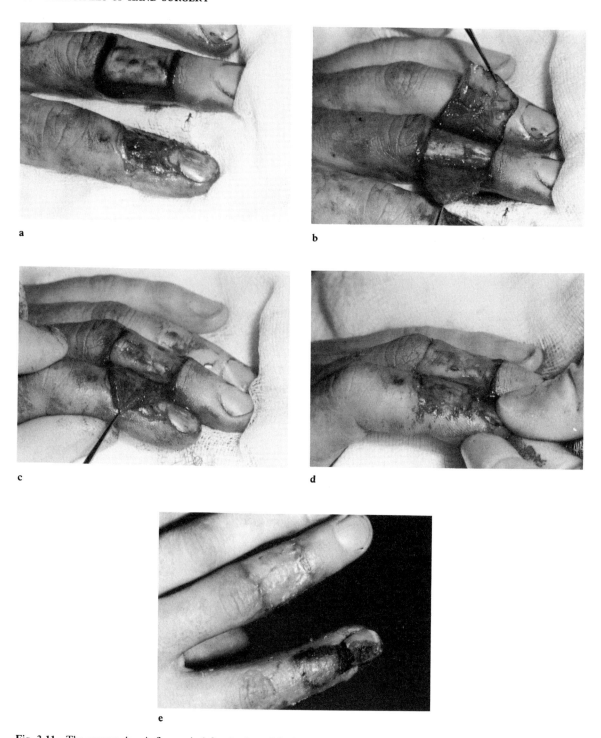

**Fig. 3.11** The reverse dermis flap. **a** A defect in the nail-bed area requiring a reverse dermis flap. The reverse dermis flap from the middle finger is being de-epithelialised. **b** The epithelium has been elevated and its attachment maintained to the ulnar side of the finger. The reverse dermis flap is then lifted from the paratenon and folded over. **c** A reverse dermis flap is now being applied to the defect on the adjacent index finger and the epithelial graft is repositioned over the paratenon of the donor finger. **d** A graft is then applied over the reversed dermis flap. **e** The result some 4 weeks later

## Proximal phalangeal area

These defects are best covered using a flag flap from the adjacent finger. The flag flap is elevated, comprising the whole cosmetic unit of the proximal phalangeal skin, but preserving the paratenon overlying the extensor tendons, and transposed to its new site where it is immediately inset. The flag flap can be used to cover the dorsal or volar surface of an adjacent digit, the volar surface of the same digit, or to create a web space (Fig. 3.12). This flap is more reliable on the index and middle fingers. The pedicle must be wide enough to contain the termination of the dorsal metacarpal artery as well as adequate venous drainage and normally should be at least a third of the width of the flap itself. Foucher has modified this using a wider pedicle as an island flap (Fig. 3.13). This flap requires considerable technical expertise. Extensive loss (two phalangeal

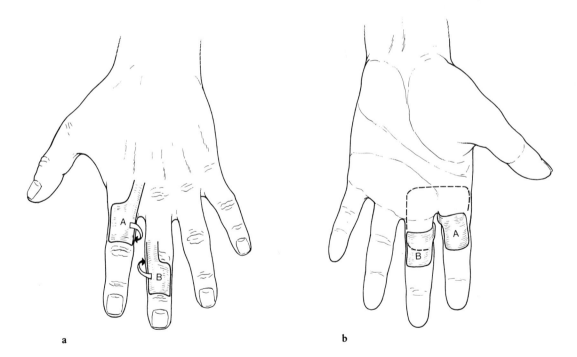

**Fig. 3.12** The flag flap. **a** The flag flap can be used from the dorsum of the middle phalangeal area where its venous drainage appears to be axial but its arterial in-flow is usually dermal, or it can be taken as an axial flag flap from the dorsum of the proximal phalangeal areas. In this site it is based on the terminal branch of the dorsal metacarpal arteries. It can be rotated to cover the volar surface of the finger, as seen in **b** or the volar surface of an adjacent finger

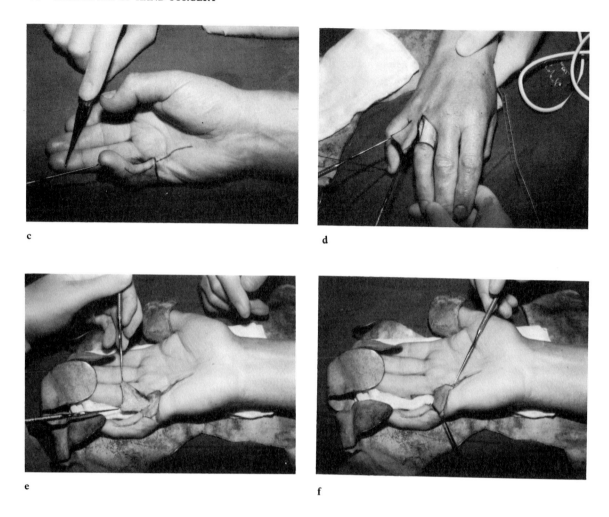

**Fig. 3.12**  **c** Release of Dupuytren's band. **d** Elevation of an axial flag flap. **e** Flag flap delivered and ready to cover the volar defect. **f** Flag flap about to be sutured into the defect

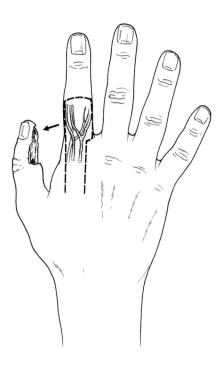

**Fig. 3.13**    The Foucher flap

areas) cannot be covered by local skin from adjacent fingers which would involve the exposure of at least one joint dorsal surface. *For extensive defects, the use of an adjacent digit as a donor site is contraindicated; distant flap cover is required.* The groin is the donor area most easily disguised. Some patients have rather thick subcutaneous fat in this area but if the flap is elevated medial to the anterior superior iliac spine it is usually reasonably thin (Fig. 3.14). The positioning may be difficult and the use of a chest flap taken from the infra-mammary area, at about the level of the anterior axillary line, can provide a useful alternative, as

the fat may be thinner than in the groin (Fig. 3.15). Cross-arm flaps produce the best thin skin cover but are rarely used because of the difficulty in immobilisation.

Multiple dorsal digital defects cannot be treated with local flaps from adjacent digits. The choice lies between syndactylising the defect with the use of one single flap for cover or multiple flaps to cover individual defects. If multiple flaps are to be used the easiest donor area is the groin. If the defect is to be syndactylised a free flap may be used to provide cover, allowing immediate mobilisation.

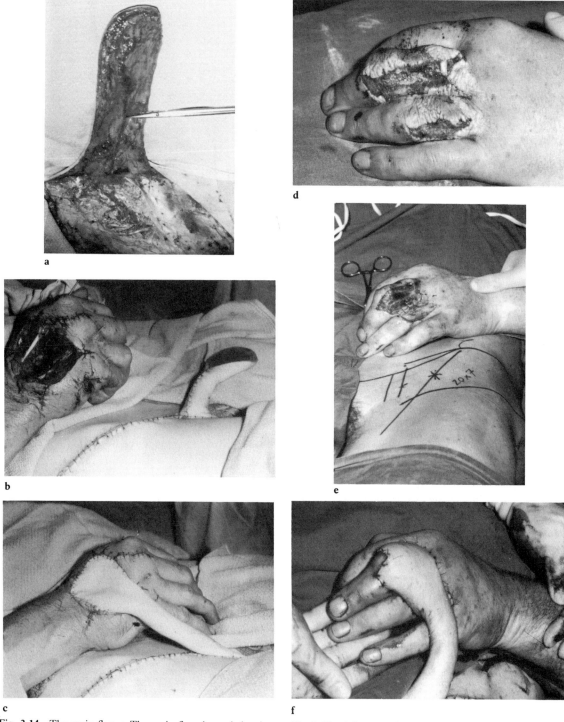

**Fig. 3.14**    The groin flap. **a** The groin flap elevated showing the superficial circumflex iliac artery. **b** A gunshot wound of the hand. The groin flap has been elevated and is applied to the defect. **c** The long pedicle allows the patient to exercise all the joints of the upper limb.

**Fig. 3.14**    **d** An extensive digital defect affecting two digits and exposing tendons. **e** Design of the flap. **f** Application of the groin flap to the defect. This will require subsequent division and later, desyndactylisation.

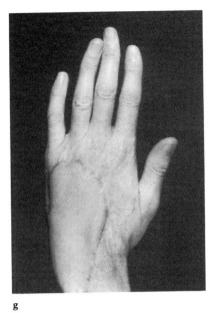

g

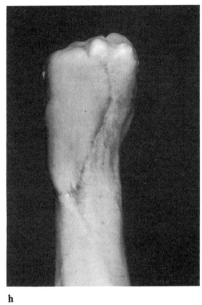

h

i

**Fig. 3.14** **g** Result of a groin flap after 2 years. **h** No restriction of flexion.
**i** Good wrist flexion

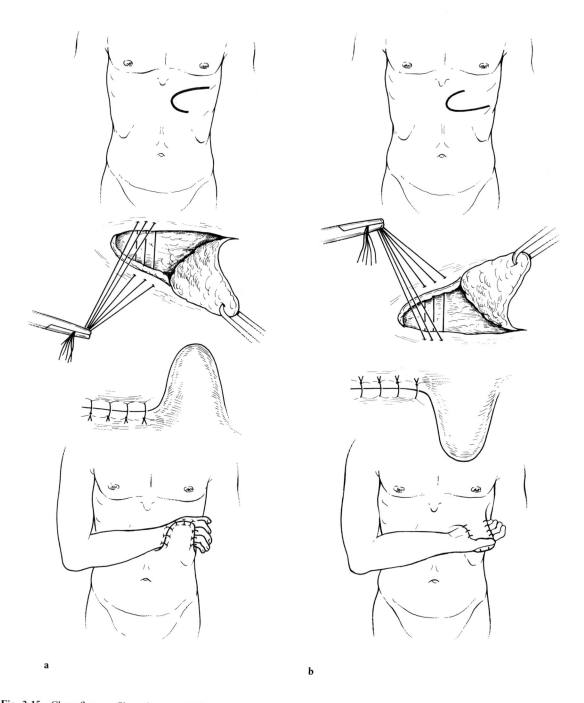

**Fig. 3.15** Chest flaps. **a** Chest flaps should be designed with eccentric limbs so that they can easily rotate, either into a superiorly or inferiorly based direction. In this illustration, when the secondary defect is closed after elevating the flap, the flap automatically transposes so that its undersurface faces superiorly. It can be seen applied to the dorsal surface of the hand. **b** By designing the eccentric limbs differently, the flap can be rotated into position to point inferiorly, and here is shown covering the volar surface of the hand

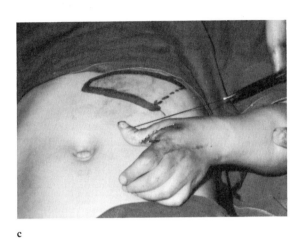

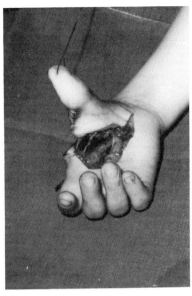

c

d

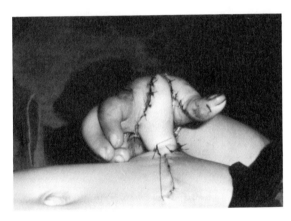

e

**Fig. 3.15** **c** A young child with congenital absence of the extensor tendons and a first web space contracture. **d** Release of the first web space. **e** Application of a chest flap

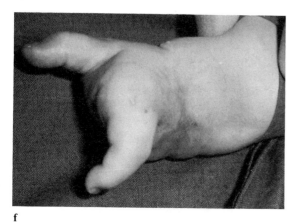

f

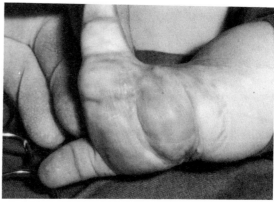

g

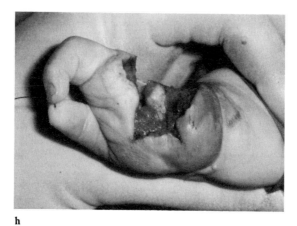

h

**Fig. 3.15  f** Loss of the ulnar three digits in a premature child, as a result of extravasation of intravenous feeding materials. The index finger is pulled in an ulnar direction. **g** A volar view of f. **h** Release of the scar contracture and approximation of the index finger to the thumb-tip shows the extent of the defect

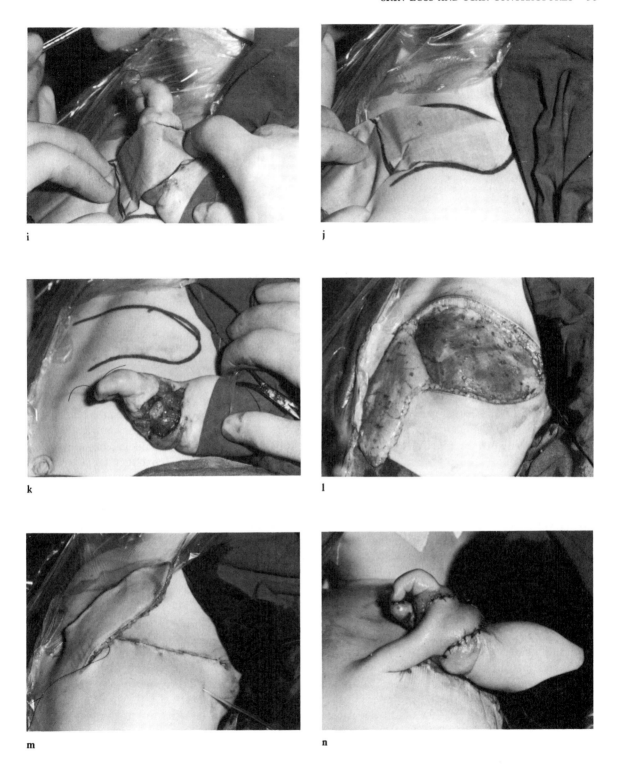

**Fig. 3.15** **i** A chest flap is planned in reverse. **j** The chest flap is then marked out on the child. **k** Proposed flap, and the defect for which it is intended. **l** Elevation of the flap. **m** Closure of the secondary defect. **n** Application of the flap

## Palmar digital defects affecting the proximal and middle phalangeal areas

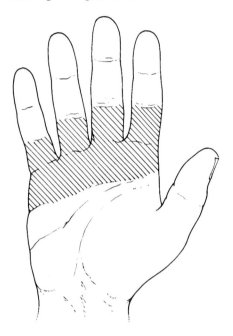

## Distal palmar defects

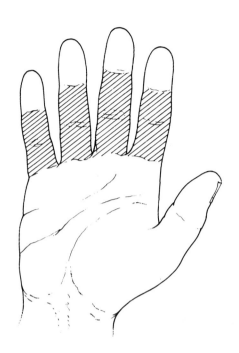

It is unusual for these defects to exceed the confines of a single phalangeal area. They can, therefore, be adequately covered by cross-finger flaps (Fig. 3.16).

Extensive loss of skin (two phalangeal areas in a single digit) from the volar surface should not be treated by a large cross-finger flap as this would involve exposure of the dorsum of the proximal interphalangeal joint in the donor finger leading to some restriction of movement.

Most commonly, these defects are covered by the use of distant flaps. The priority in choosing a donor site must be the provision of thin skin.

The radial artery fasciocutaneous forearm flap may be used to cover the entire volar surface of multiple digital injuries if the injury is syndactylised. Later interdigital division may be required. When the radial flap is used in a retrograde fashion problems have been encountered with venous drainage and in cases of doubt the use of a venous anastomosis should ensure an adequate circulation. The resulting donor site following the use of this flap is, however, cosmetically unacceptable to many patients and in particular it should never be used in young women.

Skin loss in this area may be associated with burns or the resection of Dupuytren's contracture with involved overlying skin. If underlying fat is lost, flap cover is required. In congenital deformities there may be distal migration of the web space, requiring insertion of an adequate amount of skin. Skin grafts provide no tactile adherence and may not withstand the normal trauma of everyday use but they are of necessity routinely used in the primary treatment of large burns. Numerous local flaps are available to cover this area and these provide some degree of tactile adherence, an important consideration in this part of the palm which plays a key role in strong grip. If limited cover is required in the distal palmar area the flag flap is raised from the proximal phalangeal area. The flap is elevated superficial to the paratenon and passed through the interdigital cleft to be inset into the volar defect.

The seagull flap is useful to deepen the web space and simultaneously cover distal palmar defects. This flap is really two flag flaps in which the flag poles have been combined (Fig. 3.17).

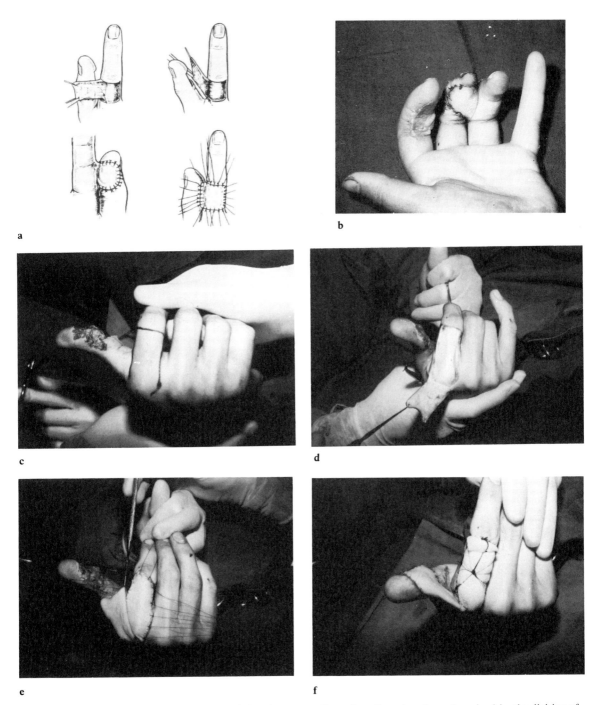

**Fig. 3.16** Cross-finger flap. **a** The principles of elevating a cross-finger flap. Extra length can be gained by the division of Cleland's ligaments. **b** A cross-finger flap having been applied to a volar defect on the middle finger. **c** A cross-finger flap designed from the dorsum of the index finger, proximally based to cover a defect resulting from a circular saw injury to the thumb. The flexor pollicis longus had been badly damaged and initially skin cover was obtained before allowing this patient to undergo a secondary tendon graft. **d** Elevation of the flap designed in **c**. The paratenon has been carefully preserved over the underlying extensor apparatus. **e** A full thickness skin graft has been applied to the secondary defect in **d**. **f** A tie-over dressing has been applied to keep the skin graft in place and a cross-finger flap has been sutured into place on the recipient site

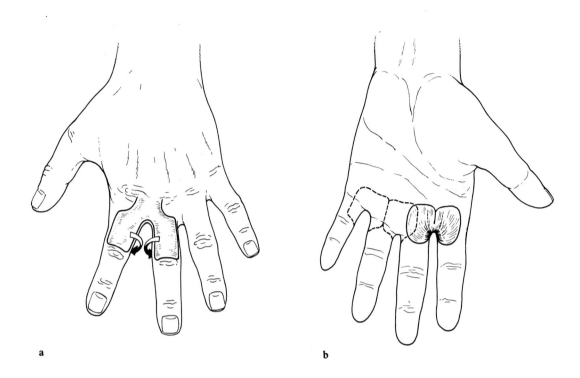

a                                                    b

**Fig. 3.17**   The seagull flap. **a** This is really a combination of two axial flag flaps. It is useful in covering the volar surface of the metacarpophalangeal joint area, after release of contractures or in the presence of skin loss, as in **b**

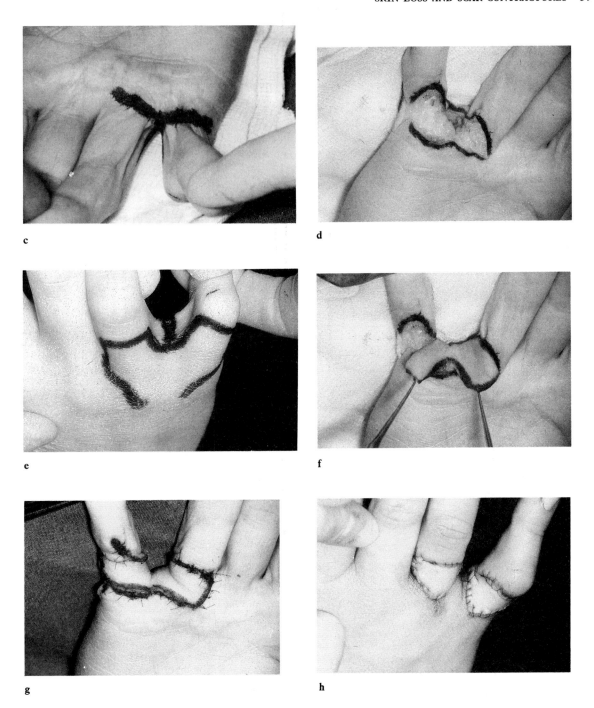

**Fig. 3.17** **c** Planned release of contractures affecting the metacarphophalangeal joint area. **d** Defect following release of contracture. **e** Proposed plan of seagull flap. **f** Delivery of flap from the dorsum. **g** Flap having been sutured into place. **h** Full thickness grafting of dorsum. Note the excellent web space that is obtained using this technique

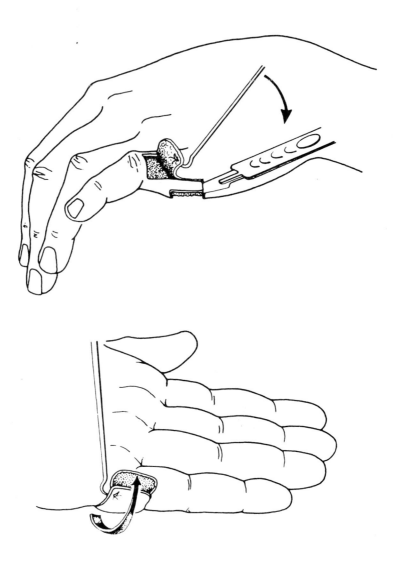

**Fig. 3.18**  The dorsal transposition flap. Reproduced with permission from Rob & Smith, Operative Surgery — The Hand, 4th edn, Butterworth & Co. (Publishers).

The dorsal transposition flap is a longitudinally orientated flap taken from the dorsal aspect of the proximal phalangeal area. Having been elevated it is transposed around the side of the digit and inset into the region of the flexion crease of the metacarpophalangeal joint. This flap needs to be inset in a lax fashion, otherwise a circular constricting scar is formed on the lateral aspect of the digit. This may interfere with venous drainage and compress the neurovascular bundle supplying the ulnar aspect of the finger. The flap is particularly useful in the little finger (Fig. 3.18). Metacarpophalangeal joint immobilisation for a period of about 2 weeks is necessary in the position which takes tension off the pedicle. Rest is required to allow adequate take of the full thickness skin grafts which have been applied to the secondary defects. Provided the patient is subsequently rapidly mobilised, no ill-effects are encountered.

Extensive cover of distal palmar defects requires distant flap cover as in the case of the proximal palm.

## Proximal palmar dorsal metacarpal and wrist area defects

Free tissue transfers are the method of choice in the treatment of these proximal areas (Fig. 3.19). If such a service is unobtainable, random abdominal flaps or chest flaps from the inframammary area may be used. The hand is of necessity positioned close to the donor site in such a way as to prevent a full range of movement being obtained in all the joints of the upper limb (in particular at the metacarpophalangeal joints). A stiff hand is common after the application of these flaps. Vigorous physiotherapy is required to achieve normal function.

The use of the groin flap avoids these problems. The secondary defect leaves a linear scar in an area which is well hidden. It is raised so that it always has a 10-cm long pedicle. Distal to this a paddle of skin can be inset into the defect. It is thus possible to mobilise the upper limb more effectively.

The 10-cm pedicle allows motion of the shoulder, elbow, wrist and hand joints without fear of dislodging the flap or pulling the hand away from the body. Supination and pronation of the wrist are possible. Minimal strapping is required, which is discarded within 24 hours of application of the flap. The patient is then encouraged to mobilise and immediate rehabilitation of the injured hand is therefore possible (Fig. 3.14).

The groin flap can be elevated without any prior delay to a length of 25 cm almost irrespective of the width of its pedicle. The pedicle must be placed over the known course of the superficial circumflex iliac artery (Fig. 3.20). It is wise to use sufficient width to allow tubing of the pedicle without tension as congestion of the flap may result. The donor defect is closed directly, if less than 10 cm in width. The hip is flexed to reduce tension on this wound. The proximal portion of the groin flap is then tubed and the distal paddle can be inset. Division of the pedicle is undertaken at about 3 weeks. If the pedicle is to be used in further reconstruction an initial delay is necessary. This is undertaken by dividing the superficial circumflex iliac artery and vein as close to the base of the pedicle as possible. A formal division of the flap is then undertaken a week later. Details of the elevation of groin flaps are to be found in texts concerned with technique. One point, however, should be made. The fascia at the medial border of the sartorius muscle must be elevated along with the flap. At this point the superficial circumflex iliac artery changes from its position deep to this fascia to become more superficial in the subcutaneous tissues. If this fascia is not elevated the arterial supply is inevitably kinked at this point. Elevation of the fascia allows an extra 5 cm to be added to the flap.

If cover is required simultaneously for both proximal palmar and dorsal metacarpal areas the Y-shaped hypogastric groin flap may be used. This is a combination of a groin flap and hypogastric flap on a common pedicle (Fig. 3.21).

The radial forearm flap (Fig. 3.22) is an alternative source of skin cover in the hand.

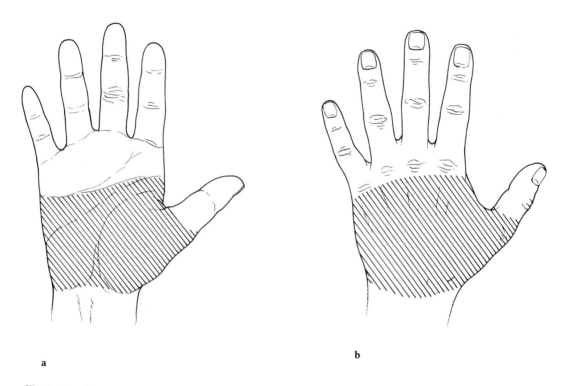

a

b

**Fig. 3.19   a** Palmar skin loss, proximal to the distal palmar crease. **b** Dorsal skin loss in the metacarpal area

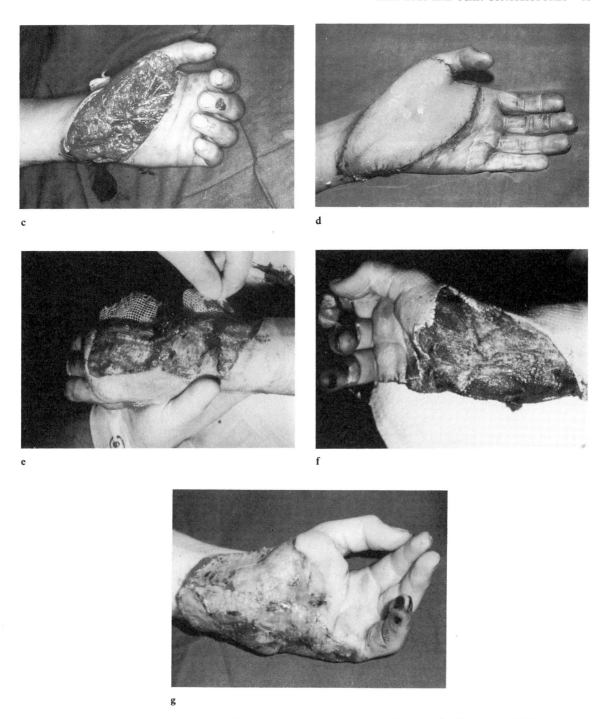

**Fig. 3.19   c** A palmar degloving injury, exposing tendons and neurovascular bundles requiring flap cover. **d** A free vascularised groin flap used to produce immediate skin cover using microvascular techniques. Immediate mobilisation can be commenced. **e** Severe crushing injury producing dorsal skin loss and volar skin loss as seen in **f**. It should be remembered that simple split skin grafting and positioning of the hand in the appropriate position may often be all that is required. **g** Skin grafting of these defects

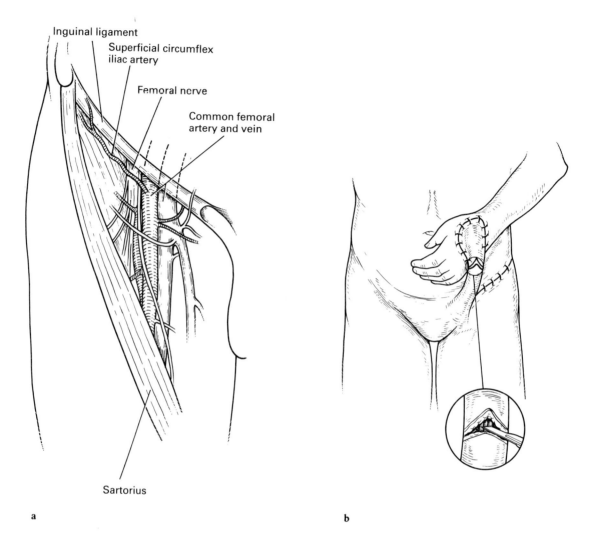

Inguinal ligament

Superficial circumflex
iliac artery

Femoral nerve

Common femoral
artery and vein

Sartorius

a

b

**Fig. 3.20   a** The superficial circumflex iliac artery is the axial basis of the groin flap. It runs below and parallel to the inguinal ligament. **b** Occasionally it is necessary to divide the pedicle of a groin flap and use the pedicle in reconstruction. This is particularly important when a thumb is being reconstructed. If the pedicle is required in reconstruction, a delay must be performed by incising the base of the pedicle locating the vessels, and dividing them.

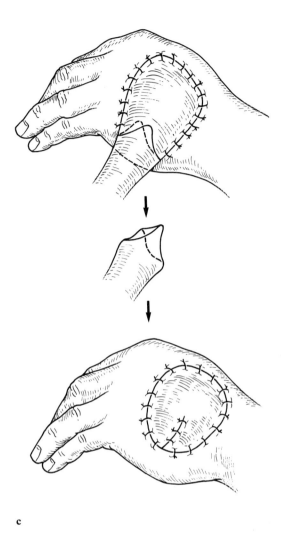

c

**Fig. 3.20**   c If only the distal portion of the flap is being utilised for reconstruction, no delay is required and the flap can be immediately inset as illustrated

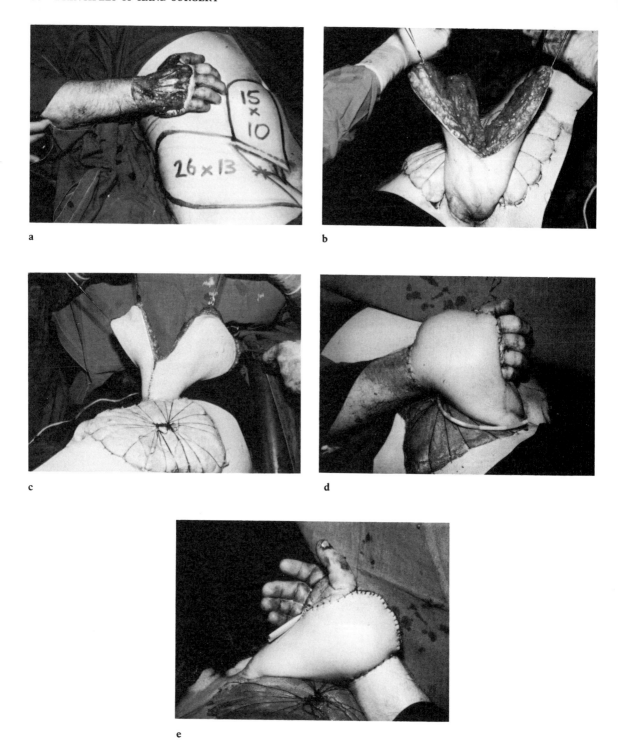

**Fig. 3.21** **a** The design of the Y-shaped hypogastric groin flap used to cover a volar and palmar skin defect with exposed underlying tendons. **b** After elevation of the Y-shaped flap, the pedicle is tubed, producing two flaps which oppose each other, into which the hand can be inset. **c** The view from above. **d** Application of the Y-shaped hypogastric groin flap to the hand. **e** A view of the volar application of the flap

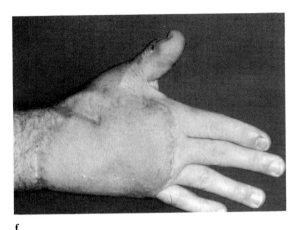

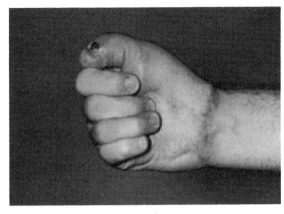

f

g

**Fig. 3.21** f Result after one thinning procedure showing full extension of the fingers and thumb. g Result after one thinning showing full flexion of the digits

## Forearm defects

Extensive flap cover of forearm defects is rarely required unless further reconstructive efforts are to be undertaken at a later date. Skin grafts are perfectly adequate for the provision of cover to the proximal two-thirds of the forearm. In the distal third of the forearm, flap cover of tendons is preferable. To cover the whole of the forearm, more skin is required than can reliably be provided by the groin flap (which will not extend sufficiently far up the arm). It is safer to use random abdominal flaps (Fig. 3.23).

In using random flaps certain principles need to be borne in mind. The design of such flaps is undertaken in the operating room with the patient anaesthetised. Under such circumstances the forearm can be supinated with ease. However, the natural position of the forearm in the alert and conscious patient is that of semipronation and flaps should be designed in this position. The design of the skin flap system should give a completely closed system with no raw areas to granulate and provide a bed for infection with saprophytic organisms. Where there is underlying bone exposed this is a matter of considerable importance but even in its absence such infections will delay wound healing.

The design should be such that gravity will increase the application of the flap to the defect. In general inferiorly based flaps are preferred because the natural tendency of the forearm to become more dependent will increase the wrap-around effect of the abdominal flap upon the defect. Superiorly based flaps tend to detach from the defect if the limb drops inferiorly. However,

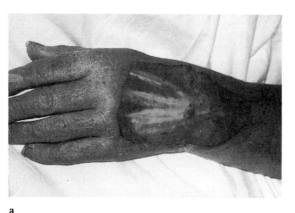

a

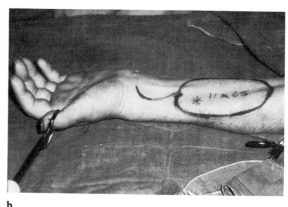

b

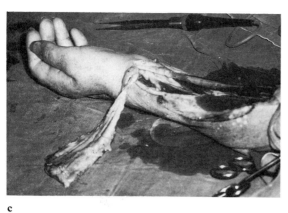

c

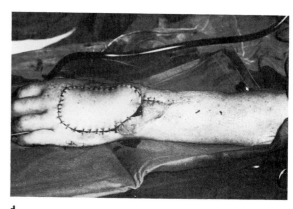

d

**Fig. 3.22   a** The radial flap, used to reconstruct a dorsal defect resulting from extravasation of intravenous dextrose in a patient suffering from diabetes. **b** Outline of the radial flap. **c** Elevation of the radial flap, distally based. **d** Suture of the flap in place

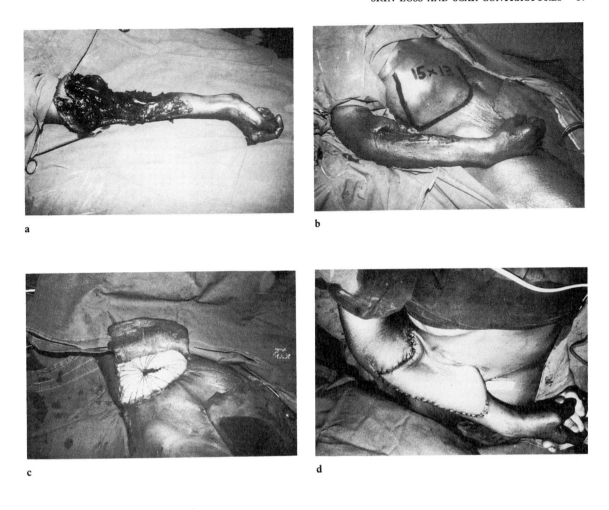

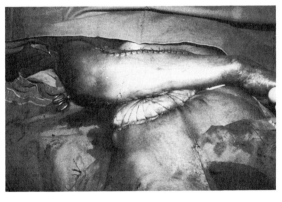

**Fig. 3.23** **a** Extensive damage of the forearm caused by being pushed through a plate glass window, devascularising the hand; complete destruction of all the muscle tendon bellies which were avulsed and of the median and the ulnar nerves and the radial nerve. This patient required immediate skin cover and at a later date had tendon transfers and a wrist fusion performed. **b** Proposed outline of a random abdominal flap. **c** Elevation of the flap. Grafting of the secondary defect and grafting of the bridge portion of the pedicle. **d** Application of the flap to the defect. **e** Flap applied, view from below

for dorsal forearm defects, a superiorly based flap is more easily applied since it has a shorter pedicle. For volar defects an inferiorly based flap would be aided in its application by the effect of gravity. The pedicle base however, although initially satisfactory, may be turned through 180° by the effect of gravity. The choice of which flap to use depends on the siting of the defect and upon the mobility and length of each patient's limb. The technical elevation of such flaps is relatively simple, but much experience is required in their planning. Their postoperative supervision requires the attention of specialised nursing staff.

### Tissue expansion

Tissue expansion involves the use of an expandable prosthesis placed in the subcutaneous tissues. Gradual inflation of this increases the amount of overlying skin and mitotic figures have been noted in the basal layers of the skin in response to such expansion. It seems that new skin may therefore be generated and not the existing skin merely stretched. It is possible to expand skin adjacent to a defect and then upon removal of the expander to use the increased amount of skin for cover. The technique of tissue expansion is likely to play an increasing role in the management of upper limb skin loss. However, it is more useful as a preliminary to the elective surgical excision of an area of tissue. If an open wound exists, it is better to graft it and use an expander as a secondary procedure.

# SKIN CONTRACTURES

Superficial dermal wounds will normally proceed to healing within 2 or 3 weeks by epithelialisation from dermal islands. Full thickness loss of dermis, however, will heal by secondary intention if left ungrafted, producing abundant scar tissue and later contractures. Delayed wound healing, with infection or unopposed contraction following injury or operation, will produce similar results. In all of these contractures a sheet of scar tissue develops.

Linear contractures, which consist of a tight band of skin, can be seen as the result of poor scar placement in relation to the relaxed skin tension lines. They arise from poor planning of surgical incisions with unsatisfactory placement of flap or graft marginal scars.

Such contractures, whether of the linear or sheet variety, can arise from primary problems in the skin. If they are allowed to become longstanding, secondary changes occur in the underlying structures. Tendons may become shorter, the fascia overlying muscle may become thickened and shortened and peri-articular joint adhesions may lead to fixed joint deformities. The converse is also true: thus a failed primary tendon repair, an intra-articular fracture with a volar plate injury, a muscle infarct, or paralysis after nerve injury may all lead to deformity which, if uncorrected, produces secondary skin shortening.

Reconstruction of such contractures depends not only on whether they are linear or sheet but also upon the presence of associated deformities of underlying structures. All aspects of a contracture must be released to produce a longstanding correction. Early scar tissue is composed of immature collagen which is metabolically a very active tissue. It is in a dynamic state undergoing constant replacement and is capable of responding to external stresses. The scar may be lengthened and collagen reorientated at this stage. Postoperative splintage is therefore of great importance in the maintenance of a correction. Splintage is certainly required for the first few weeks after contracture release and night splintage should normally be continued until collagen maturity. At the time of surgical correction adequate skin cover should be provided. Prior to surgical release preoperative splintage will often partially correct the deformity. An end-point is reached where no further progress is made and surgical intervention is then indicated. Occasionally it is possible to straighten a flexed digit by releasing contracted structures in the palm (for example Dupuytren's contracture). In other circumstances, the cause of the contracture lies within the flexed digit itself. Problems may be encountered if a midlateral approach is chosen as the previous surgeon may have used a volar incision such as that described by Bruner. Long-established contractures are a pitfall for the unwary. It is important to realise that collagen is freely deposited in a finger which has been held in flexion for a long period of time, not only around the joints but also around the neurovascular bundles. The vessels become embedded within a collagen framework and surgical release, allowing full extension of the digit, may compress or even tear the vessels rendering the digit ischaemic. Lack of distal perfusion is usually apparent immediately upon release of the tourniquet. If perfusion remains poor in extension the finger should be allowed to flex for this may improve the circulation. The use of dynamic extension over succeeding weeks will usually regain extension. If digital flexion does not produce improved circulation, urgent exploration of the digital vessels should be undertaken and vein grafts will be required. The patient should be warned of this possibility pre-operatively.

## LINEAR CONTRACTURES

These contractures present as scars which cross the flexor surfaces of joints or web spaces.

### The Z-plasty technique

The technique is used where there is a scar running across a joint or concavity, producing a linear contracture. There must be laxity of the skin on either side of the scar contracture as its release and gain in length is at the expense of the tissues on either side. There are numerous variations in the technique of Z-plasty and their use depends upon the amount of lengthening required in releasing the contracture, and the amount of laxity present in adjacent tissues (Fig. 3.24). The presence of previous scars may determine the type of Z-plasty release undertaken. Fundamental to the success of a Z-plasty are:

1. The release of the underlying contracture, and
2. The transposition of two flaps so that the central limb of the Z-plasty is more favourably placed.

If step 1 is achieved successfully, step 2 follows automatically. When a Z-plasty will not transpose with ease the contracture may require further release or the original planning of the procedure has been incorrect. The length and angle of the limbs may be varied. Both of these factors influence the ease of transposition of the flaps as well as the percentage increase in longitudinal skin length. A 60° Z-plasty with equal length limbs will produce a 75% lengthening. It is important to note that the outer limbs of a Z-plasty never move — only the central element transposes. Thus in the initial planning of the Z-plasty, particularly in scar revisions, the limbs should be planned to be as nearly parallel as possible to the relaxed skin tension lines. The longer the limbs the more difficult it is to transpose the flaps and the smaller the angle between the limbs and the central element the less lengthening occurs upon transposition. The flaps must be thick enough to include both dermis and subcutaneous tissue to ensure adequate vascularity. Occasionally this is a problem if a linear exposure is used in Dupuytren's and converted to a Z-plasty. If there is a shortage of lax tissue on either side of the contracture a simple Z-plasty may not be possible. However, a multiple Z-plasty can give the same degree of lengthening without the need for transposition of large adjacent skin flaps. In the release of web space contractures previous scarring may prejudice the outcome of a single large Z-plasty and the four-flap Z-plasty or double reversed Z with central Y–V may be required to producce lengthening of the web (Fig. 3.25).

## SHEET CONTRACTURES

Sheet contractures may affect the first web space or the volar surface of the digit. Replacement of the skin defect may require the use of full thickness skin grafts or of a flap. Where a whole area of skin requires replacement complete skin cover should be obtained at the time of the release so that there are no raw areas producing granulation tissue and therefore excessive scar tissue. At the lateral aspects of joints the skin cover should reach the midaxial point of the joint to prevent any tendency towards marginal scarring producing flexion contractures. Once the contracture has been released this position needs to be maintained

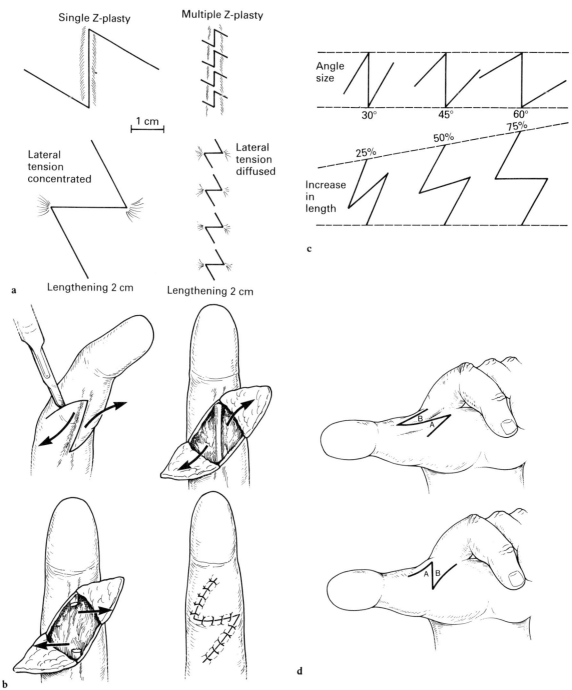

**Fig. 3.24** **a** In a contracture treated by a single Z-plasty, it should be noted that only the central limb transposes. If the tissue laxity on either side of the contracture is insufficient to allow a large Z-plasty, the same degree of lengthening can be obtained by a multiple Z-plasty, as shown on the right. **b** Illustration of a clinical problem with scar contracture crossing the flexion crease of a digit at right angles, producing a linear contracture and flexion deformity. The proposed Z-plasty is planned so that the resulting central limb will eventually lie in the flexion crease of the digit. The flaps are elevated, the underlying contracture band is removed and the flaps automatically transposed upon extension of the digit. **c** Altering the angle of the Z-plasty increases the length gained up to a maximum of about 60°, after which the difficulties of transposing the flaps cannot be surmounted in order to capitalise on the intended increase in length. **d** A large Z-plasty used to deepen the web space and release a contracture of the first web space. This is the one situation where the angle can be increased to 90° and flap transposition can still occur

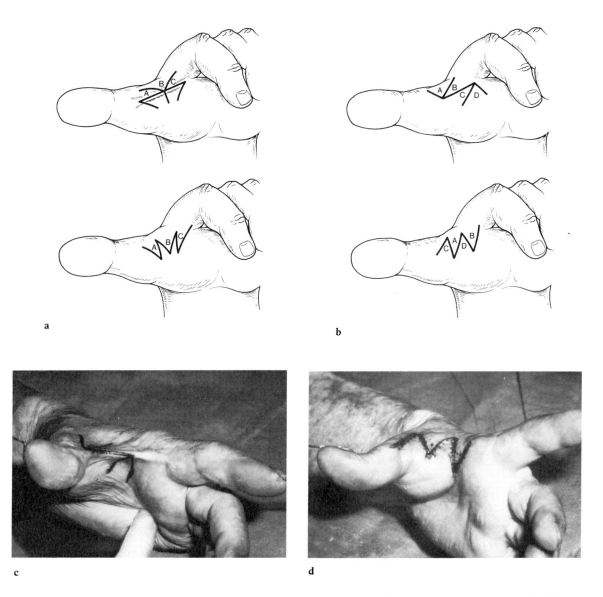

**Fig. 3.25 a** Occasionally the presence of scarring in the web space may be such that a large Z-plasty is impossible. Flaps may therefore have to be designed to take into account the distribution of existing scars. A double opposed Z-plasty with a central Y to V plan is shown in this illustration. **b** Another alternative plan is the use of the four flap Z-plasty, as shown above. This gives excellent increase in length for minimal availability of transposable tissue on either side of the contracture. **c** A clinical case of the four flap Z-plasty showing the plan. **d** Result after transposition of the flaps

while wound healing occurs. If necessary Kirschner pins may be required to maintain the digits in full extension while a full thickness graft takes to the underlying bed, or the first web space may require splinting in abduction to assist in flap application. *Prolonged night splintage for several months is required to ensure maintenance of correction during collagen maturation.*

## SUMMARY

Wound healing by secondary intention must be avoided in the hand. It is a malignant physiological process leading to scar deposition and the elimination of loose areolar tissue planes. As a result, the hand becomes encased in scar tissue, restricting mobility and suppleness. Months of rehabilitation may be necessary prior to secondary reconstructive procedures and valuable time is thus lost. Skin cover changes the pace of repair by allowing primary wound healing and immediate rehabilitation. Free tissue transfers, where appropriate, represent the most efficient means of achieving these aims at the present time.

# 4. Fingertip injuries and amputations

*Principal authors:   P. J. Smith, F. D. Burke*

## FINGERTIP INJURIES

The fingertips represent the final frontier between man and his hostile environment. As he explores his surroundings, they act as sensory probes which are so richly innervated that they have been called the eyes of the upper limb. Their other function is as the final effector mechanism of a motor system capable of precise manipulation and great dexterity. This explains their anatomical complexity, which is such that even a relatively trivial injury will fundamentally alter their specialised functions. This dual role exposes them to noxious stimuli and mechanical dangers which account for the frequency with which they are injured. There is no satisfactory substitute for this sophisticated tissue (Fig. 4.1).

Injuries to the fingertips are among the most frequent seen in the casualty department. It is therefore inevitable that they are treated by the least experienced members of staff. Poor management can lead to prolonged or permanent disability but appropriate treatment should lead to a rapid return of function. It is the responsibility of the hand surgeon to establish clear assessment methods and reliable guidelines of management for the local emergency department.

Every injury in which tissue is amputated presents the surgeon with the choice of recon-

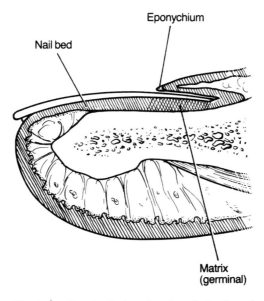

**Fig. 4.1** a Longitudinal section through the fingertip

struction or terminalisation. In such circumstances there are ideal levels of shortening at which the digit functions best. If exposed tendon insertions are intact, reconstruction by soft tissue coverage may be indicated.

## ASSESSMENT

In assessing any patient with a fingertip injury, a precise appreciation of both the *mechanism* and *anatomy* of the injury is essential before formulating a plan for management. The *patient's general health* may also influence the decision to reconstruct or terminalise and may influence the choice of reconstructive technique.

### Mechanism of injury

The mechanism of injury is the key factor in determining the site and extent of injury and the surgeon must therefore determine how the accident occurred. The wounding instrument may indicate whether tissues have been cut, crushed or avulsed. Blunt trauma, producing crushing injuries, leads to compression of the nail-bed and pulp against the phalanx. The less compressible structures are disrupted leading to stellate lacerations of the nail-bed overlying comminuted fractures of the terminal phalanx. Haematoma may develop subungually as well as in the pulp subcutaneous spaces. In severe cases, the pulp bursts open. A superimposed avulsion injury may occur when a finger is trapped by a door or between other objects; sudden withdrawal of the digit as a reflex action adds avulsion to the crushing injury.

Injuries with sharper objects, such as industrial guillotines, lead to differing patterns of tissue loss. In such injuries, damage is localised to the site of injury and reconstruction may be undertaken using adjacent tissues. Where the mechanism of amputation involves rotating machinery, damage may be more extensive than is at first apparent. The vascular tree undergoes a traction injury with intimal disruption proximally. This is particularly important should replantation be considered. The time since injury and the degree of contamination must also be determined as they may influence

whether the wound is closed primarily or delayed and whether or not deep structures are repaired (see Ch. 1).

### Anatomy of the injury

Examination of the fingertip will determine the *level and direction of tissue loss, the particular digit involved and whether there is multiple digital damage.* Oblique injuries to the fingertip may involve predominantly volar or dorsal loss, each requiring different methods of reconstruction (see below). In general where soft tissue injury occurs alone, skin grafts may be appropriate, but if bone is exposed, flap cover is required. Nail-bed injuries require careful treatment to minimise subsequent deformity. Transverse amputations proximal to the nail-bed may spare tendon insertions making reconstruction desirable, or may be associated with tendon loss making terminalisation appropriate.

The particular digit involved influences management. Stiff interphalangeal joints are less disabling in the thumb and index than in the ring and little fingers. On the radial side of the hand, restoration of sensation is the main aim but on the ulnar side preservation of power grip is more important. The maintenance of sensitive skin at the tips of the index finger and thumb is important if precision pinch is to be retained. In the index middle pinch area, consideration must be given to innervated flaps to provide sensation. Multiple digital involvement may remove the option of using skin from adjacent digits and if flap cover is required, the surgeon may be forced to use more distant donor sites.

### The general health of the patient

The *age* of the patient is crucial. In young children conservative management with appropriate dressings is likely to produce a more acceptable result than surgical reconstruction. This technique utilises the child's ability to partially regenerate amputated tissue. The degree of bony exposure is often used as the deciding factor in choosing conservative or surgical management. Major disproportion with extensive bone exposure requires skeletal shortening. However, lesser degrees of bony exposure do not require reconstruction in children. A tulle gras dressing is applied and should be left undisturbed until the dressing spontaneously separates, as in a healing skin graft donor site. Occasionally the dressing may become caked by blood and it may be felt desirable to remove it. If so, it should be soaked off gently while the child is under adequate sedation. There is no justification for the avulsion of such dressings in the fully alert child; a more compassionate approach maintains the child's confidence in his medical attendants as well as retaining regenerating epithelium. The young adult is primarily concerned with cosmesis and this should be taken into account in determining the method of management for this group of patients. In the elderly, the simplest technique appropriate for good wound healing should be chosen. Awkward positions of immobilisation for cross-finger flaps may lead to stiff digits in this group. Simpler reconstructive techniques should be used or terminalisation may be preferred to permit rapid rehabilitation.

The general health of the patient is of importance. Diabetes, impaired circulation due to vasculitis or exacerbated by smoking, vitamin deficiencies, hypoproteinaemia, immune deficiencies or the use of systemic drugs such as steroids, may all impair wound healing and influence the choice of technique in the management of the patient with the fingertip injury. The occupation of the patient may also significantly influence management. It may be appropriate to reconstruct a pianist's fingertip using complex techniques, but inappropriate to do so for the same injury in a manual labourer who has simpler requirements and wishes to return to work as rapidly as possible. The patient's recreational needs must also be considered as these may be more demanding than their occupation. Labourers may also be amateur woodworkers or musicians.

## TREATMENT

The aim in the management of fingertip injuries is to produce a durable pulp with good sensation which is stable on its underlying structures. Scars on the volar pulp should be avoided. If present, they should not adhere to underlying bone. The bone should be well padded with ample subcutaneous tissue. Divided nerve ends should lie in these well-padded areas. If the nail can be preserved and distal volar curvature avoided, it is useful. If not, it is troublesome and the germinal matrix should be ablated.

## Management of tissue disruption

### Subungual haematoma

Some authors advocate removal of the nail and the repair of the underlying nail-bed disruption. If the nail has not been displaced, it implies that the underlying disruption is minor. Treatment may be required if there is great discomfort. The haematoma can be evacuated by using a hot paperclip.

### Nail-bed disruption

In the management of any acute nail-bed injury, adequate splintage to maintain the eponychial fold and lateral nail fold is essential to minimise adhesions which may lead to later deformity. The treatment of established nail-bed deformities is unsatisfactory. It is therefore preferrable to reduce their incidence by careful primary treatment. If the nail is available it makes an excellent splint. If not, metal foil from a suture pack or folded tulle gras can be used (Fig. 4.2). A splint should be retained for 2 weeks. It should not be removed in error by nursing staff when the first dressing is changed. Nail-bed injury may be associated with a comminuted fracture of the terminal phalanx. Such fractures do not usually require specific treatment unless a fragment of bone penetrates the nail bed (see Ch. 6). In such circumstances, the fracture must be carefully manipulated into position or if necessary the protruding fragment should be levelled to allow adequate nail-bed reconstruction (see below). The nail-bed itself may be dislocated from the proximal nail-fold and this may be associated with an epiphysial injury in children. It is simply remedied by replacing the proximal germinal matrix deep to the eponychial fold (Fig. 4.3). Stellate lacerations of the nail-bed should be repaired under magnification with 6/0 plain catgut. The wound edges are often friable and the sutures tend to tear out (Fig. 4.4).

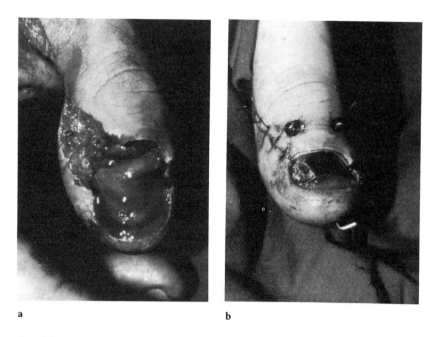

a                                                      b

**Fig. 4.2**  **a** Reconstruction of a nail-bed injury and reinsertion of an extensor tendon.
**b** The nail-fold is retained by the use of a folded piece of aluminium

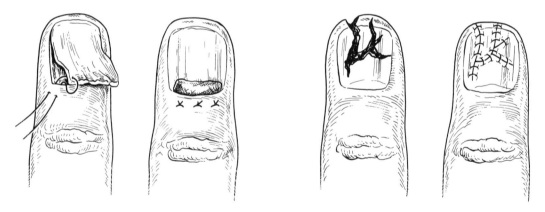

**Fig. 4.3**   Nail-bed dislocation                **Fig. 4.4**   Stellate laceration of the nail-bed

*Pulp disruption*

If the pulp is disrupted due to a bursting injury,
it may normally be closed primarily but undue
tension should be avoided. In the rare case where
gross swelling prevents primary closure, the
wound should be cleaned and débrided and the
limb elevated, allowing the fingertip to heal spontaneously. If conservative management is
undertaken, it is particularly important to ensure
that the healing pulp is not displaced laterally
leaving the distal phalanx without adequate
cushioning. Significantly displaced pulp tissue
may require repositioning.

## Management of tissue loss

### Soft tissue loss without bone involvement

These isolated pulp injuries remove the full thickness of the skin and expose the underlying subcutaneous fibrofatty tissues. Treatment is governed by the size of the defect. If the defect is less than 1 cm in diameter, wound contracture should be encouraged to diminish the size of the resulting scar. For these defects, an extremely thin split skin graft may be applied or the wound may be allowed to contract spontaneously. This graft will contract to diminish the size of the defect thus producing a smaller area of sensory abnormality on the terminal pulp. If the defect is greater than 1 cm in diameter, the aim is to replace it with tissue as similar as possible to the normal structures. A hypothenar graft is useful in this situation but care must be exercised as the donor site can prove troublesome. The amputated portion of the pulp, if present and suitable, may be defatted and applied as a full thickness graft. In general, in these circumstances hypothenar grafts give better results (Fig. 4.5).

### Fingertip injury with bone exposure

Management is determined by the direction of tissue loss which may be either transverse or oblique. If oblique, the volar pulp or nail-bed may be the predominant tissue lost. A different method of reconstruction is required for each of these types of injury.

The extent of the nail-bed injury should be assessed. If the proximal half of the nail-bed remains, the germinal matrix is viable and a new nail will eventually grow. If less than half the nail-bed remains and there is no distal phalanx to provide support for the regenerating nail it may develop a pronounced curvature. In such circumstances, consideration should be given to ablating the remaining nail-bed to avoid subsequent problems.

### Volar loss with bone exposure

The cross-finger flap is the ideal method of reconstruction for this defect. The flap can be based transversely, proximally or distally. The trans-

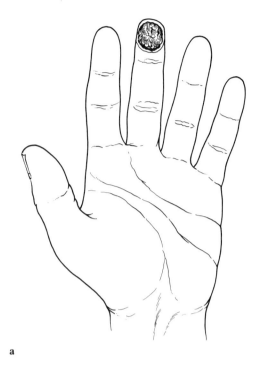

a

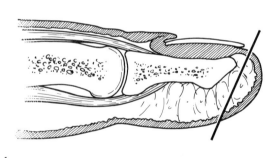

b

**Fig. 4.5** Hypothenar graft to the finger tip. **a** Showing the soft tissue exposure alone. **b** Diagram illustrating soft tissue injury to the pulp alone. This is suitable for a graft

versely based cross-finger flap is most commonly used. The donor finger should lie beside the injured digit with ease and there should be no tension in the flap. Consideration should be given to the resulting cosmetic defect on the dorsum of the hand. This can be minimised by raising the flap as a complete cosmetic unit stretching from proximal to distal interphalangeal flexion/extension creases and from midlateral line to midlateral line. After reconstruction with a full thickness graft, the donor defect looks more acceptable than an oblique or rounded defect. Although contour may be satisfactory using this technique the problem of graft pigmentation remains. The flaps are elevated under tourniquet control and care is taken to preserve the paratenon overlying the extensor tendon. The flap is reflected until Cleland's liga-

ments, which lie dorsal to the neurovascular bundles, are visible. If an increase in length is required to approximate the flap to the defect, this can be achieved by the division of Cleland's ligaments. An extra 3–5 mm of skin can be obtained by this method. The flap is then trimmed to fit the defect, the tourniquet is released and haemo-

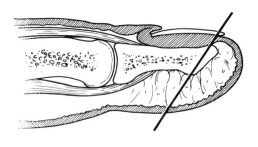

a

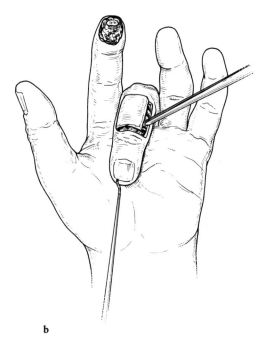

b

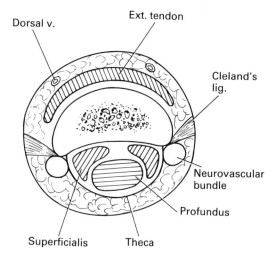

c

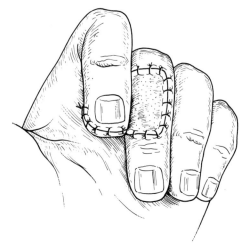

d

Fig. 4.6  a Volar loss with bone exposure. Ideal for cross-finger flap coverage. b Elevation of a cross-finger flap. An incision is made in the dermis. The vessels are coagulased and the flap is raised superficial to the paratenon covering the extensor tendon. c Transverse section through the digit showing the relationship between the extensor tendon and the phalanx and the flexor tendons, the neurovascular bundles, and Cleland's ligaments. The paratenon over the extensor tendon must be preserved in elevating a cross-finger flap. Cleland's ligaments may be divided at the base of the cross-finger flap to gain extra length. d Cross-finger flap applied to the tip of an index finger defect with grafting of the donor finger

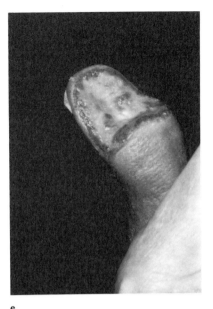

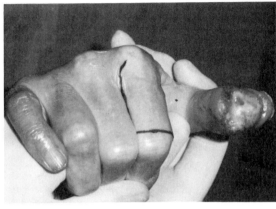

e

f

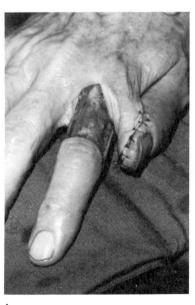

g

h

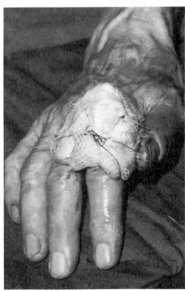

i

**Fig. 4.6  e** A cross-finger flap used to reconstruct the thumb defect resulting from an infection. **f** The proposed cross-finger flap outlined on the index finger. It is a proximally based flap. **g** Elevation of the cross-finger flap, leaving the paratenon intact. **h** Application of the cross-finger flap to the recipient site. **i** A tie-over dressing applied to the skin graft on the dorsum of the index finger. A splint is then applied to immobilise the hand

stasis achieved. The flap is sutured in place and a full thickness skin graft is applied to the secondary defect. A plaster cast should be used to protect the repair by immobilising the adjacent digits (Fig. 4.6).

Division is undertaken 10–21 days after application of the flap. The timing depends on the area of the inset, the width of the pedicle and the age of the patient. The inset of the flap is the contact area which has been established between the flap and the recipient bed. The more extensive this is, the more likely that the recipient bed will have revascularised the flap and be capable of maintaining its viability upon division of the pedicle. The width of the pedicle gives an indication of the flap's dependency on the blood supply from the donor site. The wider the pedicle, the larger is the blood supply and the more dominant it is in

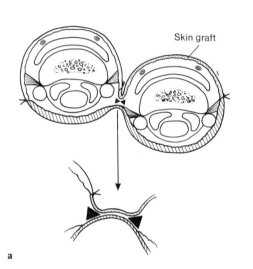

Skin graft

a

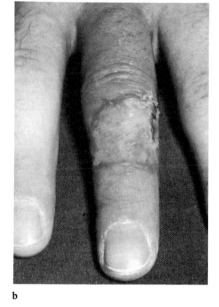

b

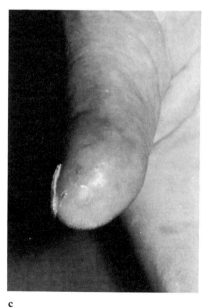

c

**Fig. 4.7   a** The Recipient and donor fingers are bridged by the cross-finger flap and a skin graft applied to the secondary defect. At the point of bridging, two triangular areas of fibrous tissue develop which must be removed at the time of division. **b** The donor site after division. **c** The result of a cross-finger flap applied to the tip of the thumb after division

relation to the blood supply from the recipient bed. A wide pedicle may therefore need to be divided in stages, whereas a narrow pedicle in the presence of an extensive inset can be divided in one stage. The quality of the final result is influenced by the care taken during division of the cross-finger flap. It should always be performed under tourniquet and the wound should be inspected prior to surgery to ascertain if conditions are suitable for the operation to proceed; there should be no infection, maceration or flap separation. The inset must be extensive enough to maintain flap viability upon division. The flap is divided leaving more on the recipient site than on the donor site. This leaves two raw wide edges, one on the side of the recipient finger and the other on the side of the donor finger. These raw areas are the apex of a triangular wedge of scar tissue which develops at the points of reflection and inset of the skin flap (Fig. 4.7). These triangular areas should be excised in order to allow complete inset of the flap in its recipient site as well as closure at the margin of the donor defect. The fingers are mobilised 48 hours after division.

*Transverse loss with bone exposure*

These injuries may be suitable for management using a cross-finger flap or a *thenar flap* (Fig. 4.8). Proximally based thenar flaps have a tendency to pull away from the recipient site. Distally based flaps by contrast tend to have their apposition to the recipient site increased as the finger extends. However their pedicle base is folded through almost 180° to achieve cover. Transversely lying thenar flaps can be elevated by using distally based flaps with eccentric limbs. The flap will turn towards the longest limb to cover volar defects and such flaps can also be used to cover dorsal defects around the eponychial fold. All thenar flaps should be taken from the metacarpophalangeal flexion crease area at the base of the thumb. Care must be used in their elevation to avoid injuring the digital nerves to the thumb. The main problem with thenar flaps is that they tend to produce stiffness in the proximal interphalangeal joint of the recipient digit due to the position of immobilisation that is necessary and the length of time that it has to be maintained.

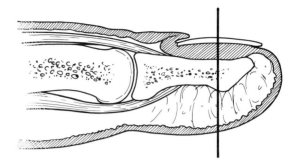

a

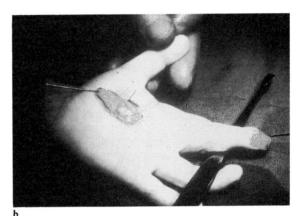

b

Fig. 4.8 a Transverse loss with bone exposure b Illustration of a thenar flap

They are thus most useful in young children and should not be used in the elderly.

*Dorsal loss with bone exposure*

Dorsally oblique injuries exposing bone remove a large percentage of the nail-bed matrix (Fig. 4.9).

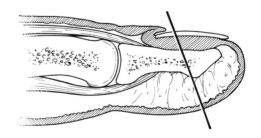

Fig. 4.9 Dorsal loss with bone exposure. Note the amount of nail-bed damage that may occur

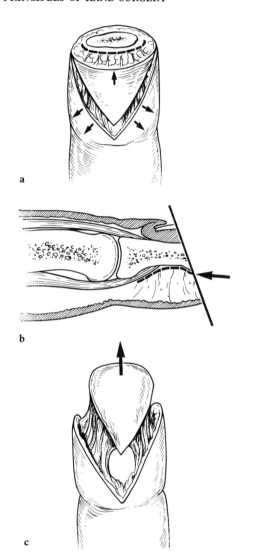

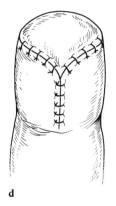

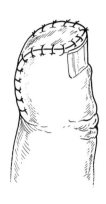

**Fig. 4.10** The design of the Atasoy V–Y advancement flap. **a** The visor-shaped flap is advanced to cover the tip of the finger by undermining it so that it is purely dependent on neurovascular pedicles on either side. **b** Showing the fibrous septae which would anchor the flap. **c** Advancement of the flap to cover the tip of the finger. **d** The result of the V–Y advancement flap

It is more common therefore to have to ablate the residual nail-bed in these injuries. The *V–Y advancement flap* popularised by Atasoy is the ideal method of reconstruction for this kind of injury (Fig. 4.10). It can also be applied to vertical injuries provided that a minimal amount of bone shortening is undertaken.

The principle behind the design of this flap is that it swings like a visor or hood to a more dorsal situation. Its viability and sensation is maintained through the volar branches of the terminal trifurcation of the neurovascular bundles on either side.

It is similar to a child's swing with the seat representing the flap and the rope on either side representing the neurovascular input. It is clear therefore that subcutaneous tissue on either side needs to be preserved to maintain the viability and sensibility of the transferred skin flap. If the volar cortex of the terminal phalanx presents an acute angle this can be rounded off. A triangular flap is designed with the base of the triangle placed distally along the volar edge of the fingertip defect. The apex of the triangle is placed proximally at the flexion crease of the distal interphalangeal joint. The narrower this angle the easier it is to close the secondary defect once the flap is advanced. An incision is made along the sides of the triangle through dermis only. As soon as subcutaneous tissue is reached, the knife is placed parallel to the overlying dermis and used to undermine in a proximal and lateral direction. In order to mobilise the flap, attention must now be directed to the fibrous septae as they attach to the periosteum on the volar surface of the distal phalanx. These are then divided at their bony insertion and it should be possible to elevate the base of the flap and advance it to the dorsal edge of the defect, suturing it in place. The secondary defect which was originally a V is now closed as a Y. There should be no tension. If there is evidence of tension, it implies that mobilisation of the flap has been unsatisfactory. Stitches should be left in place for 3 weeks. If removed earlier, as with all V–Y techniques, there is a tendency for the flap to return towards its original position. This is an elegant method of reconstruction which provides virtually normal pulp tissue with normal sensation. It must, however, be performed with care for if the flap fails through poor technique or inadequate postoperative management, the specialised pulp tissue is irretrievably lost. As with all flap surgery these patients require early inpatient monitoring of flap circulation and the technique should only be undertaken by experienced surgeons.

*The Kutler technique* which involves using smaller triangular flaps from the lateral portion of the stump produces a less satisfactory result because of the vertical scar which it creates at the centre of the pulp. If there is some dehiscence of the wound, then a wide and insensitive scar results. If the volar V–Y advancement technique retracts, the resultant granulation tissue and scar is placed on the distal portion of the nail-bed and may contribute to a curved nail but the pulp itself will still retain its desirable characteristics of laterally placed scars and normal sensation.

### Bone exposure proximal to the nail-bed

Treatment is governed by the level of vascular damage in a clean-cut amputation (Fig. 4.11). If the vessels have been divided just proximal to the

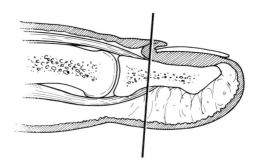

**Fig. 4.11**  Bone exposure proximal to the nail-bed

neurovascular trifurcation it may be feasible to replant the fingertip and such cases give the best results in replantation surgery. Should the part be unsuitable for replantation, then treatment is governed by the presence of the profundus insertion. If present, attempts should be made to preserve it in order to retain grip strength. In such circumstances, cross-finger or thenar flaps may be required. If the profundus insertion is disrupted, then stump closure with minimal bone shortening is undertaken, with contouring of the middle phalangeal condyles.

### The thumb

The same principles of management apply to the thumb as to the other digits. *The preservation of sensation and adequate length are of paramount importance.* Pulp loss associated with bony shortening or exposure may necessitate the use of innervated flaps to import sensation to this crucial area. The exposed bone ideally requires cover with pulp-like tissue. Cross-finger flaps do not provide the necessary subcutaneous tissue to re-create a normal pulp and fail to import adequate sensation, although some sensibility develops after 2 years. Pedicled neurovascular island flaps from the ring or middle finger will provide innervated pulp tissue but are associated with the problem of transference — sensation in the thumb perceived as in the donor digit. More extensive innervated cover may be achieved by the use of a radially innervated flap from the dorsum of the index finger. Free transfers of pulp tissue from the toes allow early one-stage reconstruction avoiding many of the complications associated with other methods. Their immediacy and safety has made them the method of choice in many centres.

### Free innervated flaps

Using microsurgical techniques it is possible to transfer the pulp from the great toe or web space skin, based on its digital vessels, and to suture these to the recipient vessels in the thumb. The plantar nerves are sutured to recipient nerves (Fig. 4.12). Such transfers avoid the 'crossover' problems associated with median and radial neurovascular island flaps. However, they do insert a nerve repair between the peripheral receptors and the central nervous system and so sensation is necessarily impaired, but they provide specialised pulp tissue without associated damage to other digits in the hand.

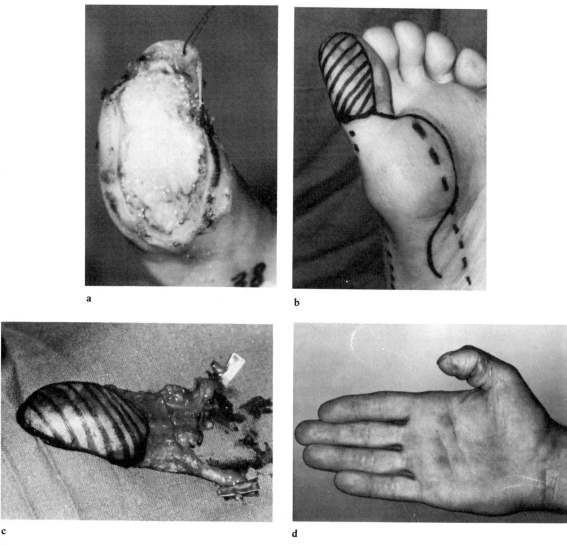

**Fig. 4.12**  Free innervated pulp flap to cover the thumb. **a** Amputation of the tip of the thumb exposing bone and requiring flap cover. **b** Neurovascular free pulp transfer, outlined on the sole of the foot. **c** Free pulp transfer having been elevated, neurovascular pedicles outlined and vessels clamped. **d** Result of free pulp transfer, with the patient actively flexing the thumb. Innervated two-point discrimination is 4 mm compared with 2 mm in the contralateral pulp

*The flag flap or radially innervated neurovascular flap*

The axial flag flap may be raised from the proximal phalangeal area of the dorsum of the index finger and is based on a pedicle running towards the second web space. The pedicle must be at least one-third of the width of the flap to maintain its viability and contains a terminal branch of the dorsal metacarpal artery, the dorsal venous drainage and one or more dorsal terminal branches of the radial nerve. The flap is elevated just superficial to the paratenon and is transposed and inset to the area of volar loss on the thumb. The pedicle may be de-epithelialised. This flap is versatile and its use for other defects is described in Chapter 3. Foucher has modified the technique and raises the skin from the dorsal phalangeal area of the index finger as an island. This is supplied by a wide subcutaneous pedicle. The arc of rotation of this flap is such that it may not cover the tip of a thumb of normal length but is adequate for an injured and shortened thumb.

*The median nerve neurovascular island flap*

The ulnar hemi-pulp of the middle finger is used as the donor site. The flap and ulnar neurovascular bundle of the digit are elevated and the defect is closed using a full thickness skin graft (Fig. 4.13). Prior to elevation of the flap, the vascular anatomy in the palm should be inspected to ensure that it is normal. The flap and neurovascular bundle are then elevated starting distally and working towards the palmar arch. During elevation it is important not to denude the neurovascular bundle of surrounding subcutaneous tissues as the venous drainage of this flap is thought to run through venae comitans associated with the digital artery. Stripping the neurovascular bundle may not only impair the venous drainage but also damage the nerve. Care must be taken to ensure that there is no tension on the pedicle once the flap has been transferred and sutured in place. The flap and neurovascular bundle are tunnelled across the palm and delivered into the area of the volar defect of the thumb.

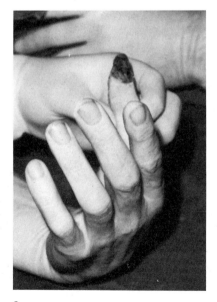 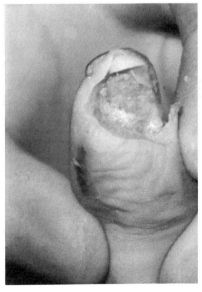

a                b

**Fig. 4.13** **a** Neurovascular island flap. A defect on the tip of the thumb. **b** Close-up of the defect shows bony exposure, and extensive pulp loss

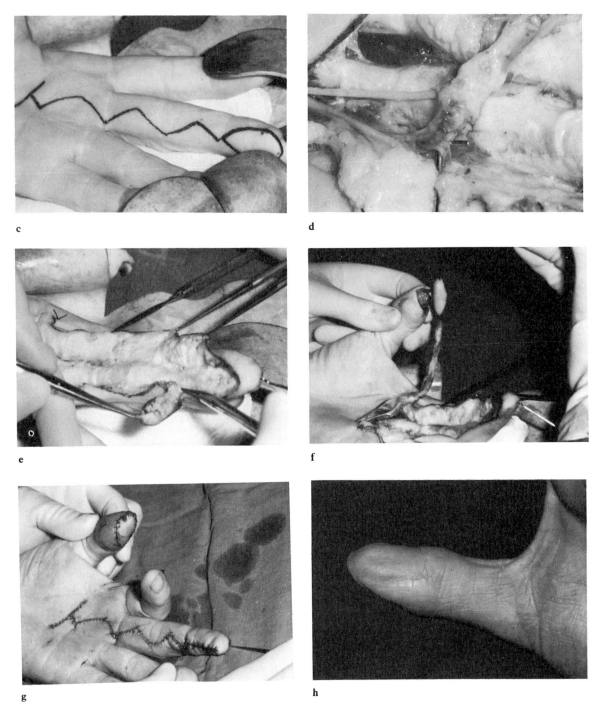

**Fig. 4.13  c** An outline of the neurovascular flap and the Bruner incision used to expose the pedicle. **d** Elevation of the neurovascular island flap is preceded by checking the vascularity of adjacent digits. **e** Once the vascularity to the radial side of the little finger and to the ring finger has been ascertained, the ulnar digital artery to the radial side of the ring finger may be divided, and the pedicle mobilised. **f** Elevation of the flap completed, with its vascular pedicle intact. **g** Transfer of the neurovascular pedicle completed and sutured into place. In this case the secondary defect could be closed directly.
**h** Neurovascular island flap in place, some months after transfer. Sensation is normal but is transferred

Although these flaps import sensibility to the reconstructed thumb, it is always interpreted as coming from the original flap donor site. Thus injury to the thumb is felt as if it had occurred to the donor finger. In younger patients, such 'cross-over' is less troublesome. It is less obvious in radial than in median innervated neurovascular island flaps. This problem can be overcome by dividing the donor nerves and suturing them to the thumb digital nerve stumps or by using neurovascular free flaps from the foot.

# AMPUTATIONS

We have restricted the use of the term 'amputation' to the purposeful shortening of a digit at a site of election. 'Terminalisation' describes wound closure in trauma which may require minimal bone shortening. Neither should be the first resort of the technically destitute, but should be undertaken by a surgeon thoroughly familiar with other reconstructive methods.

## INDICATIONS

Amputation or terminalisation should be considered in the primary management of severe injuries when the damaged tissues are no longer useful for reconstruction of the involved area or any other simultaneously damaged area. This is likely to occur when extensive crushing has produced a devitalised digit. If replantation is considered undesirable or can no longer be considered because of too great a time-lapse, terminalisation must be undertaken or a level of more proximal amputation must be chosen.

Stiff and insensitive digits may be amputated with overall improvement of hand function. In a patient with poor motivation, amputation may be preferable to reconstruction. Pain is not an indication for amputation of a digit. Amputation as a method of treating neuroma pain in an otherwise satisfactory stump is contraindicated. Amputation may be required for the removal of a malignant tumour, to remove an extra digit in congenital deformities, or for the treatment of established digital gangrene.

## AMPUTATION TECHNIQUE

The aim when undertaking an amputation is to produce *a well-padded, durable and pain-free stump of adequate length and normal sensation*. This should allow unrestricted use of the digital stump. Volar skin is therefore best, as this is glabrous, secreting sweat and thus aiding grip. Scar placement should be such that the scar does not impinge upon the contact surface. The scar should be free of the underlying structures and not adherent to tendon or bone. A pain-free stump may be obtained by ensuring that the digital nerves are shortened so that they lie in ample subcutaneous tissue. It has been suggested that bipolar coagulation of the nerve ends reduces the subsequent incidence of neuroma formation.

The flexor and extensor tendons should be divided under tension and allowed to retract. They should not be sutured together over the bony stump for this would produce a restriction of flexion due to tethering of the extensor tendon. It also risks reducing function in adjacent fingers; the profundus muscle and tendons are incapable of independent motion in the middle, ring and little fingers; tethering of one tendon will prevent full excursion of the remainder — *the Quadriga Effect*. In amputations where the distal profundus insertion is divided (such as those proximal to the distal interphalangeal joint level) there is the possibility of *a lumbrical plus finger* developing. This is a deformity resulting from flexion forces being directed through the lumbrical as the profundus contracts producing paradoxical extension at the proximal interphalangeal joint. Division of the lumbrical has been advocated when amputating at this level.

The level of amputation should be such as to allow maximum use of the finger. The shorter the finger the less useful it is. Amputation proximal to a flexor tendon insertion further diminishes grip strength in the hand. If possible, even a small remnant of distal phalanx should be retained if the profundus insertion is intact, in order to maintain grip strength. It may be useful to attach flexor tendons distally to the fibro-osseus sheath to preserve flexion power, but if tensioning is incorrect, there is the risk of producing the Quadriga effect. After ensuring that haemostasis is adequate upon release of the tourniquet, the skin flap should be closed without undue tension.

In traumatic amputations at fingertip level, before proceeding to bone shortening and stump closure the question should always be asked 'is this the best technique available or are there other reconstructive methods which would preserve length, function and sensation?' Methods used for preserving length at the fingertip level may also be applied to more proximal injuries.

## THE PROBLEMS OF PARTICULAR DIGITS

### The index finger

The index finger is concerned with fine manipulative tasks. Patients will transfer thumb/index pinch to the middle finger after even minor injuries to the index tip, thereby excluding it. Amputation of the index leads to loss of precision handling skills and less power is available for their control. Permanent damage to the index fingertip which prevents its normal use in pinch is the functional equivalent of an amputation, however the finger will still contribute to power grip. Total amputation of the index finger will reduce grip strength by 20%. At the level of the middle phalanx preservation of the superficialis is useful. Even a small proximal phalanx stump with weak flexion is of benefit in the control and use of hammers and other tools. Amputation through the proximal phalanx allows this although the cosmetic aspect is less satisfactory. Amputation may be performed at metacarpophalangeal joint level, bevelling the metacarpal head to round off the corner of the palm. Control of hammers and similar tools is decreased compared to more distal amputations but the appearance is improved. Manual workers may prefer to maintain the width of the palm. Resection of the index ray may be performed near the metacarpal base; the first dorsal interosseous should be re-attached to the radial side of the middle finger. This produces a satisfactory cosmetic appearance, but a narrow palm and reduced control over tool handles. Great care must be taken to preserve the palmar branches of the digital nerves, or a significant number of patients will develop a disabling area of hyperaesthesia at the base of the web space.

### The middle and ring finger

Preservation of the proximal phalanx will prevent objects falling through a gap in the hand. The stump may play some part in grasp and the palm remains broad. The stumps of middle and ring fingers are less troublesome than border digit stumps which may be inadvertently snagged. However, metacarpophalangeal joint flexion in these digits may lag behind adjacent normal fingers due to the lack of any long flexors. The sublimis tendon may be sutured to the A2 pulley in an attempt to avoid this.

If amputation is performed through the metacarpohalangeal joint there is no stump, the grip is weakened, but the palm remains broad. Coins and other objects slip through the gap between the fingers — a persistent irritation to the patient. The cosmetic appearance is poor, there being an obvious gap between the fingers. This is the least satisfactory level from both the functional and cosmetic point of view. In this type of 'battlement hand' co-ordinated finger function is difficult.

A more extensive procedure involving ray excision produces an excellent cosmetic appearance and closes the gap between the fingers. However, the palm is narrowed — a disadvantage to heavy manual workers. The procedure can be performed in two ways. The simplest technique is to excise the involved ray, close to the base of the metacarpal. The adjacent rays may be drawn into correct alignment by strong unabsorbable sutures to the deep intervolar plate ligaments. Further sutures through drill holes in the metacarpal shafts may be used to strengthen the repair. A palmaris longus tendon graft can be used instead of sutures to provide a permanent biological fixation. The border metacarpal should be held sufficiently firmly to allow early vigorous physiotherapy for maximum mobility of the remaining fingers. Zig-zag dorsal and volar incisions with trimming of skin edges will produce a very satisfactory cosmetic appearance. If the adjacent metacarpals are too rigid at the bases to permit satisfactory alignment distally, then a lateral release of the carpometacarpal joint may be required.

Ray transposition is a more complicated technique involving transfer of the adjacent border metacarpal on to the base of the excised ray. The involved ray is excised as previously described, leaving 1–2 cm of proximal metacarpal. The adjacent border metacarpal is divided at the same level and transposed on to the remaining metacarpal base. Fixation is achieved by Kirschner wires with interosseous wiring or a small AO plate. Firm fixation is advised so that early mobilisation may be permitted to overcome any tendency towards intrinsic contracture resulting from interosseous muscle damage.

### The little finger

Being involved principally in grasp rather than precision handling, every effort should be made to preserve distal tendon insertions. The levels of elective amputation are similar to the index finger.

### The thumb

Amputation stumps at or distal to the interphalangeal joint level will provide satisfactory function for many patients although the specialised pulp is lost. In traumatic amputations involving the distal phalanx, efforts should be made to preserve flexor pollicis longus function. This tendon contributes greatly to grip strength. Its preservation may require the judicious use of reconstructive techniques with skin flaps. If more proximal amputation of the thumb has occurred immediate reconstructive efforts are required to preserve length and function. Thumb replantation has been one of the most successful aspects of microvascular surgery, and where feasible, should always be considered. Thumb reconstruction is discussed in Chapter 13.

### THE CARE OF AMPUTATION STUMPS

Careful surgery is required to give good results when amputation has been undertaken. The postoperative care of the amputation stump is also important if the best results are to be obtained.

Massage will help to avoid scar adhesions to underlying bone and will soften the swollen stump and help to reduce any tendency towards sensitivity. Creams may be applied to soften the skin, thus preventing fissuring and cracking. In some patients there may be an unacceptable amount of sensitivity at the amputation stump due to a small neuroma. These may often be managed by a desensitisation programme in which the patient massages the tip and undertakes tapping and manipulation against progressively harder objects. The majority of symptoms will settle with such a programme.

### CONSEQUENCES OF AMPUTATION

The functional significance for the patient depends on his occupational and recreational demands and motivation. The more sophisticated the patient's needs, the more significant is the functional disruption produced by minor injury. Assessment of disability must take account of this and cannot be correlated with the level of amputation alone.

The amputation stump may give rise to physical symptoms such as pain, cold intolerance, paraesthesia or complaints of a phantom limb. Restriction of motion of the stump and adjacent digits can occur. Psychological symptoms may aggravate the physical disability; fear of the workplace, apprehension about the pain, and awareness of deformity.

Amputation is a social stigma which inevitably provokes comment. Aesthetic considerations are all too often ignored. Patients may attempt to disguise ugly amputation stumps by modification of hand posture; interphalangeal joint amputations are not apparent in the clenched hand. In some patients, the appearance of the three-fingered hand is aesthetically satisfactory while in others it is less pleasing and appears to depend on the balance between digital length and palmar breadth.

Realistic flexible cosmetic prostheses may be custom-made to apply over digital or palmar amputation stumps. Considerable time and expertise are required in their manufacture and application but they may be of significant benefit to certain patients.

## SUMMARY

Amputation is one of the most poorly performed operations, often being undertaken by the most junior member of staff. It should be appreciated that it is technically demanding, requires fine judgement as to its necessity and level, and professional rehabilitation to ensure that such patients rapidly return to their normal activities.

# 5. Tendon repair

*Principal authors:   D. A. McGrouther, F. D. Burke*

The hand, like a puppet, is principally controlled by cords applying force from a distance. Each tendon moves several joints and alters the balance of force vectors at others. Although muscles are distinguished by Latin names to imply an action in motion, their major role is the application of force, often in isometric contraction. Tendons provide the specialised function of transmitting tensile forces from muscle groups to the skeleton; they are therefore capable of transmitting enormous loadings while gliding over bones and through sheaths. After repair there is the dilemma of maintaining this ability to glide while limiting loading to avoid tendon rupture.

The malevolence of the healing process is such that there is no treatment plan in tendon surgery which will guarantee a successful outcome. More than in any other area, however, the results will reflect the quality of each of the three stages of management: assessment, surgical technique and rehabilitation.

Tendon is histologically composed of aligned collagen fibres with a linear orientation. Tendon is relatively acellular, the cells being mature fibrocytes, and therefore nutritional needs are minimal. On the dorsum of the hand the tendons lie in loose areolar tissue, which provides them with a blood supply via a network of small vessels in the paratenon. On the volar surface the tendons are restrained within a synovial sheath by a system of pulleys to prevent bowstringing. The synovial sheath acts as a lubricating system for the tendons; a small amount of fluid between the visceral and parietal layers allows the tendon to glide with minimal friction. The annular pulleys (Fig. 5.1)

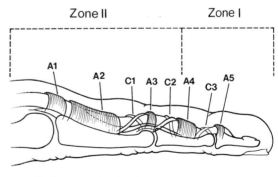

**Fig. 5.1  a, b** The arrangement of the annular and cruciate pulleys of the flexor tendon sheath

are attached to the phalanges and retain the tendon close to the digital skeleton, maintaining a constant moment arm of flexor action and allowing full digital flexion. Cruciate pulleys are situated over the joints and concertina on digital flexion. Thus functioning flexor tendons in Zone I and II are both under tensile (longitudinal) and compressive (lateral) loading which necessitates a very specialised system of nutrition; a system of microscopic internal channels within the tendon maintains an intratendinous synovial fluid circulation through the pumping action of the pulleys pressing on the tendon surface. It seems likely that during motion the tendon is wrung out like a sponge, nutrient fluids being drawn into the internal channels upon release of the compressing force. In addition to synovial nutrition, the tendons within the sheath also have a blood supply, which reaches the tendon through a constant system of long and short nutrient vessels (vinculae) situated dorsally and of sufficient length to allow tendon excursion. When these are divided, there is considerable bleeding and granulation tissue formation. The capillary network within the tendon is more developed on the dorsal aspect.

Tendons undergo an excursion in relation to the underlying skeleton and the magnitude of this for the flexor and extensor tendons is shown in Tables 5.1 and 5.2 (see p. 111). The total excursion of a tendon at any chosen point is the sum of the individual excursions from motion of each of the joints distal to that point. On making a fist, for example, there is proximal excursion of the long flexor tendons as the fingers flex and their excursion at the level of the metacarpals is therefore considerable (35 mm). The wrist, however, extends on making a fist and this joint motion

means that in the forearm the flexor tendon excursion is very much less than at the level of the metacarpals. The reduced excursion of the forearm flexor tendons allows the application of maximal power by the muscle units. A very much greater excursion is necessary in moving the hand and wrist from the position of full extension to full flexion, but the total excursion is rarely required in everyday use. The tenodesis action of the wrist (flexion on digital extension and vice versa) forms an important regulator of tendon power and excursion. This valuable form of fine adjustment of digital function is lost if an arthrodesis of the wrist is performed.

### Theories of tendon healing

It has been shown experimentally that tendon has an *intrinsic* ability to heal, even in the absence of a blood supply, provided that cellular viability is maintained by adequate synovial fluid perfusion. Free tendon fragments will heal in a rabbit's knee joint. There is, however, an inevitable *extrinsic* tendon healing process, due to cellular proliferation and fibrous tissue deposition, which arises from the healing process in the surrounding tissue layer. It has been argued that the extrinsic healing process is required to restore the strength of tendon union. All layers of the wound, therefore, contribute to the healing process and tend to envelop the healing tendon ends, tethering them to surrounding structures by rigid adhesions.

The postoperative management programme can encourage one or other of these different healing mechanisms. Mobilisation promotes intrinsic healing and will also mould surrounding adhesions in a favourable way; long loose adhesions will allow adequate excursion. Immobilisation by

**Table 5.1**   Excursion of flexor tendons expressed in mm for every 10° of joint motion.

| | Thumb | Index FDP | FDS | Middle FDP | FDS | Ring FDP | FDS | Little FDP | FDS |
|---|---|---|---|---|---|---|---|---|---|
| 10° DIP | | 1.0 | | 1.0 | | 0.95 | | 0.84 | |
| 10° PIP | 1.3 | 1.3 | 1.3 | 1.4 | 1.4 | 1.2 | 1.2 | 1.0 | 1.0 |
| 10° MP | 1.6 | 2.0 | 2.2 | 2.2 | 2.5 | 2.1 | 2.4 | 1.9 | 2.1 |
| 10° wrist (flexion range) | 2.1 | 2.6 | 2.6 | 2.6 | 3.3 | 2.2 | 2.5 | 2.2 | 2.4 |
| 10° wrist (extension range) | | 2.2 | 2.1 | 2.2 | 2.4 | 2.2 | 2.3 | 2.2 | 2.3 |

contrast will allow the extrinsic process to lay down scar tissue between tendon ends and the surrounding tissues making later excursion difficult.

## FLEXOR TENDON INJURIES

Injuries of the digital flexor tendons remain one of the greatest challenges in hand surgery. However, such injuries are sufficiently uncommon that surgeons only slowly gain experience in their management.

### Diagnosis

Careful examination is required to ensure that the diagnosis of a flexor tendon injury is not missed. A history of injury involving glass or a knife should suggest a possible tendon division. The site of tendon injury may be predicted. If the outstretched hand lands on a sharp object the tendons are cut with the fingers in extension. Accidents with tools or knives often result in injury to the fingers in flexion. Inspection of the cascading posture of the fingers provides the first clue to tendon injury. In the resting hand the index finger lies in the most extended position with increasing flexion in the more ulnar digits. Thumb posture is best assessed by comparison with the contralateral hand. The pointing finger is said to indicate a flexor tendon injury (Fig. 5.2). With experience the surgeon can see at a glance what has been divided, by assessment of the hand posture at rest combined with the tenodesis test; the automatic digital flexion and extension which accompanies passive wrist extension and flexion.

Injury to flexor digitorum profundus presents as a loss of distal interphalangeal joint flexion. Flexor digitorum sublimis injury is revealed by an altered cascade, with undue extension at the involved proximal interphalangeal joints. In addition, there is loss of independent finger flexion. The patient is instructed to flex his fingers one at a time while the remainder are held in extension by the examiner's hand (Fig. 5.3). This test relies on the anatomical fact that the flexor profundus is a common muscle unit to the middle, ring and little fingers. The index flexor digitorum profundus usually has an independent muscle

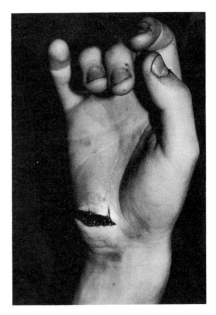

Fig. 5.2 The pointing finger indicates a flexor tendon injury. The posture of the little finger is noted to be much more extended than its normal resting position indicating flexor tendon injury. The ring finger is also partially extended due to division of the flexor digitorum sublimis

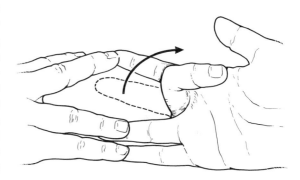

Fig. 5.3 Testing for the function of the flexor digitorum sublimis. The middle finger can be flexed independently when the other digits are immobilised in extension. This test is not accurate for the index finger which has independent profundus action. In some patients, independent action of the sublimis of the little finger is not possible

belly, whereas flexor sublimis has an independent belly to each digit. Independent flexion of one digit is therefore a function of flexor digitorum sublimis. In suspected tendon injury *power testing is contraindicated* for fear of converting an incomplete tendon injury to a complete separation.

Nerve and vessel injuries should also be noted and the hand X-rayed to exclude skeletal damage.

## Treatment

In relation to the timing of operative intervention, the terms 'primary', 'delayed primary' and 'secondary' have proved unhelpful, as there is little agreement on the corresponding time intervals (see Ch. 1)

*The ideal treatment programme is immediate surgery performed by an experienced surgeon.* This may be difficult to achieve as the surgeon or theatre may not be available or the diagnosis delayed. It is logistically more satisfactory in most cases to have an appropriate theatre session available once in each 24-hour period when such complex cases can be treated by an experienced hand surgeon.

Where such a service is not available, cross-referral to a hospital specialising in hand surgery should be considered. The laceration should be gently cleaned and dressed with paraffin and moist dressing gauze. The hand should be immobilised in a plaster of Paris back slab in moderate wrist flexion. Cross-referral is limited more by the surgeon's pride, the administrator's purse, or the desire of junior doctors to 'have a go', rather than true geographical constraints. The referring doctor should discuss the injury with the hand surgeon over the telephone. This allows a plan for repair to be set in motion. The principle is to bring together the patient and an experienced surgeon, with full back-up facilities (postoperative supervision and rehabilitation), in an unhurried and well-equipped theatre within 24 hours of injury.

If delay exceeds 24 hours, the risk of infection (see Ch. 1)) will have reached a level which may prevent a satisfactory outcome. Skin suture at the referral centre is therefore indicated and antibiotics should be administered if a delay of more than 24 hours seems likely. Hand oedema will also increase and the tendon will become softer and more friable.

Primary repair of flexor tendons can only be undertaken when certain strict wound criteria are met. The tendon laceration must be clean cut and the chance of infection low. If the wound is liable to become infected, thorough débridement is necessary and the patient must be treated with antibiotics for much will be lost if infection supervenes. In some cases this will necessitate prolonged inpatient treatment. Primary repair inevitably increases local tissue damage with scarring. If the primary repair should fail, secondary reconstruction surgery is always made more difficult, a fact not always appreciated by the inexperienced emergency surgeon. *Failed primary repair is worse than doing nothing at all.*

The problems of technique and rehabilitation are multiplied when more than one digit is injured or where repair of associated nerve and vessel injuries is also required. The four-finger injury needs many hours of skilled primary surgery and has the potential to cripple the hand.

If there has been a delay the tendon ends will retract, soften and later develop an outgrowth of immature scar tissue at the stump. The empty tendon sheath will collapse and the pulleys become friable, so that after the initial wound healing period, it will not be possible to bring the retracted tendon ends back within a normal sheath.

The management of flexor tendon injuries depends on the level of division. There is a convention by which these injuries are classified into Zones (Fig. 5.4).

### Zone I

Distal to the sublimis insertion, the flexor profundus alone is divided. Access for repair is difficult in the area of the A4 pulley and it is preferable to repair the tendon through a window in the cruciate sheath, either proximally or distally. With the more distal injuries the proximal end may be advanced and re-attached to bone, but suture to the stump of profundus is more usual. Postoperatively the choice of rehabilitation policy lies between static immobilisation and dynamic splintage. Results are variable, with some stiffness of distal and proximal interphalangeal joints frequently resulting.

### Zone II

Zone II has been aptly termed 'no-man's land' by Sterling Bunnel. It corresponds to the part of

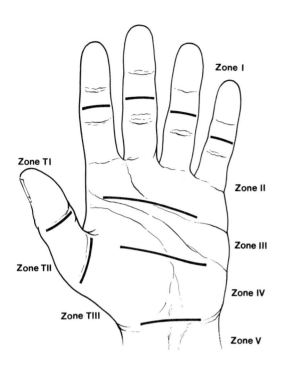

**Fig. 5.4** Zones of flexor tendon injury

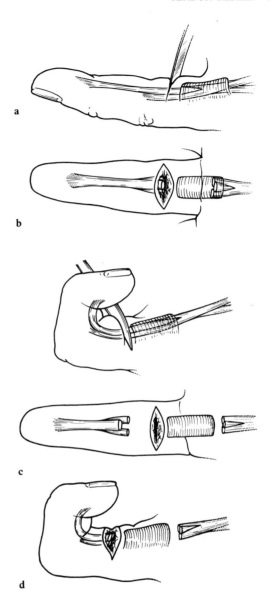

**Fig. 5.5** The level of tendon injury depends on the posture of the finger at the moment of division. **a** If the digit is injured in extension, **b** distal tendon ends are found in the wound, but the proximal end will retract. **c** If the finger is injured in flexion the tendon ends will be found distal to the wound as the injured finger will extend, **d** the tendon ends can be delivered to the wound by re-creation of the posture which was present at the moment of injury

the flexor sheath system containing both flexor tendons. It extends from the flexor sublimis insertion to the proximal end of the pulley system (the proximal interphalangeal joint skin crease and the distal palmar crease are the commonly accepted landmarks). As two tendons with different excursions lie within the pulley system, this Zone provides the greatest challenge to successful tendon repair.

The actual level of the tendon transection within the sheath can vary widely, depending on whether the laceration occurred in flexion or in extension (Fig. 5.5). In the more proximal part of the sheath, there are two discreet tendons lying one upon the other. Further, distally, the sublimis decussates around the profundus, taking up a dorsal position at the level of the proximal interphalangeal joint. The flexor sublimis, therefore, lies in two separate slips, lateral to the profundus over the proximal phalanx, but more distally it is a flat sheet dorsal to the profundus. A clearer picture of the levels of injury can be obtained by re-creating the posture which was present at the moment of injury.

The levels of tendon injury can be related to the sheath injury by flexing the proximal interphalangeal joint until the sublimis cut lies at the level of the sheath injury. The distal interphalangeal joint is then flexed until the profundus injury coincides with the others. From this knowledge of the posture of the digit at the time of injury, it is possible to appreciate the relative movement occurring between the repair lines in the tendons and sheath during the rehabilitation period.

It is also worthwhile noting whether the sublimis is one tendon or two at the site of division and whether the vinculae are intact. This information provides a complete picture of the tendon injury and permits a more precise prognosis to be made, for some Zone II injuries have a better outlook than others. It is possible that Kleinert's postoperative regimen (see p. 103) will favour flexor tendons cut in extension, whereas the Strickland regimen (see p. 103) will favour those cut in flexion, as the tendon repair sites will be maximally offset by these choices of rehabilitation.

### Zone III

In the midpalm, tendon repairs have a better prognosis. Dynamic mobilisation may be undertaken in co-operative patients and those whose rehabilitation can be closely supervised. The final recovery time may be shortened by this programme. Alternatively, static immobilisation may be used for a period of 3 weeks; later mobilisation will be rendered more difficult by adhesions, but a satisfactory range of motion can be regained.

### Zone IV

In the carpal tunnel the wrist should be splinted in a neutral position to avoid bowstringing. The rehabilitation choices are similar to Zone III, but there is a greater tendency for motion to be restricted by adhesions.

### Zone V

Above the wrist, suture of the muscle units is difficult, but it may be possible to retrieve the tendon from the centre of the muscle. Mattress sutures are required. Static immobilisation is usual.

### Incisions for flexor tendon repair

The traumatic skin wound associated with a flexor tendon division is generally transverse or oblique. Extension of the wound will be necessary to allow sufficient exposure for repair, and in planning the incision three principles must be followed:

1. Skin must not be devitalised by the design of unsafe flaps.
2. Continuous longitudinal volar scars should be avoided as these will cause later contractures.
3. Consideration must be given to possible future surgical treatment.

The wound may be extended by conversion into a Bruner incision or by using midlateral (neutral line) incisions (see Ch. 1) proximally on one side of the digit and distally on the other. Proximal extension is always necessary. Distal extension may be limited when the tendons have been cut in extension. Care must be taken where there is a digital artery injury to avoid raising a flap with a poor blood supply. Skin flaps can be elevated by either of these techniques and retracted to allow exposure of the tendon sheath. The neurovascular bundles must also be carefully protected. Midlateral incisions are better should tenolysis be required later.

Rarely, both proximal and distal tendon ends will be visible at the level of the sheath laceration. If the digit has been cut in extension, the distal end will be in view, but if the digit has been cut in flexion, the distal end will slide distally as the finger extends after division. Proximal tendon ends will always retract, but the vincula may remain intact if the tendon was not under great tension when cut. Tendons are often divided under tension and they may retract proximally for considerable distances, tearing the vincula. When the tendon sheath has been exposed the digit should be flexed to reveal the cut distal tendon end. A laceration in the tendon sheath requires extension to visualise and allow room for repair, but the annular pulleys must not be divided. Where the tendon has been divided in the centre of an annular pulley it is probably better to plan to undertake the repair proximally or distally in the region of the adjacent pulleys by making a window which can later be closed. This will be facilitated by opening the sheath using an 'S'-shaped incision, leaving a cuff of cruciate sheath on the volar plate to allow later suture placement. The A2 and A4 pulleys must be preserved in the digits and in the thumb the oblique pulley is the most important.

The retracted proximal tendon ends may be difficult to retrieve, particularly if the profundus has retracted through the sublimis decussation. Rarely it may be possible by external massage ('milking') to deliver the tendon ends to the incision site. More frequently, the retracted ends remain out of view. Plunging into the sheath with blunt gripping instruments is contraindicated, for this will damage the sheath and cause adhesions. The least traumatic way of delivering the retracted proximal end is to make a small incision at the distal palmar crease to expose the flexor tendons at the mouth of the A1 pulley (Fig. 5.6). The cut ends will not be seen and the tendons are not removed from the sheath. A fine Silastic cannula can be introduced into the proximal sheath at the A1 pulley, alongside the tendons. The cannula is passed distally through the sheath until it appears within the wound. The proximal end should be sutured side to side to the tendon in the palm and distal traction on the cannula will deliver the tendon stumps to the laceration site. The core stitch can then be placed in the tendons leaving the ends long. After placement of this stitch, the tendon is allowed to retract into the sheath until the side-to-side suture between cannula and tendon is again visible in the palm. This stitch is removed and the cannula is extracted leaving the proximal tendon end available for delivery into the wound by means of traction on the core stitch. The proximal tendon stump can then be held at the repair site by transfixing tendon and sheath with a fine needle (Fig. 5.7a), allowing the tendon repair to be completed.

## Technique of flexor tendon repair

The principles are:

1. There should be a core stitch to transmit longitudinal tension.

2. A fine peripheral stitch is placed to achieve the best possible matching of the opposed tendon ends, thereby producing a smooth outer gliding surface. This stitch also transmits longitudinal tension.

3. Pulleys must be preserved.

4. Closure of the sheath is desirable.

The delicate layer of cells which surrounds the flexor tendon can easily be damaged by trauma and this will increase subsequent adhesions. During repair, the tendon should be kept moist and handled solely at its cut surface, so that the gliding surface is disturbed as little as possible. Both tendons should be repaired. The alternative technique of suturing the profundus and excising the sublimis leaves a dead space which fills with scar tissue and, in addition, the profundus vincular blood supply is further compromised. A core stitch of braided material (Ethibond 4/0 for example) is used to transmit limited longitudinal tension (Fig. 5.7). This stitch should be placed towards the volar aspect of the tendon so as to cause minimum disruption to the blood supply. The bite should not be less than 1 cm from the cut surface. It must not be overtightened as this will cause bunching which may lead to triggering. It must be placed so as to grasp some tendon fibres within the loop to avoid slippage and elongation of the repair during loading in the early healing phase (Fig. 5.8). The Kirchmeier/Kessler suture has the greatest resistance to pullout, but must be correctly inserted to grasp tendon fibres. After insertion of the core suture, a continuous peripheral monofilament stitch (8/0 or 6/0 nylon) is placed to ensure a smooth outer surface. The finger should be passively wound up several times after repair while inspecting the repair site. This *provocative test* will reveal any tendency for the tendon repairs to trigger on cruciate pulleys or the edge of the window, or on one another, and any such tendency must be corrected. The best means of doing so is by sheath repair, but this is difficult as the synovial sheath is flimsy. If this is not possible, it may be permissible to create a large window in the sheath, with preservation of annular pulleys proximally and distally. With careful planning, the window may allow the repair to glide through an adequate excursion without triggering. Large windows carry a risk of bowstringing and increased adhesion formation.

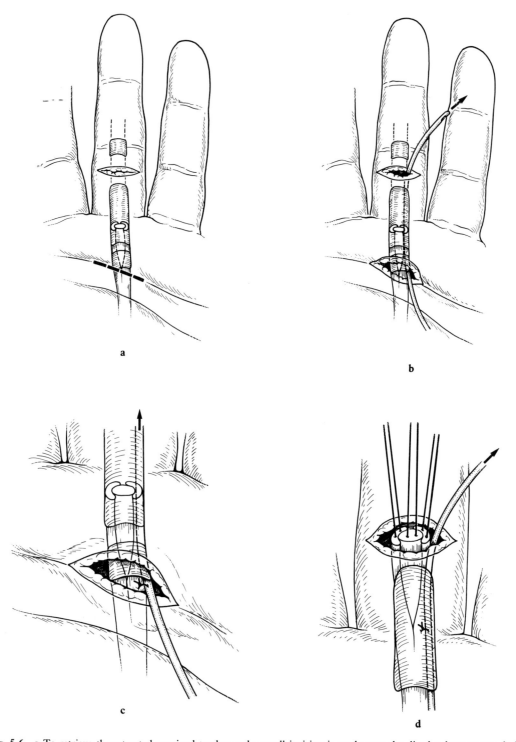

**Fig. 5.6** **a** To retrieve the retracted proximal tendon end a small incision is made over the distal palmar crease. **b** A paediatric feeding tube is inserted from the proximal end into the tendon sheath and delivered at the wound. **c** The feeding tube is stitched side-to-side to the tendon or tendons. **d** By traction on the distal end of the suture the tendon ends can be delivered in the wound and core stitches inserted

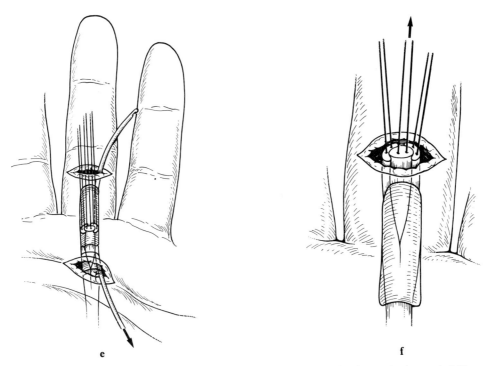

e The feeding tube is again pulled proximally and the side-to-side suture removed in the proximal wound. f The cut tendon ends can now be advanced to the wound by traction on the core stitch to allow completion of tendon suture

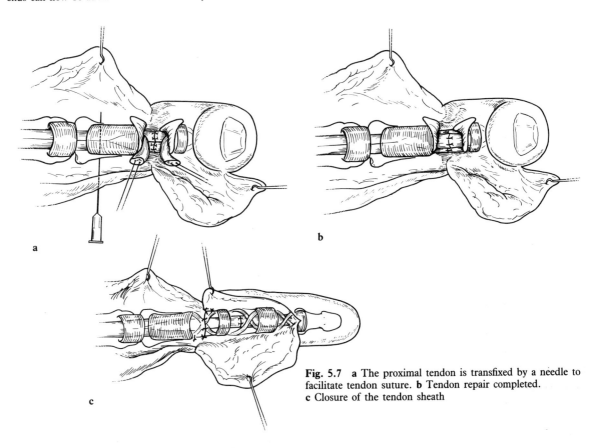

Fig. 5.7  a The proximal tendon is transfixed by a needle to facilitate tendon suture. b Tendon repair completed. c Closure of the tendon sheath

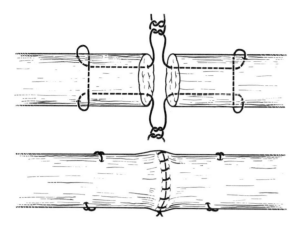

**Fig. 5.8** Detail of the core stitch and peripheral continuous stitch

## Postoperative rehabilitation after flexor tendon repair

A precise rehabilitation programme is essential to achieve a satisfactory result and patient motivation is of considerable importance. None of the repair techniques in common usage is strong enough for immediate active use.

The aim of rehabilitation is to prevent failure of the tendon repair, either through rupture or adhesion.

Early failures are due to rupture from technically inadequate repair or excessive use, causing separation of the repair. The patient may feel a snap and the finger becomes flaccid in a more extended position. A more gradual pulling apart due to the stitch cutting through the soft tendon end also may occur.

Later failure comes from repair elongation or attenuation. It has been shown by serial radiographic measurements of wire marker stitches that a poor clinical result may be correlated with an elongated repair. Although some lengthening occurs in all repairs, there seems to be a critical point beyond which it is associated with a poor result. The primary event may be adherence of the repair at or distal to the suture line. During the healing phase, the tendon repair is gradually gaining tensile strength, but the peritendinous adhesions are also gaining strength. The outcome of subsequent passive stretching of the digit will depend on the relative strengths of the tendon repair and surrounding adhesions. In the early stages, if the tendon repair is stronger, the adhesions will mobilise on passive stretching. If on the other hand the adhesions are stronger, the tendon will attenuate. At a later stage (approximately 8 weeks), it may still be possible to mobilise the adhesions. If the adhesions are stronger, however, the tendons will be stuck fast. The timing of the application of passive force after tendon repair is therefore a mixture of science and art. It seems unwise to apply strong extension force until 6–8 weeks after repair. Adherence and rupture/attenuation may therefore be seen as different stages of the same process.

The rehabilitation options are:

### Static immobilisation

Static immobilisation is the simplest regimen and is possible in areas where the tendon lies in a loose connective tissue network, as in Zone V. Tethering is not significant. Static immobilisation may also be the chosen technique in Zone II injuries in the patient unlikely to co-operate with a more complex regimen. It must be appreciated that immobilisation does not prevent isometric muscle force which may disrupt the repair. Three to five weeks' immobilisation is usual.

### Controlled mobilisation

Where tendons pass through tight fibrous tunnels, they are likely to form a firm bond to surrounding structures during the healing phase, limiting function. *A controlled range* of mobilisation during healing is therefore desirable, so that any adhesions which form should be sufficiently long and mobile to permit normal excursion of tendons, both relative to each other and the adjacent sheath. Some mobility of the tendon during the healing phase will promote the development of long loose adhesions. *A controlled load* on the tendon repair will also promote stronger union. Tension is therefore a 'happy mean' situation. Too little or too much is unsatisfactory. The best compromise between the risks of early rupture or later adhesion is to introduce a programme which avoids active use, yet permits

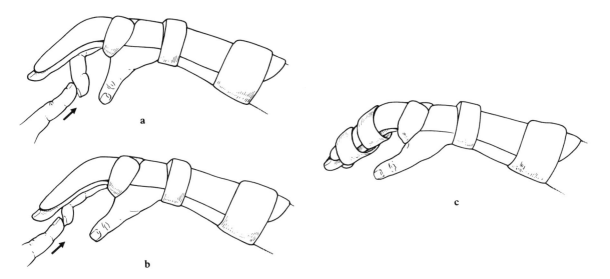

**Fig. 5.9** Technique of flexor tendon mobilisation by intermittent passive motion. **a** The proximal interphalangeal joint is passively flexed by the therapist or by the patient working under supervision. **b** Passive flexion of the distal interphalangeal joint. **c** The resting position between exercise periods

a limited and controlled amount of passive use. *Strickland* suggests a regimen whereby the digits are held in the optimal position for immobilisation, and the wrist is held in flexion to relax the flexor tendons (Fig. 5.9). The digits are passively flexed twice daily, initially by the therapist and later by the patient. This regimen attempts a limited programme of mobilisation, but should the treatment fail, the digits are in a favourable configuration for secondary reconstruction (proximal interphalangeal joint extended).

*Kleinert's* dynamic mobilisation regimen allows the patient to actively extend the digits, but passive flexion is achieved by the recoil of elastic bands using the splint shown (Fig. 5.10a, b). The musculotendinous unit is maintained at less than its physiological resting length by flexion of the wrist and metacarpophalangeal joint. This system, however, tends to encourage motion of all joints in the digits and, as the fingers stiffen from postoperative oedema, there is a tendency for the system to favour metacarpal joint motion rather than movement at the more distal joints. Metacarpophalangeal joint motion is not associated with tendon excursion at the repair site in the digits. In theory there is a good case for immobilisation of all joints proximal to the repair site

to ensure the best chance of distal joint movement and therefore satisfactory excursion of the repair. Specific additions to the regimen must be made to encourage distal interphalangeal joint motion, which is the only joint whose motion contributes to excursion between the two adjacent repaired tendons. A palmar bar may be added to the splint to increase distal interphalangeal flexion (Fig. 5.10c, d). Motion of the metacarpophalangeal joints may be blocked by a spatula or finger, thereby encouraging full interphalangeal joint extension. The splint requires correct fitting and frequent monitoring to ensure that it is achieving the desired effect. The dynamics of the rubber bands will affect the range of joint motion achieved. A disadvantage is that the hand spends all night and long periods of the day in a position of flexion which is not the ideal position for immobilisation of the proximal interphalangeal joints (see Ch. 2). It is not appropriate in the hand with interosseous paralysis as interphalangeal joint extension is weak and the hand will become fixed in a claw position. Dynamic mobilisation can be disastrous in children, mentally defective patients or drug addicts.

It is of central importance to the success of tendon surgery that the prescribed movement

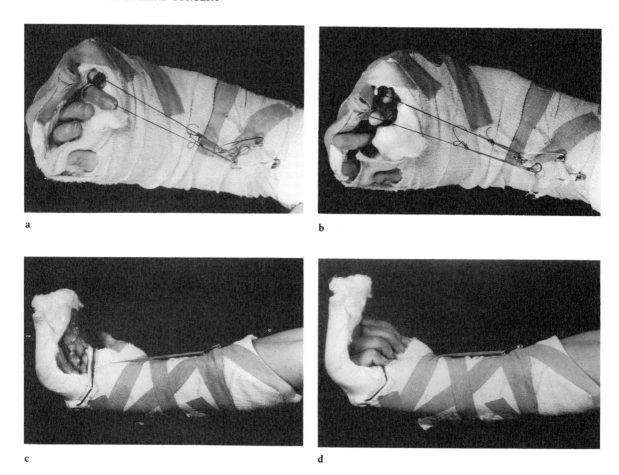

**Fig. 5.10  a, b** Kleinert splint. Active extension is performed by the patient against the resistance of rubber bands. Recoil of the elastic achieves a range of flexion. **c, d** The addition of a palmar bar increases the distal interphalangeal joint flexion range and therefore encourages excursion of FDP relative to FDS

programme should be followed exactly. The patient should be kept under observation daily until it is certain that he is achieving the appropriate range of joint motion, whether by the Kleinert or Strickland regimen. The patient who moves well during the rehabilitation phase is at risk from rupture of the repair, while the patient who moves little may develop dense adhesions. Where there is poor compliance, it may be necessary to keep the patient in hospital until the desired motion is achieved.

*Active motion*

After replantation, or other severe injuries, active mobilisation may be chosen in spite of the risk of rupture. There is considerable research interest in the development of a suture method which will allow the wider application of early active use.

**Unsatisfactory results following flexor tendon surgery**

*Early (days/weeks)*

1. Rupture
   — poor repair
   — poor rehabilitation
2. Infection
   — inadequate wound management
   — desiccation
3. Flap necrosis — inappropriate incisions

*Late (weeks/months)*

1. Attenuation/adhesion (late rupture)
2. Joint contracture
   — position unsatisfactory during early splintage
   — secondary to adherent tendon
3. Bowstringing

## Secondary tendon reconstruction

Secondary tendon reconstruction may be required if primary repair has failed or no repair has been performed. If all of the variables likely to affect the outcome of primary surgery are favourable, a satisfactory result will only be achieved in 60–80% of tendon injuries in no man's land (Zone II). If function has not been restored, the choice lies between secondary reconstruction or acceptance of the functional loss. On occasion, only one operation is required, but it may be necessary to move through a staged series of procedures before acceptable function is achieved. *Further tendon surgery is governed by the Law of Diminishing Returns where the potential gain from each operation will become less and less.* The operations may be considered in the following order:

1. Secondary repair.
2. Tenolysis where a repaired tendon is intact, but adherent to surrounding structures.
3. Tendon grafting by a one-staged technique, where sheath and pulley damage is minimal with satisfactory joint mobility and an unscarred tendon bed.
4. Staged tendon grafting, where there is significant damage to the pulleys or joint releases are required (i.e. a *'poor bed'*).
5. Tenolysis of the tendon graft.
6. Salvage procedures: tenodesis or arthrodesis to stabilise the distal interphalangeal joint.
7. Amputation.

### 1. Secondary repair

In the palm, or at the wrist, later tendon repair can sometimes be undertaken after a delay of many weeks without too much difficulty. Although it is not a policy of choice, late presentation of the patient does not always indicate a need for tendon excision and grafting.

### 2. Tenolysis

Tenolysis is the freeing of the repaired tendon from surrounding scar tissue. Prerequisites for tenolysis are:

a. An intact adherent tendon where active motion is less than the passive range.
b. Good passive range of motion.
c. A hand which is soft and supple.
d. A highly motivated patient.

The prognosis in tenolysis is related to the length of the adherent area. A short scarred area can be successfully released, but longer areas may rupture and further adhesions are likely. The ideal time is 6–9 months after repair, when scars have matured. Earlier intervention leads to a summation of induration in the hand, as described by Bunnel.

The adherent area may restrict tendon function completely or partially. All adhesions to the pulleys, adjacent tendon or underlying phalanges and volar plate must be released (Figs. 5.11 and 5.12). The annular pulleys must be preserved to prevent bowstringing. A realistic view must be taken of what can be achieved; if both flexor tendons have become adherent, the restoration of full function is difficult. It may be preferable to free the tendons en masse from surrounding tissue as far as the middle phalanx, and rely on a common action of the conjoined tendon at the proximal interphalangeal joint, accepting the tenodesis of the distal joint.

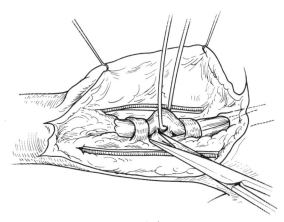

**Fig. 5.11** Technique of tenolysis

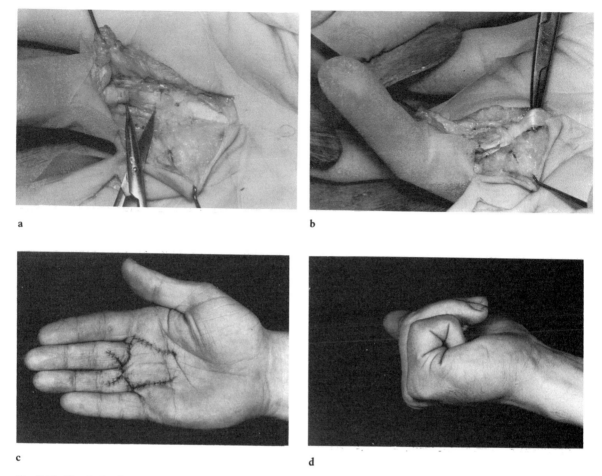

**Fig. 5.12** Tenolysis of repaired flexor tendon. **a** The points of the scissors indicate the degree of attenuation and adhesion of the tendon repair. **b** The two tendons were densely adherent and were freed en masse. The A1 pulley has been reconstructed. **c** The extension range achieved. **d** The flexion range 1 week after operation. After 3 months, the fingertips could flex to the palm. There was no active distal joint flexion

## TECHNIQUE

A midlateral incision is best, but it will be necessary to use the same incision as has been used for the primary tendon procedure. There are advantages in performing the operation under local anaesthetic nerve blocks at the wrist. In this way, the gain in active motion can be demonstrated to surgeon and patient during surgery. The disadvantage is the difficulty of obtaining good tourniquet control for what may be a prolonged operation requiring a good visual field.

The rehabilitation programme must be designed to achieve an effective excursion at the tenolysis site. This may require splintage of uninvolved joints (especially proximally).

*A tendon freed from surrounding adhesions is often attenuated and always devascularised and therefore prone to rupture in the postoperative rehabilitation phase.* It should therefore be protected from excessive tensile loading while movement is encouraged.

An intensive inpatient course for 2–3 weeks may be necessary to capitalise on the excursion won at surgery.

Strickland has suggested a 'frayed tendon rehabilitation programme' after tenolysis. Initially the hand is immobilised in the position of desired functional improvement; generally it is hoped to improve the flexion range and the hand is immobilised in flexion in the immediate postoperative period. The rehabilitation programme consists of assisted active motion. The digits are flexed to the palm by a therapist and the patient is asked to hold the digits in this position. No exercises against resistance are performed and it may be necessary to protect the pulleys by wearing thermoplastic rings. Further local anaesthetic blocks or infusions may facilitate rehabilitation.

### 3. One-stage tendon grafting

Prerequisites for tendon grafting are:

a. Full passive joint mobility. There may, however, be apparent joint limitation which is due to the presence of the distal end of the flexor tendon pistoning within the sheath and blocking passive flexion.

b. The hand should be soft and supple.

c. Intact pulleys.

d. Good skin cover.

e. The presence of an adequate motor muscle.

f. Interosseous muscle function should be intact. Where tendon grafting is performed in the presence of interosseous dysfunction, a claw hand will result. Immobilisation in the postoperative period will result in fixed deformity. Such patients require restoration of metacarpophalangeal flexion by tendon transfers prior to flexor tendon reconstruction.

g. Tendon grafting is contraindicated in the very old or very young. In young children, the procedure should be deferred for several years, until the child is old enough to co-operate with rehabilitation.

If the pulleys are in good condition, the damaged flexor tendons may be excised and replaced by a tendon graft at one operation.

**Pulley reconstruction.** If a vital annular pulley has been completely divided by the injury, direct repair is not adequate. Pulley reconstruction is therefore necessary, using a strip of tendon, fascia or extensor retinaculum. It may be possible to attach this to the insertion of the previous sheath on the phalanges (Fig. 5.13), 'the ever-present rim', but this is not always sufficiently robust and

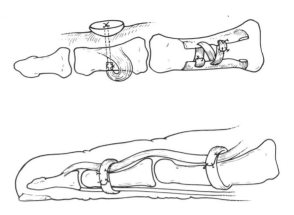

**Fig. 5.13** Techniques of pulley reconstruction

the tendon may need to be passed around the bone. It is passed superficial to the extensor apparatus over the middle phalanx, but deep to the extensor apparatus when reconstructing a pulley over the proximal phalanx to minimise interference with intrinsic function.

In the digits, the A2 and A4 pulleys are the most important to prevent bowstringing (Fig. 5.14) by keeping the tendon in close apposition to the corresponding phalanges. In the thumb, the oblique pulley (over the base of the proximal phalanx) must be preserved or reconstructed.

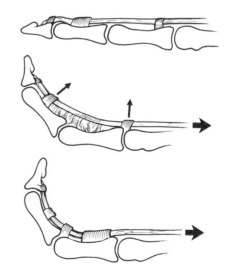

**Fig. 5.14** Bowstringing on flexion due to inadequate pulleys

The distal sublimis is left in place as a gliding surface. The aim is to restore one motor to the digit, and either the sublimis or profundus may be chosen depending on which has greater amplitude. The sublimis musculotendinous unit has an advantage as the motor because of its independent action, but may have retracted further. Donor tendons suitable for grafting must be long and slender. The palmaris longus, the extensor digiti minimi or a toe extensor are suitable. Plantaris is more difficult to remove and is not always present. The palmaris longus is frequently used, but suffers the disadvantage that it may be too short to extend from the distal phalanx to the wrist. It is, however, satisfactory when a short graft is used distal to the palm. In general, for a single digit an upper limb donor site is best, but for multiple digits it seems wise to choose the foot (extensor digitorum longus gives three or four tendons). Care must be taken in wound exposure and closure when harvesting tendon grafts to minimise the secondary deficit.

A simple transverse incision may be made over palmaris longus at the wrist and care must be taken not to inflict any injury to the median nerve. From this distal incision, the dissection can be continued proximally subcutaneously, using blunt-nosed dissecting scissors and, perhaps, a tendon stripper with great care. A fibre-optic cold light Aufricht nasal retractor may help visualisation. The graft is best handled by application of an artery forcep to its end, that part of the tendon later being sacrificed. Unnecessary contact is avoided as this is thought to increase the chance of adhesions. The tendon must be kept moist. It is not known whether it is better to remove or preserve the paratenon.

The distal insertion is by suture to the profundus tag or distal phalanx (Fig. 5.15). Proximal insertion is by a weave fishmouth suture at either the distal palm or above the wrist (Fig. 5.16). Adhesions at these sites are more yielding, allowing later mobilisation. There should be sufficient space for excursion of the junction without triggering, but careful planning is necessary in the palm to ensure that the fishmouth does not impinge on the A1 pulley, limiting full extension. Either the proximal or distal end of the graft may be sutured first. The graft must be

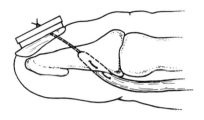

**Fig. 5.15** Suture of the distal end of the tendon graft

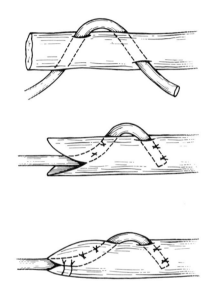

**Fig. 5.16** Fishmouth weave (Pulvertaft technique) for suture of proximal end of tendon graft

placed under the correct tension by observing the tenodesis action of the wrist, i.e. on rocking the wrist backwards and forwards the digits are seen to extend as the wrist flexes and vice versa. Alternative rehabilitation programmes of rest or early passive motion are possible. The patient may be re-admitted for physiotherapy after 4–6 weeks.

*Thumb.* Tendon grafting produces good functional results in terms of power grip and key pinch, but the range of joint motion may be limited. Pinch and grip can be quite satisfactory even if only a small part of the interphalangeal flexion range is preserved. The act of gripping also helps to correct any bowstringing which may be present. Alternative techniques of thumb flexor tendon reconstruction are by transfer of the flexor

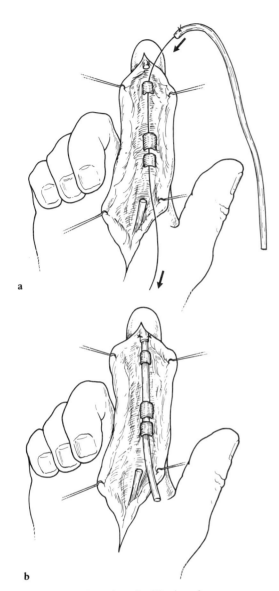

**a**

**b**

**Fig. 5.17 a, b** Insertion of a Silastic rod

sheath is created or maintained by the insertion of a Silastic rod (Fig. 5.17). A rod 4 mm in diameter is generally satisfactory. Larger rods may buckle and loosen at the distal attachment during passive mobilisation. Rods may either be of soft Silastic or of a more rigid type (that described by Hunter). These rods maintain a suitable dead space surrounded by a pseudo-sheath for the later re-insertion of a tendon graft, but permit passive mobilisation of the digit in the meantime (Fig. 5.18). At the first stage a long incision is necessary to identify or reconstruct the annular pulleys. The scarred flexor tendon is excised. A motor is selected and sutured side by side to a wrist flexor. Where a short graft is to be inserted to the midpalm, the motor may be sutured to the palmar fascia at the first stage to prevent retraction and shortening of the muscle. At the second stage, at least 3 months later, it is only necessary to expose the ends of the rod and the tendon graft may be pulled through the new sheath by suturing its end to the end of the rod (Fig. 5.19). The distal incision should lie beyond the distal interphalangeal joint to reduce adhesions over the middle phalanx.

Complications of the first stage are:

    a. Infection.
    b. Synovitis — a sterile inflammatory reaction.
    c. Detachment and proximal migration of the rod.
    d. Skin breakdown and exposure of the rod.

sublimis of the ring finger or step lengthening of the flexor pollicis longus tendon.

***Bridge grafts.*** A short bridge graft in the palm may obviate the need for excision of a relatively unscarred distal tendon from its sheath.

### 4. Two-staged tendon grafting

When the pulleys are damaged, a first-stage operation is necessary to reconstruct pulleys and a

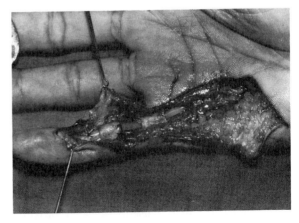

**Fig. 5.18** Silastic rod in situ

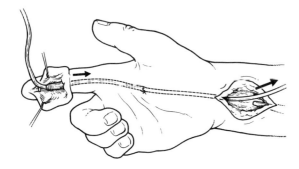

**Fig. 5.19** Replacing the Silastic rod by a tendon graft

Complications of the second stage are:

a. Flexion deformity due to adhesions.

b. Rupture. Detachment may occur at either the proximal or distal end. Such cases should be left for 6 months and then regrafted.

c. Bowstringing due to inadequacy or stretching of pulleys.

d. Sheath contracture.

e. A graft which is too long or too short.

f. The lumbrical plus deformity (scarred lumbrical or overlong graft). The profundus may pull through the lumbrical tendon, or scar, extending rather than flexing the proximal interphalangeal joint.

g. Swan-neck deformity due to loss of the sublimis tendon.

*5. Tenolysis of the tendon graft*

An adherent tendon graft may require tenolysis. Care must be taken to avoid damage to the pulleys.

*6. Salvage operations*

A number of patients will not have a satisfactory wind up of the digit after these procedures and stabilisation of pinch may be achieved by tenodesis of the distal interphalangeal joint or arthrodesis. Alternatively, these procedures may be indicated at an earlier stage if the patient decides against tendon surgery. They are particularly indicated where a useful range of proximal interphalangeal joint motion is preserved. Amputation may be indicated if a digit has little active or passive motion and interferes with the function of adjacent fingers.

## Flexor tendon grafting in the presence of an intact sublimis

In the patient with an intact sublimis, reconstruction of distal joint flexion by a tendon graft may be considered. A thin graft (e.g. plantaris) must be used. The tendon graft may be introduced through the flexor digitorum sublimis decussation regaining distal joint flexion. It is necessary to select a patient who is 'determined to seek perfection' (Pulvertaft), as existing function is at risk. Early mobilisation is indicated to maintain proximal interphalangeal joint function.

## Avulsion of the flexor digitorum profundus insertion

This is most common in the ring finger, proven to be the weakest profundus insertion on mechanical testing. It often follows a sporting injury, especially rugby. The tendon may rupture at its insertion or avulse a fragment of bone which may be visible on X-ray. This usually disrupts the articular surface of the distal interphalangeal joint. When the tendon has retracted into the distal palm, there is often a palpable lump. It is necessary to re-route it through the flexor sheath. This can be achieved by passing a cannula through the sheath and pulling the tendon back through the sublimis decussation. This will only be possible in the early stages. On occasion, particularly where there is a large bone fragment avulsion, the tendon may retract for only a short distance and it may be located within a cruciate pulley in the digit. Re-attachment of the tendon or bone fragment is performed with a wire in the same manner as the distal end of a flexor tendon graft. The rehabilitation programme is as for tendon repair.

## EXTENSOR TENDON INJURIES

The extensor apparatus is particularly vulnerable over joints. A Zone classification is not in common clinical usage. Division over the distal interphalangeal joint constitutes an open mallet finger which requires repair and splintage, often with a Kirschner wire across the extended distal joint. Application of a mallet splint may result in skin necrosis where there has been an open wound. The wire should, however, be removed as soon as the wound edges are stable and replaced by a padded mallet splint (see below).

Division of the extensor apparatus over the proximal interphalangeal joint results in division of the central slip. The significance is frequently missed in emergency departments. The finger initially has a normal posture, but there is gradual distortion of the extensor apparatus as the lateral bands slip sideways and volarly to become flexors. The classical boutonnière deformity develops which is similar to that seen in rheumatoid arthritis (see Ch. 16) with proximal interphalangeal flexion and distal interphalangeal hyperextension. If recognised at the outset, this injury requires immediate repair and splintage. Wounds in this area may cause septic arthritis of the proximal interphalangeal joint. If diagnosis is delayed and a boutonnière deformity becomes established, repair of the flimsy middle slip is not possible and a reconstruction is necessary, using a tendon graft with a bony attachment to the middle phalanx. Alternatively, one of the lateral bands may be transferred to reconstruct the middle slip (Matev procedure).

Distal to the metacarpophalangeal joints, the extensor apparatus is a thin sheet composed of numerous delicate bands with different functions. As in the case of injuries over the proximal interphalangeal joint, injury to this delicate sheet may be apparent in the posture of the finger (boutonnière), but deformity may only manifest itself after a delay, due to gradually increasing deformation of the extensor aponeurosis. Over the metacarpophalangeal joints, diagnosis of tendon injury may be difficult, as the junctura tendinae and the adjacent tendons may achieve satisfactory digital extension. On occasion, unrepaired extensor tendons at this level may recover spontaneously as retraction is limited. The significance of open wounds in this area is discussed in relation to human bite injuries (see Ch. 11). Proximal to the metacarpophalangeal joints, the extensor tendons exist as discreet structures which may be repaired using the same techniques as for flexor tendon injuries.

The extensor tendons at wrist level lie within tight fibro-osseous tunnels and adhesions to the tunnels are likely. This may be prevented by early mobilisation or, in a severe injury, partial or total excision of the extensor retinaculum may be indicated.

When examining the patient with extensor muscle damage in the forearm, injury to or compression of the posterior interosseous nerve should always be considered.

The usual rehabilitation programme after extensor tendon injury is to immobilise the hand statically. Dorsiflexion of the wrist relaxes the extensor tendons to such an extent that the position of the metacarpophalangeal and interphalangeal joints is not critical. Generally, the interphalangeal joints are straight and the metacarpophalangeal joints are held in mid-flexion. Dynamic splintage may also be used.

### Tendon ruptures

The commonest closed tendon rupture is the *mallet* finger. The thin extensor apparatus is particularly vulnerable over the distal interphalangeal joint. The diagnosis is readily apparent with a flexion deformity of the distal interphalangeal joint. There may be an associated swan-neck deformity due to the pull of the extensors being concentrated on the middle slip. Treatment is by closed splintage which should hold the distal joint in a neutral position or mild hyperextension. The Stack polypropylene splint is a popular method of fixation, or alternatively a padded aluminium splint (Zimmer). The fitting must be

**Table 5.2** Excursion of extensor tendons expressed in millimetres for every 10° of joint motion

|  | Thumb | Index | Middle | Ring | Little |
|---|---|---|---|---|---|
| 10° DIP | — | 0.6 | 0.8 | 0.6 | 0.6 |
| 10° PIP | 0.9 | 0.8 | 0.8 | 0.8 | 0.6 |
| 10° MCP | 1.2 | 1.5 | 1.5 | 1.5 | 1.0 |
| 10° Wrist | 1.5 | 2.0 | 2.0 | 2.0 | 1.4 |

careful to achieve the correct joint positioning without undue pressure from any part of the splint. The splint should be attached by adhesive or Velcro strapping and the fitting checked after a few days when swelling has subsided. It should then be worn constantly for 6–8 weeks. The intelligent patient can be advised on how to remove the splint for cleaning, holding the distal joint in hyperextension by pinching against the thumb. If the patient can not comprehend this, the splint should be worn constantly. Failures are due to poor compliance with this regimen or an inadequate splint.

The boutonnière deformity may also arise from a closed rupture of the middle slip of the extensor apparatus at the proximal interphalangeal joint. Splintage is less likely to be successful than in the case of a mallet injury. Static splintage in extension is required, using an aluminium splint or a Link polypropylene splint. After 6 weeks of immobilisation a dynamic Capener splint should be worn for a further 6 weeks. If this is unsuccessful, reconstruction will be necessary (as above).

Rupture of the extensor pollicis longus may occur in rheumatoid arthritis or following a minimally displaced Colles' fracture. Repair is not possible as the tendon is attenuated. Transfer of extensor indicis proprius is indicated. Secondary tendon repair of the extensors in the distal forearm is often unrewarding and tendon transfers may be required.

By contrast with the flexor surface of the forearm, extensor tendon repairs have a much better prognosis. This is not due to more favourable extrinsic or intrinsic healing properties, but to the paucity of pulleys and the powerful flexors which will overcome adhesion around the extensor system.

## Tenovaginitis stenosans

De Quervain's syndrome is an inflammation of the tenosynovium of the extensor tendons at the base of the thumb where the abductor pollicis longus and extensor pollicis brevis pass through the retinaculum in the first dorsal compartment. The extensor pollicis longus travels in the third compartment and is not involved. The patient has a positive Finkelstein's test (ulnar deviation of the carpus with the thumb adducted and flexed across the palm) provoking pain over the first dorsal compartment. The test may produce mild discomfort in the normal wrist and comparison with the uninvolved wrist is always desirable. Crepitus over the compartment on movement of the involved tendons is less common, but diagnostic. Tenovaginitis can also involve the wrist extensors in the other dorsal compartments. The condition is frequently associated with compensation claims and caution should be exercised in the application of this diagnosis.

The differential diagnosis is from degenerative conditions in the underlying joints (usually first carpometacarpal arthritis and, more rarely, trapezioscaphoid arthritis or scaphoid non-union), or, on occasion, irritation of the terminal sensory branches of the radial nerve, arising from laceration or contusion. Tenovaginitis is often provoked by unaccustomed activity of the hand or wrist (for example, spring cleaning, or home improvement projects). Repetitive production-line employment may also cause synovitis around the extensor tendons as they travel through the first compartment.

The condition may resolve with a short period of immobilisation in a plaster cast or treatment with non-steroidal anti-inflammatory agents. If the symptoms have not settled within 3 weeks, further splintage or medication is unlikely to be of benefit. Intermittent prolonged periods of splintage should be avoided. A steroid/local anaesthetic injection accurately placed within or at the mouth of the first compartment may relieve symptoms or, at least, obtain a remission. The choice of steroid is of some importance. Subcutaneous steroid injection may cause local depigmentation and fat atrophy, with significant cosmetic deformity. The problem seems most common with the depot-type steroid preparations, and shorter-acting steroids are advised for all subcutaneous injections, particularly in females.

Patients who do not obtain lasting relief from either a short period of immobilisation or steroid injection require surgical decompression. This is performed through a transverse or oblique incision, taking particular care to identify and preserve the major sensory branches of the radial nerve which overlie the first extensor compartment. Damage to, or tethering of these nerves is an all too frequent complication which may give rise to persistent discomfort and prolonged disability. The abductor longus and extensor brevis are fully released by incising the overlying retinaculum. Anomalies of the extensor tendons are common and care must be taken to ensure that there are no extra slips of tendon travelling through a separate compartment, which might remain compressed.

## Triggering of fingers and thumb

Nodules may form in the flexor tendon at any age. A minority are rheumatoid in nature. The thumb or ring finger are most frequently involved. Non-rheumatoid trigger finger in adults is a perplexing condition. On occasion, a nodule on the tendon is evident, but more frequently no abnormality is seen yet the patient is unable to readily extend the finger from a flexed position. Extension is accompanied by a click and discomfort. The patient often considers that the problem lies in the proximal interphalangeal joint, but careful palpation will reveal a nodule at the level of the A1 pulley. Mild cases may resolve with an infiltration of steroid around the mouth of the tendon sheath, but more severe cases merit surgical release limited to the A1 pulley. Release of the pulley system more distally is contraindicated as it would give rise to bowstringing of the flexor tendons.

# 6. Bone and joint injuries

*Principal author:   F. D. Burke*

In many parts of the body, fracture management emphasises the need for bony union. Non-union is rare in the hand. Complications are more likely to arise from malalignment of the fracture or, more frequently, stiffness in the surrounding joints and loss of tendon excursion. Hand function relies on mobility of the digits. The ultimate objective of fracture management is to obtain a pain-free, stable and mobile hand.

## FRACTURES IN CHILDREN

Salter and Harris have classified epiphyseal injuries into five categories (Fig. 6.1):

*Type I* involves displacement restricted to the level of the epiphysis. There is no fracture and the joint surface is not involved. The base of the distal phalanx and the lower end of the radius are most frequently involved in the upper limb. Reduction is easily achieved in the first few hours but the epiphysis will soon adhere in its new position, rendering manipulative reduction difficult. Subsequent growth abnormality is uncommon.

*Type II* differs in that a fragment of the metaphysis remains with the epiphyseal portion. This represents the commonest variety of epiphyseal injury and is most frequently seen at the base of the proximal phalanx (often involving the little finger). Early manipulative reduction is advised and growth disturbance is rare.

*Type III* injuries involve the articular surface but the fracture does not extend beyond the epiphysis. Accurate reduction of the fragment reduces the risk of subsequent osteoarthritis and growth disturbance. The condition is fortunately uncommon.

*Type IV* injuries are an extension of the previous, with the fracture crossing the epiphysis. The condition is rare also. There is the risk of joint incongruity (with subsequent arthritis and the possibility of tethering of a portion of the growth plate with progressive deformity at the joint). Accurate reduction and fixation are advised.

*Type V* injuries are usually diagnosed in retrospect. There is damage to a portion of the epiphysis without fracture. Premature partial

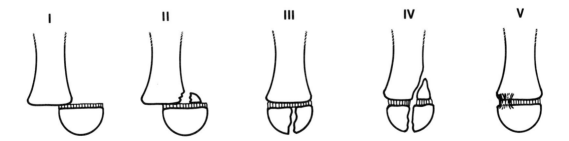

**Fig. 6.1**  The Salter–Harris classification

epiphyseal closure follows with progressive angular deformity. Corrective osteotomy may be required.

## ADULT FRACTURES

### Conservative management

Some fractures in the hand are stable and unlikely to displace if mobilised early. A certain amount of experience is required before confidently predicting which fractures are stable; they are minimally displaced and often present as oblique cracks. There is no indication to immobilise a stable fracture upon a splint beyond 3–4 days for relief of the initial discomfort. Early movement will increase the chance of full mobility of the hand.

The majority of unstable fractures can be treated by resting the hand upon a splint in the correct position for 3–4 weeks to permit clinical union. However splintage in this manner runs the risk of stiffness developing in the adjacent joints. The injury to the tissues frequently results in oedema of the involved portion of the hand. Fibrin is laid down in the soft tissues by the oedematous exudate and may restrict subsequent motion. This is most commonly seen around the metacarpophalangeal and interphalangeal joints. If oedema is allowed to diffuse around the collateral ligaments in a lax position, the effect of the subsequent fibrin deposits will be to shorten them. This is particularly important at the metacarpophalangeal joint, where the ligaments are lax in extension and tighten progressively when flexed (Fig. 6.2). If oedema of the hand is anticipated, it is important to splint the hand with the joints in such a position that their collateral ligaments are under tension. This reduces the chances of subsequent stiffness of the hand due to shortening of the collateral ligaments. Clinical experience and anatomical dissection indicate that the most favourable position in which the fingers may be placed is 90° of flexion at the metacarpophalangeal joint and virtual full extension of the interphalangeal joints. The thumb is held extended at metacarpophalangeal and interphalangeal joints and abducted from the palm to avoid contracture of the first web space. The metacarpophalangeal

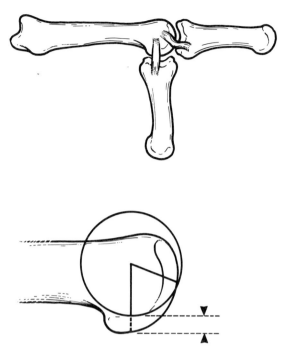

**Fig. 6.2** Collateral ligaments of the metacarpophalangeal joint

joints of the fingers are the most difficult to maintain in the optimal position for immobilisation. Palmar oedema tends to force them into an unfavourable semi-extended position.

The position of metacarpophalangeal joint flexion and interphalangeal joint extension is perhaps best maintained with the use of a volar splint. A single roll of 10 cm plaster of Paris is unwound and folded three times, such that there are eight thicknesses of plaster in a strip approximately 30 cm long. Plaster wool of similar width and slightly greater length is laid upon the hand and forearm, with the wrist extended. This is most easily achieved by resting the supinated wrist on a 10-cm rolled bandage. The plaster slab is then immersed in water and excessive liquid removed. It is laid upon the volar aspect of the forearm and hand and ridged over the wrist to increase strength in that area. As the plaster dries, the metacarpophalangeal joints are flexed and the interphalangeal joints extended. A crepe bandage is then applied proximally to distally and 2.5-cm Elastoplast used to draw the proximal phalanges firmly onto the splint (Fig. 6.14)

## Operative management

If the fracture cannot be manipulated and maintained in satisfactory alignment on a volar slab, consideration must be given to internal fixation. The decision is not taken lightly and should be performed by an experienced surgeon in an operating theatre with adequate instruments, illumination and assistance. The least invasive manner is to pass Kirschner wires through the skin, transfixing one bone fragment to the other. The procedure is best performed using image intensification. It is difficult to achieve accurate reduction of intra-articular fractures by this means.

A small fragment can be sutured back to the main portion of the bone by passing the wire through the major fragment (Fig. 6.23c).

### Crossed Kirschner wires

Crossed Kirschner wires have frequently been used in the past for the management of transverse shaft fractures (Fig. 6.3). The wires need to be passed at a very oblique angle and are not easy to insert. There is a tendency for the bone ends to become slightly distracted during the procedure. The tips of the wires frequently lie close to the adjacent joint, restricting early postoperative motion. This has been superseded to some extent by a more modern method.

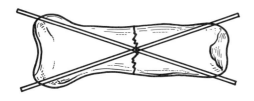

**Fig. 6.3**  Crossed Kirschner wires

### Intraosseous wiring

This is a good technique for transverse fractures and offers greater stability (see below, 7. The transverse midshaft fracture). It is not applicable to the more oblique fractures. Insertion of Kirschner wires is best performed with the use of a power drill. Accurate positioning of the wire will only be obtained if a small portion of the wire is protruding from the drill. If a large portion of wire is protruding, the control over the direction of the tip of the wire is significantly reduced.

### Intrafragmentary screw fixation

This technique is applicable to oblique fractures. The quality of cortical bone in the hand is excellent and very firm fixation can be obtained. The fracture is usually exposed through a lateral incision, preserving periosteal attachments. Haematoma and debris are cleared from the fracture surface with fine curettes. The fracture is reduced and held with bone-holding forceps. Both cortices are drilled with a drill bit of small diameter and the depth gauge identifies the appropriate screw length (Fig. 6.4) Both cortices are tapped and the more proximal cortex overdrilled with a larger diameter drill bit. The screw thread slips through the proximal cortex but engages firmly in the distal one. As the screw is tightened, the shoulder of the screw engages the proximal cortex, producing direct compression between the bone fragments. Minifragment plates may be used on metacarpal fractures but are rarely indicated more distally.

Internal fixation should be stable enough to permit early vigorous motion. Open reduction increases the soft tissue injury, may further devascularise the bone fragments, and changes a closed wound to an open one. These potential disadvantages are only acceptable if adequate stability is achieved so that early movements are feasible.

### External fixation

External fixators are infrequently used in hand injuries but may be of value in the management of metacarpal or phalangeal fractures, in association with skin loss. They provide fracture stability and yet permit access to the area of skin loss.

## Articular fractures

Fractures may involve the articular surface of a joint. An accurate reduction of the bone fragments

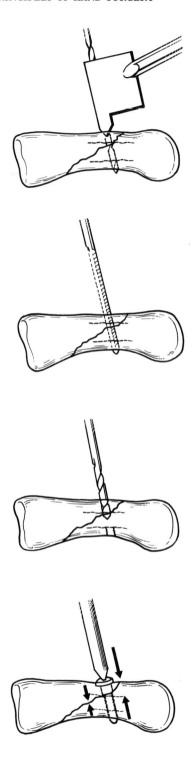

with optimal congruity of the joint surface will minimise the chance of subsequent degenerative arthritis. In addition, early movement of such cases reduces the risk of joint stiffness and may provide more satisfactory fibrocartilaginous healing in the area of the fracture. These objectives may best be attained by exploration, accurate reduction of the bone and internal fixation of the fragments. If such treatment is performed, it is very desirable that the fixation should be sufficiently rigid to permit early mobilisation of the fracture.

## FRACTURES OF THE DISTAL PHALANX

The numbers adjacent to the fractures discussed in this section indicate the area of injury in Figure 6.5.

### 1. Tuft fractures

These fractures are commonly associated with a crush injury of the fingertip. The fracture normally settles with the soft tissues. Splintage is not required and the fracture receives no specific treatment.

### 2. Shaft fractures

These are usually minimally displaced and are splinted by the adjacent nail. Damage may occur to the nail-bed. Accurate repair offers the best prospect of satisfactory subsequent nail adherence (see Ch. 4). Sufficient stability is usually obtained

**Fig. 6.4**  The lag screw technique of interfragmentary compression

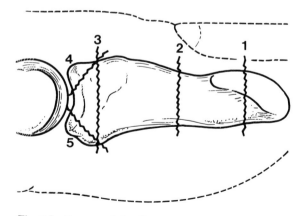

**Fig. 6.5**  Fracture of the distal phalanx

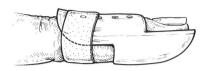

**Fig. 6.6**  The Stack mallet splint

with the use of either a mallet-type finger splint (Fig. 6.6) or a Zimmer metal/foam rubber variety. The fracture is immobilised for 3 weeks. Internal fixation is only required where there is marked angulation of the fracture, with instability. A longitudinal Kirschner wire may be passed proximally from the fingertip, stopping short of the distal interphalangeal joint.

### 3. Salter–Harris Type I epiphyseal injury (Seymour)

This injury is characterised by a flexion of the distal portion of the phalanx. The displacement may dislocate the germinal matrix of the nail, such that it lies superficial to the skin. Reduction of the phalanx is readily achieved if the injury is recent, but like many epiphyseal injuries it becomes more difficult if delayed beyond 24–36 hours. The fingertip should be held in extension in a mallet-type splint for 2 weeks and then mobilised. The germinal matrix will not reduce spontaneously and needs to be introduced back under the eponychium. Failure to reduce the germinal matrix results in superficial infection that may progress to osteomyelitis of the distal phalanx (Fig. 6.7).

Similar fractures near the base of the distal phalanx occur in adults. They are also treated by reduction of the nail-bed and a mallet finger splint for 3 weeks.

### 4. Extensor insertion fractures

The fracture usually follows compressive loading of the distal interphalangeal joint. As the load increases, the middle phalanx condyles split the base of the distal phalanx, as shown in Figure 6.8. The fragment includes the insertion of the extensor tendon and a mallet finger deformity develops with an extensor lag at the distal interphalangeal joint. Management depends on the size

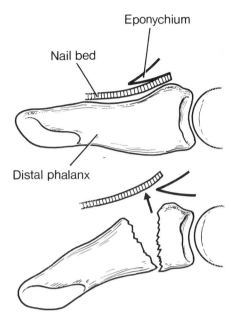

**Fig. 6.7**  Dislocation of the proximal nail-bed

of the bone fragment and the percentage of the articular surface involved. If the fragment of bone is small with minimal involvement of the articular surface, conservative management is recommended. Treatment in a mallet-type splint for 6 or 8 weeks will usually result in mild extensor lag and excellent distal interphalangeal joint flexion. Operative re-attachment of small fragments may improve extension at the risk of a loss of distal interphalangeal joint flexion. If the fragment of bone is large and involves more than a third of the articular surface, there is a strong case for internal fixation. A large fragment is easier to re-attach and open reduction produces a smooth articular surface, with perhaps less chance of subsequent degenerative joint disease. If more than a third of the articular surface is involved, the entire stability of the joint is threatened and the distal

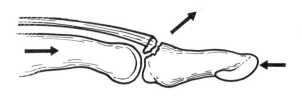

**Fig. 6.8**  Extensor insertion fracture

phalanx may drift into volar subluxation. The fragment is held in a reduced position most rigidly by an interfragmentary screw. Kirschner wires may be used, or the fragment drawn into place by a wire suture passed through the distal phalanx and tied over a button on the pulp. If sufficient stability is achieved, early mobilisation is advised to reduce the risk of stiffness at the distal interphalangeal joint. Intermediate-sized fragments may be managed by either conservative or operative means. Conservative management is favoured for the majority of these cases, particularly if the fracture is comminuted.

## 5. Flexor insertion fractures

The fracture may arise by a compressive loading of the digit, or represent an avulsion of the profundus tendon with the entire bony insertion separating from the remainder of the distal phalanx. (Fig. 6.9)

Although the insertion of the extensor tendon is limited to a small area on the dorsal lip at the base of the distal phalanx, the flexor profundus insertion is much more broadly based and extends over the proximal third. If the articular portion of the fracture exceeds a third of the joint surface, dorsal subluxation of the distal phalanx may occur. This can be overcome by maintaining the distal interphalangeal joint in 30/40° of flexion. A comminuted fracture of this type may be managed in an extension block splint for approximately 4 weeks. A large single fragment may be reduced and held with a minifragment screw and interfragmentary compression. The profundus tendon may then be mobilised at an early stage with the best chance of a satisfactory range of motion at the distal interphalangeal joint. Kirschner wires, or a wire suture tied over a button on the nail, may be used but the fixation is less rigid.

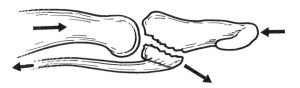

**Fig. 6.9** Flexor insertion fracture

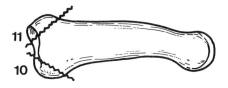

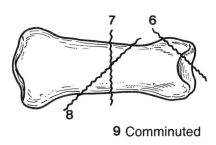

**9 Comminuted**

**Fig. 6.10** Fractures of the middle phalanx

## FRACTURES OF THE MIDDLE PHALANX

The number adjacent to the fractures discussed in this section indicates the area of injury in Figure 6.10.

## 6. Condylar fractures

These are particularly difficult to manage. The fragment involves the articular surface and is frequently displaced. This increases the risk of stiffness and degenerative arthritis. In addition, significant displacement will produce angular deformity at the joint. If the fragment is large and displaced, open reduction and fixation, using an interfragmentary screw, offers the best prospect of sufficient stability to allow early movement. There is often conflict between adequate exposure and devascularisation of the fragment. Extensive dissection of the fragment reduces an already precarious blood supply. The screw may be supplemented with a Kirschner wire to control rotation (Fig. 6.11).

Kirschner wire fixation may be preferred, particularly if the fragment is small, but produces no significant compression at the fracture site. The

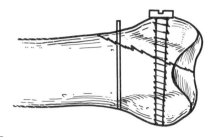

a

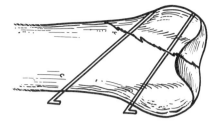

Fig. 6.12 Kirschner wire fixation of a condylar fracture

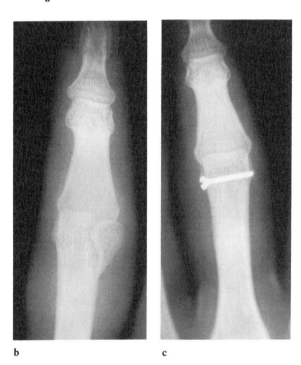

b                    c

Fig. 6.11 Lag screw fixation of a condylar fracture. **a** A lag screw inserted with additional Kirschner wire for increased stability. **b** Radiograph of a displaced condylar fracture of the proximal phalanx. **c** Stable reduction obtained with a single screw with interfragmentary compression

fracture should be reduced and two non-parallel wires passed through the fragment and middle phalanx (Fig. 6.12). The wires pass out of the opposite side of the finger between the digital vessels and the extensor tendon. The ends of the wires are then drawn through until flush with the outer aspect of the fragment. It is prudent to have the other ends of the wires some distance from the adjacent joints. The tips of the wires may be left under or through the skin. Prominent wires at the joints will cause discomfort and limit mobilisation.

If the reduction is felt to be sufficiently stable, early mobilisation is permitted. The Kirschner wires may be removed at 4 weeks and are withdrawn without the risk of distracting the healing fracture.

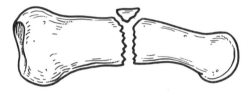

Fig. 6.13 The transverse midshaft fracture (lateral view) with dorsal fragment

## 7. The transverse mid-shaft fracture (Fig. 6.13)

### Conservative management

Manipulation and application of a volar slab will usually achieve a satisfactory reduction (Fig. 6.14). There is commonly a flake of cortical bone free on the dorsal surface and a tendency for further dorsal angulation of the fracture. Frequent outpatient review, with a true lateral radiograph on the volar slab, is advised to ensure that the reduction is maintained. There is little cancellous bone in this area of the phalanx and splintage for a full 4 weeks is advised. The finger can then be mobilised, strapped to an adjacent digit, for a further week. Failure to achieve or maintain satisfactory alignment necessitates operative treatment.

### Operative treatment

The technique of choice is intra-osseous wiring. The fracture is exposed from a lateral incision and

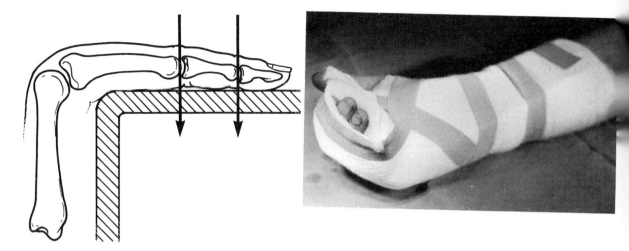

**Fig. 6.14** The optimal position for immobilisation using a volar slab

the bone ends mobilised. A transverse drill hole is made in the cortical bone 3 mm proximal and distal to the fracture. The hole is made slightly volar to the midaxial line of the phalanx (Fig. 6.15). This is particularly important if there is a dorsal flake of bone producing a tendency to recurrent angulation. It is then usually possible to pass a 24-gauge wire through the holes without a further incision in the opposite side of the finger. This is achieved by angulating the bone ends so that they face into the incision (Fig. 6.16). An appropriate sized Kirschner wire, sharpened at both ends, is then used to supplement stability. The wire is best introduced through the fracture line and passed obliquely, distally through the cortex within the area of the skin incision. The fracture may then be reduced and the wire passed proximally into the opposite cortex. The intraosseous wire is then tightened to achieve compression at the fracture site and laid flush against the bone.

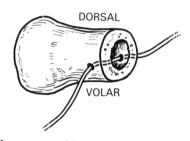

**Fig. 6.15** Intraosseous wiring technique: the site of the wire

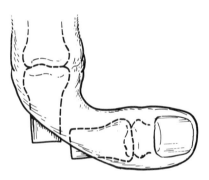

**Fig. 6.16** Intraosseous wiring technique: presenting the bone ends through a single incision

The Kirschner wire may either be cut off distally, flush with the bone, or left protruding for later removal (Fig. 6.17). The hand is rested on a volar splint for 3–5 days and then mobilised.

If an early mobilisation of a finger is planned following internal fixation of a fracture, it is important to achieve excellent coaptation of the skin edges. Special care must be taken in the placement of sutures. Any gaping of the skin in the early postoperative period will be uncomfortable for the patient and reduce the mobility of the digit.

## 8. Oblique shaft fractures

A minority are spiral fractures with a rotational component. Shortening at the fracture will result

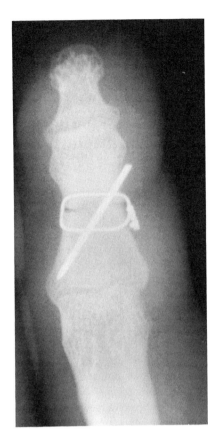

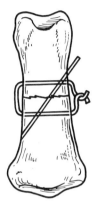

Fig. 6.17   Intraosseous wiring technique: after reduction

in a rotational deformity. Minimally displaced spiral fractures may be treated on a volar slab but constant vigilance is required lest shortening and therefore rotation supervene. Rotatory deformity can be appreciated by inspecting the fingertips end on (Fig. 6.18). Any malalignment of the plane of the nail will indicate rotation at the fracture site. If difficulty is experienced controlling the fracture, open reduction and fixation, using interfragmentary screws, is preferred. The aim is to produce excellent stability, which will permit rapid postoperative mobilisation.

Similar principles apply to the management of the commoner oblique fractures without rotational deformity. There is a broad area of fracture surface (unlike the transverse midshaft fractures) and clinical union is rapid. Stable oblique cracks may be mobilised immediately and strapped to the adjacent finger that offers most support (Fig. 6.19). Less stable fractures should be rested on a volar slab and then mobilised at 3 weeks, strapped to the adjacent finger. If difficulty is experienced

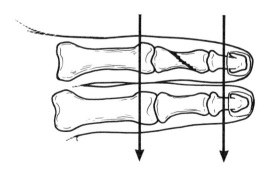

Fig. 6.19   A stable oblique fracture

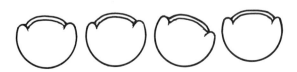

Fig. 6.18   Rotational deformity

controlling the fracture on a volar slab, an open reduction and internal fixation with interfragmentary screws is indicated.

## 9. Comminuted fractures of the middle phalanx

The fractures should be manipulated into the most favourable position and rested on a volar slab. Internal fixation is unlikely to achieve sufficient stability to permit early mobilisation and plays a limited role in these cases. The use of several Kirschner wires may be of value to improve the alignment of the fragments.

## 10. Volar rim fractures of the middle phalanx

The fracture may result from a longitudinal compressive loading of the digit or a hyperextension injury to the proximal interphalangeal joint. If less than one-third of the articular surface is involved and displacement is minimal, the finger may be rested on a volar slab for a few days and then mobilised strapped to the adjacent digit. The strapping permits rapid mobilisation without the risk of hyperextension of the proximal interphalangeal joint. If the fracture involves more than one-third of the articular surface of the base of the middle phalanx, there is a risk of joint subluxation. The majority of the collateral ligaments will insert onto a fragment of that size and the middle phalanx, without ligamentous support, will drift into a dorsal position. The subluxation is reduced by proximal interphalangeal joint flexion. If the fragment is in reasonable alignment, an extension block splint may be a satisfactory form of treatment (Fig. 6.20).

The splint blocks the last 40° of extension but permits full flexion. Early movement is achieved without the risk of joint subluxation. Open reduction and internal fixation is made more difficult by the presence of the flexor tendons and the volar plate. On occasion fixation with wire sutures or Kirschner wires may be appropriate, but it is difficult to achieve true stability. If the fracture is comminuted, an extension block splint offers the best prospect of a satisfactory result.

## 11. Dorsal rim fracture of the middle phalanx

This fracture involves the insertion of the central slip. Large fragments result in subluxation of the proximal interphalangeal joint, with the middle and distal phalanges dropping into a volar position. If there is a single large fragment, open reduction and fixation with a single interfragmentary screw achieves excellent stability and permits early movement (Fig. 6.21). A smaller single fragment may be reduced and held with fine wire sutures or the use of Kirschner wires. Management of a comminuted fracture is less rewarding. The fragments may be held reduced with several fine Kirschner wires, but early mobilisation risks loss of the position and joint subluxation. The fracture frequently unites with some volar subluxation of the middle phalanx and limited motion at the proximal interphalangeal joint.

## FRACTURES OF THE PROXIMAL PHALANX

The number adjacent to the fractures discussed in this section indicates the area of injury in Figure 6.22.

Types 12 , 13, 14, and 15 are managed in the manner described for the middle phalanx.

## 16. Fractures of the lateral border of the phalanx base

These are most commonly seen in the thumb and represent a ligamentous injury to the metacarpophalangeal joint. The fragment of bone includes the insertion of the collateral ligament. If the fragment is not reduced, joint instability may occur. Management depends on the size of the fragment. Large fragments require open reduction and

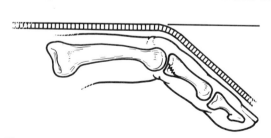

**Fig. 6.20** An extension block splint. A foam and aluminium splint is taped to the proximal phalanx of the finger to limit proximal interphalangeal extension

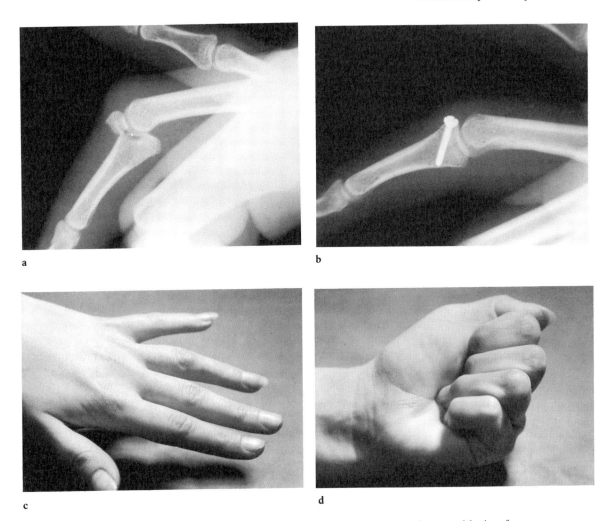

**Fig. 6.21**   A dorsal rim fracture at the base of the middle phalanx with joint subluxation treated by interfragmentary compression with a single screw and early mobilisation. **a** Lateral radiograph of the fracture subluxation. **b** Lateral radiograph confirming satisfactory reconstruction of joint. **c, d** A satisfactory range of movement regained after early mobilisation

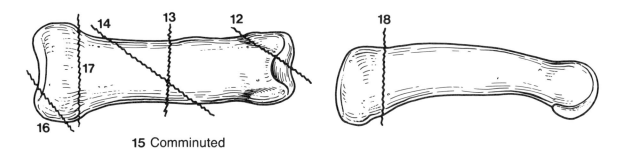

**Fig. 6.22**   Fractures of the proximal phalanx

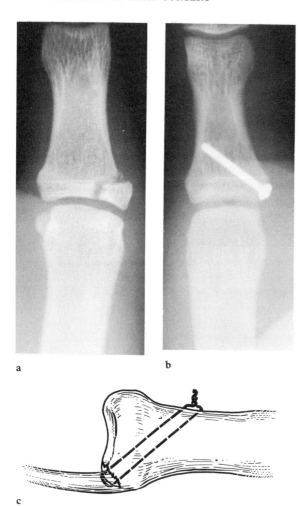

a                              b

c

**Fig. 6.23   a, b** Minifragment fixation of an ulnar collateral ligament bone fragment at the metacarpophalangeal joint of the thumb. **c** For smaller fragments a wiring technique is preferred

fixation with a single minifragment screw, using interfragmentary compression (Fig. 6.23a, b). The digit should be mobilised early. If the fragment is small, it can be wired back in place using a transosseous wire (Fig. 6.23c).

Failure to appreciate the significance of such fractures results in chronic pain and instability at the joint. The injury is particularly disabling when the ulnar collateral ligament of the thumb metacarpophalangeal joint is involved (the gamekeeper's thumb). Failure to diagnose and treat this condition correctly may result in loss of power pinch.

## 17. Salter Type II injury

This usually involves the little finger in children. The cortical bone on the ulnar border of the proximal phalanx is crushed with abduction of the distal fragment (Fig. 6.24). The proximity to the joint renders reduction difficult. Manipulation of the fracture, adducting the finger (flexed at the metacarpophalangeal joint) against a pencil in the fourth web space, may achieve correction but mild residual angulation is frequent. The fracture heals readily and early mobilisation of the little finger, strapped to the ring finger, is advised. Persistent significant abduction deformity of the little finger is rare.

A similar fracture may occur, with dorsal rather than ulnar deviation. This may present in children, in association with an epiphyseal injury and commonly in elderly patients, after a fall on the outstretched hand. The proximity to the joint frequently results in difficulty in achieving and maintaining a reduction of the fracture. Immobilisation on a volar slab for 3 weeks may be followed

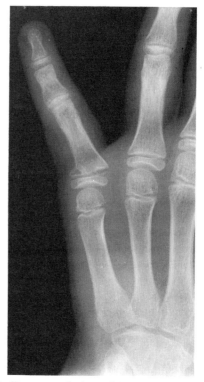

**Fig. 6.24**   Fracture at the base of the proximal phalanx of the fifth ray

by vigorous mobilisation with the finger strapped to the adjacent digit. Elderly patients frequently experience difficulty achieving full flexion of the finger after this type of injury.

## METACARPAL FRACTURES (Fig. 6.25)

Condylar fractures of the metacarpals are frequently caused by crush injuries and are often comminuted. These are difficult to stabilise sufficiently rigidly to permit early movement and conservative management is therefore indicated.

### 20, 21. Midshaft metacarpal fractures

Stable solitary fractures with minimal displacement: the fracture is supported by adjacent metacarpals. The hand may be rested on a volar splint for 3–4 days and then mobilised. If the fracture is felt to be less stable, or involves a border metacarpal, splintage on a volar slab may be required for 3 weeks. More widely displaced fractures damage the adjacent interossei. Prolonged immobilisation on the volar slab may result in tightness of the intrinsics and reduced range of motion of the fingers. This tendency to stiff fingers may be reduced by internal fixation and early mobilisation. The method of fixation depends on the obliquity of the fracture. Transverse fractures can be firmly held by small plates. Intraosseous wiring can also produce satisfactory stability although access is more difficult to the centrally placed metacarpals. Oblique fractures may be treated with interfragmentary screw fixation. If the fracture is sufficiently oblique to permit the insertion of two screws, excellent stability can be achieved.

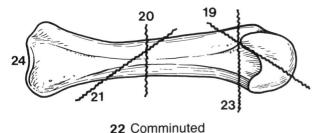

**22 Comminuted**

**Fig. 6.25** Metacarpal fractures

### 22. Comminuted fractures

Internal fixation is rarely indicated and a volar splint is preferred. On occasion the general alignment of the metacarpal may be maintained by the use of transverse Kirschner wires through the involved bone and the adjacent intact metacarpal.

### 23. Fractures of the metacarpal neck

The fifth ray is most frequently involved. The distal fragment tilts volarly. Manipulative reduction may be performed but the cortical bone is frequently crushed on the volar aspect and recurrence of deformity is frequent. Open reduction and stabilisation with Kirschner wires may be performed, but the wires frequently lie close to the metacarpophalangeal joint and impede motion. It is fortunate that fracture healing in the flexed position causes little functional disability. The involved head is less prominent when the metacarpophalangeal joints are flexed. An extensor lag at the metacarpophalangeal joint is frequently found but tends to settle over succeeding months. Rest on a volar slab for 1 or 2 weeks will permit the discomfort to settle. The finger can then be mobilised strapped to the adjacent digit.

### 24. Carpometacarpal injuries

The commonest fracture involves the first ray. The Bennett's fracture is an intra-articular injury which may result in subluxation at the carpometacarpal joint. The fragment on the volar/ulnar aspect of the metacarpal is retained by strong ligamentous attachments. The remainder of the metacarpal can sublux dorsoradially. Reduction may be achieved by longitudinal traction and mild abduction. Care should be taken to avoid hyperextending the metacarpophalangeal joint if a scaphoid-type plaster is applied. A well-moulded plaster is required. Excessive pressure over the carpometacarpal joint may cause a pressure sore, and careful padding with felt or wool is needed if this complication is to be avoided. Four weeks in plaster is sufficient to achieve satisfactory bone healing. Failure to maintain the reduction justifies internal fixation for a minority of Bennett's fractures. A large fragment may be reduced and held with a single interfragmentary screw. However, it is difficult to obtain satisfactory access to the fragment. A simpler technique is usually adequate. Reduction is obtained by the use of longitudinal traction. This is maintained while percutaneous Kirschner wires are passed from the first to second metacarpal or carpus. The pins hold the first metacarpal out to length during the healing phase and may be removed at 4 weeks when the fracture has clinically united.

## DISLOCATIONS

### Carpometacarpal dislocations

The injury is fortunately rare but easily overlooked. It is commonly associated with high-velocity injuries, frequently a motorcyclist falling from his machine at speed. The injury is probably caused by a fall on the outstretched hand and in the majority of cases the involved metacarpal dislocates dorsally. What should be an obvious deformity to the dorsal aspect of the hand is masked by soft-tissue swelling. The patient frequently has other serious injuries which may distract attention from the carpus. Anteroposterior radiographs may suggest only minimal incongruity of the carpometacarpal joint, but a true lateral view reveals the dorsal displacement of the metacarpal base. Reduction is readily achieved and maintained by a percutaneous Kirschner wire transfixing the joint. The hand is usually swollen and should be rested on a volar slab, with the metacarpophalangeal joints flexed and the interphalangeal joints extended. Active and passive movements of the fingers should be started in the early postoperative period. The capsule of the carpometacarpal joint is slow to stabilise and fixation for a period of 6 weeks is recommended.

### Metacarpophalangeal joint dislocation

The condition is not common, but may arise from a fall on the outstretched hand and predominantly involves index and small fingers. The metacarpal head passes proximal to the volar plate, with the flexor tendon to one side of the neck and the lumbrical to the other. The head is tightly wedged distally by the volar plate and proximally by the

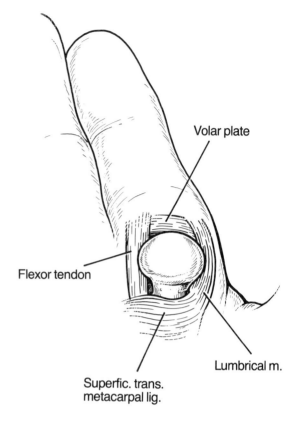

Fig. 6.26    Metacarpophalangeal joint dislocation

superficial transverse metacarpal ligament (Fig. 6.26).

Manipulative reduction is sometimes possible if the proximal interphalangeal joint is flexed to relax the intrinsic muscles. Wrist flexion relaxes the long flexors and may also be of benefit. The metacarpophalangeal joint is maintained in hyperextension while attempting to slide the base of the proximal phalanx distally on to the dorsal aspect of the metacarpal head. Hyperextension can then be corrected as the dislocation is reduced. Open reduction through a volar approach is frequently required. Release of the A1 pulley and elevation of the volar plate will allow reduction to be achieved. Joint instability is uncommon and early motion advised. Closed reduction of a dorsal dislocation of the thumb metacarpophalangeal joint is greatly facilitated by placing the first metacarpal in maximal adduction (Fig. 6.27). This

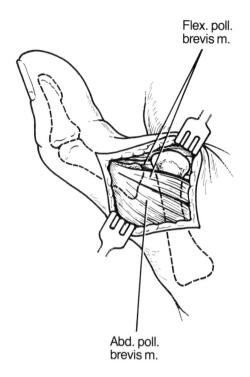

Fig. 6.27 Metacarpophalangeal joint dislocation of the thumb

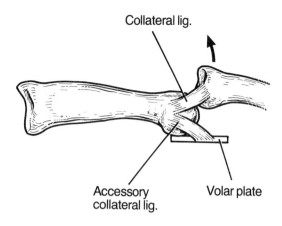

Fig. 6.28 Dorsal interphalangeal joint dislocation

manoeuvre relaxes the intrinsic muscles, which otherwise firmly grasp the metacarpal neck.

A more minor metacarpophalangeal joint subluxation can occur in which the volar plate is drawn dorsally on to the metacarpal head. Volar manipulation of the proximal phalanx base with the wrist flexed (to relax the flexor tendons) will achieve reduction. Preliminary hyperextension of the metacarpophalangeal joint must be avoided. The manoeuvre will draw the volar plate dorsally over the metacarpal head and produce a total dislocation of the joint that may require open reduction.

## Interphalangeal joint dislocation

### Dorsal dislocation

The volar plate is avulsed from its insertion into the middle phalanx and the latter dislocates dorsally. If the finger is clinically straight, both collateral ligaments have split longitudinally (Fig. 6.28). Reduction is usually achieved without difficulty with the use of longitudinal traction and initial hyperextension. Usually there is no lateral instability.

Immobilisation on a splint for 3 to 4 days will permit the major discomfort to settle and the finger may then be mobilised, strapped to the adjacent digit. Prolonged splintage reduces the prospect of a satisfactory range of motion.

### Lateral dislocation

This indicates that in addition to the above-mentioned injuries, one of the collateral ligaments has ruptured transversely. Reduction is usually obtained without difficulty and if the joint appears stable, treatment may be as previously stated. Marked instability justifies repair of the collateral ligament.

### Volar dislocation

The head of the proximal phalanx may buttonhole through the extensor mechanism between the central slip and one of the lateral bands (Fig. 6.29). Usually closed reduction can be achieved if manipulation is performed with the metacarpophalangeal and proximal interphalangeal joints in flexion, which releases tension on the lateral band. Open reduction may be required in a minority of cases, particularly if there is central slip disruption.

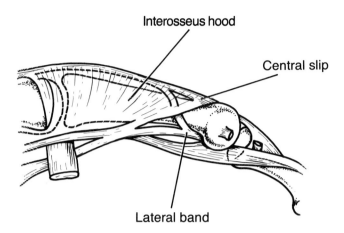

**Fig. 6.29** Volar interphalangeal joint dislocation

## PROXIMAL INTERPHALANGEAL JOINT SPRAINS

These sprains characteristically present with pain, fusiform swelling and reduced motion at the joint. Symptoms and signs may take 18 months to resolve and full motion is not always achieved. Physiotherapy is beneficial in the early stages if there is marked joint stiffness.

# 7. Carpal injuries

*Principal author:  F. D. Burke*

## INTRODUCTION

The carpus is a system of intercalated bones which transmit compressive loading from five digital rays to a pair of forearm bones, in all positions of hand circumduction. This compressive loading is balanced by strong ligaments on the volar and radial side of the wrist during power grasp which is performed in dorsiflexion and ulnar deviation. The carpus is composed of eight bones which articulate with the radius and ulna proximally and the five metacarpals distally (Fig. 7.1). The pisiform is a sesamoid bone which plays a minor role in the mechanics of the wrist. The remaining seven carpal bones are aligned in two rows. The proximal carpal row articulates with the distal end of the radius and the triangular cartilage. The latter arises from the ulnar styloid notch and inserts on the rim of the radial articular surface (Fig. 7.2). The scaphoid bone is a member of both carpal rows and acts as a strut, preventing zig-zag collapse during axial compression. Further support is provided by wrist ligaments (Fig. 7.3), which are local condensations of fibrous tissue within the wrist capsule. The majority of the ligaments lie on the volar aspect.

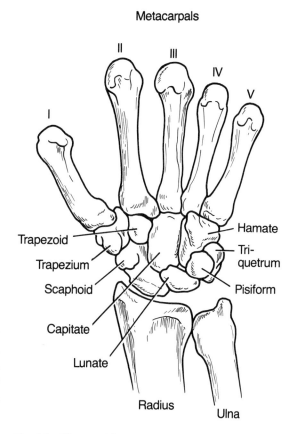

**Fig. 7.1**  The carpal bones

## EVALUATION OF THE PAINFUL WRIST

'Tenderness on the dorsal aspect of the wrist' is an inadequate assessment of an acute wrist injury. Clinical examination of the painful or injured wrist requires very precise palpation. Points of maximal tenderness should be sought and the involved underlying structure (bone, ligament, tendon or sheath) identified. This detailed examination is particularly important in acute wrist injuries where accurate localisation of tenderness will usually indicate the area of damage. The diagnostic clues provided by localised tenderness are not always available when more chronic wrist problems develop. A superficial initial assessment may permanently deprive the clinician of information.

131

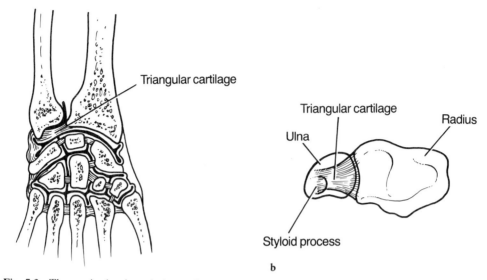

**Fig. 7.2** The proximal wrist articular surface and the triangular cartilage. **a** Anteroposterior view. **b** The radio-ulnar articular surface

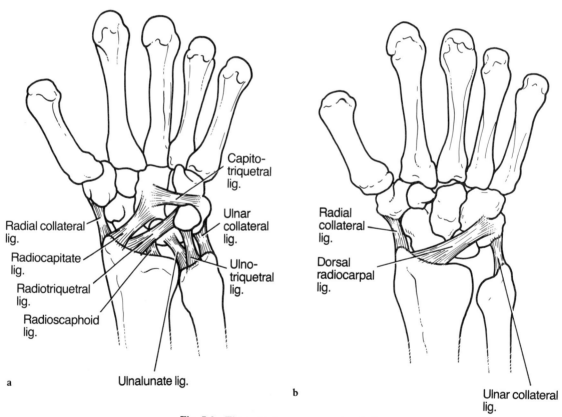

**Fig. 7.3** The wrist ligaments: **a** volar, **b** dorsal

Interpretation of radiographs of the wrist requires not only a meticulous search for fractures but also an assessment of the carpal bones' alignment. Wrist injuries may produce disability through malalignment of the carpal bones from ligamentous injury or fracture. Malalignment may be of a gross nature, as in the case of lunate dislocation, or be more subtle, requiring careful measurement of the relative axes of the carpal bones. The most informative radiograph is the lateral view in neutral position of flexion/extension, radioulnar deviation and pronation/supination. The scaphoid is obliquely aligned, the proximal pole in line with the lunate and the distal portion placed more volarly. Instability of the carpal bones affects the alignment of the lunate and the

scaphoid in particular. In neutral flexion and radioulnar deviation, the angle between the longitudinal axis of the scaphoid and the lunate should lie between 30° and 70° (Fig. 7.4a). An abnormally high or low scapholunate angle indicates a disruption of the wrist ligaments associated with carpal instability, and there are two patterns of carpal collapse. In dorsiflexion instability the lunate tilts dorsally and the scapholunate angle is greater than 80° (Fig. 7.4b,c). This has been called Dorsal Intercalated Segment Instability (DISI). The scaphoid may lie perpendicular to the longitudinal axis of the radius. This collapse pattern is caused by scapholunate ligament disruption or a scaphoid fracture. Palmar flexion instability of the lunate is less common (Fig. 7.4d): the lunate tilts volarly

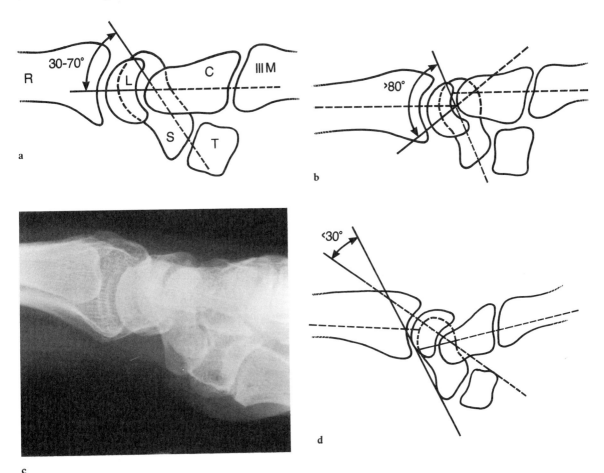

**Fig. 7.4** The scapholunate angle in normal alignment (**a**). The lunate lies on the long axis of the radius and faces the metacarpal bases. Collapse patterns DISI (**b, c**) and VISI (**d**). R, radius; L, lunate; C, capitate; IIIM, 3rd metacarpal; S, scaphoid; T, trapezium

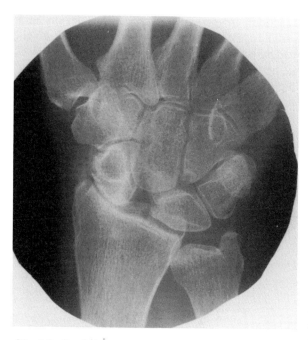

**Fig. 7.5** Scapholunate dissociation

the wrist, commonly by a fall on the outstretched hand. The scaphoid fracture has gained a reputation for being difficult to diagnose and treat. The majority of the bone surface is covered by articular cartilage and the blood supply enters principally through the distal portion. The precarious blood supply to the proximal pole, the large articular surface area and the stabilising role in the carpus together render it at particular risk of malunion or avascular necrosis.

Fractures of the tubercle probably arise by a direct blow to the palm of the hand. Pain is maximal over the tubercle in the palm rather than in the snuff-box. Distal one-third fractures have a low incidence of non-union or avascular necrosis of the proximal part. The fracture does not articulate with the radius, and if union occurs with some incongruity, consequent radioscaphoid arthritis is infrequent. Middle third fractures are the most common variety and the area of the fracture does articulate with the radius. Non-union and avascular necrosis rates are higher. Proximal pole fractures have the highest incidence of non-union and avascular necrosis of the proximal fragment.

and reduces the scapholunate angle to less than 30° (Volar Intercalated Segment Instability, or VISI). On the postero-anterior view the scaphoid and lunate bone should be separated by a gap of approximately 2 mm. If the gap is in excess of 4 mm, scapholunate dissociation is present, indicating proximal scaphoid instability with carpal collapse (DISI) (Fig. 7.5). Carpal instability frequently causes weakened grip and reduced wrist mobility. If the diagnosis is made at the time of injury the carpus can usually be satisfactorily realigned by longitudinal traction. Kirschner wires maintain alignment for 4–6 weeks while the capsule and ligaments heal. Such treatment offers the best prospect of a return to optimal wrist strength and mobility. However, the correct management of established carpal collapse is less certain. Ligament reconstruction is difficult to perform and unreliable. Limited carpal fusions may be shown to be of benefit. Early results indicate improved grip strength but with some loss of wrist mobility.

## FRACTURES OF THE SCAPHOID

The injury is caused by forced hyperextension of

### Principles in the management of scaphoid fractures

It is important to diagnose the fracture early. Delay in diagnosis and treatment reduces the likelihood of a satisfactory bone union. Differentiation from a wrist sprain may be difficult. A high index of suspicion is required by the casualty officer.

### Examination of the wrist

It is common practice to press firmly over the scaphoid in the anatomical snuff-box. Pain elicited in such a manner is thought to be indicative of a fracture of the scaphoid. If the test is employed, it is important to apply equal pressure to both anatomical snuff-boxes and demonstrate greater discomfort at the injured wrist. The terminal sensory branches of the radial nerve run across the scaphoid in the floor of the snuff-box and firm pressure against the underlying bone often causes discomfort in the absence of a carpal fracture. Pain on axial compression of the carpus or on

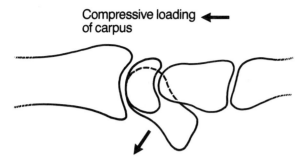

Compressive loading of carpus

**Fig. 7.6** Examination of the painful wrist

attempting to volarly sublux the carpus on the radius (Fig. 7.6) are more reliable tests. If either produces pain, a fracture of the scaphoid bone may be present.

*Radiographs of the wrist*

Radiographs must always be taken in four planes.

1. The true lateral view. A fracture of the tubercle, or the waist may be visible. The scapho-lunate angle should be carefully assessed (see above).

2. The postero-anterior view. The scaphoid lies obliquely and is not well seen in this view. However, the remaining carpal bones and their alignment are well demonstrated. If the ring sign is present (Figs 7.5, 7.7) the scaphoid is being viewed end on and is almost perpendicular to the line of the radius. This indicates that carpal collapse is present.

3. The reverse oblique or hyperpronated view. This provides an excellent demonstration of the scaphoid in the plane of its long axis. It is particularly valuable for waist or proximal pole fractures.

4. A postero-anterior view in full ulnar deviation. In maximal radial deviation the long axis of the scaphoid in a normal wrist lies almost perpendicular to the long axis of the radius. As the wrist moves into the neutral position the scaphoid rotates (Fig. 7.8). This realignment continues to maximal ulnar deviation where the long axis of the scaphoid lies close to that of the radius. Hence a postero-anterior radiograph in maximal ulnar deviation will provide a view of the scaphoid that is almost parallel to its long axis.

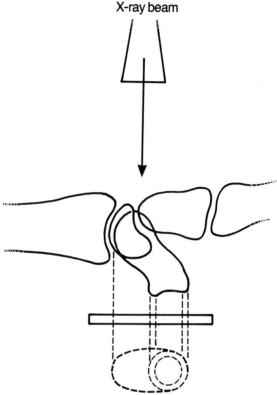

X-ray beam

**Fig. 7.7** The ring sign

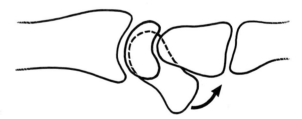

**Fig. 7.8** Scaphoid rotation on ulnar deviation

## Management of the 'possible scaphoid fracture'

If there is doubt, immobilise the wrist in a scaphoid plaster for 2 weeks, then take fresh radiographs out of plaster. A fracture is seldom revealed. However, the policy is justified on the basis of early diagnosis and treatment reducing the incidence of non-union. If doubt remains (persistent discomfort over the scaphoid without radiological confirmation of a fracture) it is necessary to continue immobilisation for a further 2 weeks. If at 1 month symptoms persist in the absence of radiological changes, immediate referral for a specialist opinion is required. The patient's management should not be allowed to drift on for several further weeks with intermittent periods of immobilisation and no clear diagnosis.

## Management of definite scaphoid fractures

### Fractures of the tubercle of the scaphoid

The fracture is rested on a scaphoid plaster for 4–6 weeks, depending on the degree of comminution. Satisfactory union is almost invariable.

### Minimally displaced fracture

There is a crack in the scaphoid but no loss of alignment of the bone and no evidence of carpal collapse. The cartilage envelope surrounding the bone is probably intact. The majority of such fractures immobilised from injury will unite satisfactorily in 6–8 weeks. Non-union rates are higher in the area of the proximal pole. Predicting the groups at risk for non-union is difficult. One method of management is to immobilise all such fractures of the scaphoid in plaster for 6 weeks. If radiographs at that stage indicate satisfactory progress to union and clinical signs have resolved, conservative treatment can be discontinued. However, where clinical and radiological signs leave doubt, immobilisation should be continued. If there is little evidence of healing in 6 weeks, internal fixation with a screw can then be performed. The improved stability and compression at the fracture will usually result in bone union. If a cavity is apparent at the fracture line, bone grafting will be required in association with internal fixation. Assessment at 6 weeks postinjury avoids the problem of a scaphoid non-union presenting after after 12–14 weeks of immobilisation. Such patients then require a scaphoid graft, which will necessitate a further prolonged period of immobilisation and may render a manual worker incapable of work for a total period of 9 months from injury.

### The widely displaced scaphoid fracture

Application of a scaphoid plaster may produce satisfactory alignment. However, if there is a persistent malalignment of the fragments, or evidence of associated carpal collapse, open reduction and internal fixation is preferred. Radiographic evidence of carpal collapse indicates significant malalignment at the fracture site and it is likely that bone union will be either delayed or inhibited completely. The volar approach gives an excellent view of the scaphoid and is preferred for all fractures except those involving the proximal pole. A dorsal approach is indicated in this group. Unheaded screws (for example the Herbert screw), which are completely buried in the bone, are particularly useful for scaphoid fractures and may be inserted through an articular portion of the bone surface with minimal damage to the joint. The curvature of the scaphoid restricts choice in the alignment of the screw and it is not always possible to cross the fracture line in a perpendicular direction. To achieve access for insertion of the screw, it is necessary to divide the radiocapitate ligament within the wrist capsule. When the screw has been placed, a careful capsular repair is performed and the wrist rested in a cast for 3 weeks.

### The comminuted scaphoid waist fracture

The bone on the volar aspect is crushed and attempts to achieve interfragmentary compression at the fracture site produce recurrent angulation. A wedge of corticocancellous bone is required to reconstitute the scaphoid length and prevent carpal collapse. Interfragmentary compression can then be achieved (Fig. 7.9).

### Trans-scaphoid perilunate dislocation

There is a dorsal dislocation of the carpus which leaves the lunate and proximal pole of scaphoid in normal alignment with the radius. Closed reduction of the dislocation is frequently possible. Internal fixation of the scaphoid is performed to stabilise the carpus.

### Scaphoid non-union

If there are minimal degenerative changes in

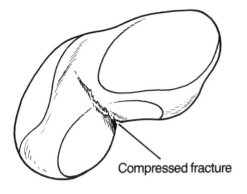

Compressed fracture

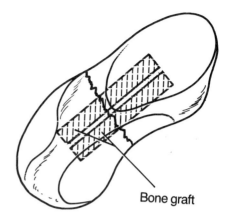

**Fig. 7.10**   The Russe bone graft

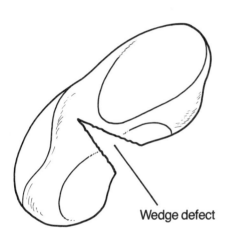

Wedge defect

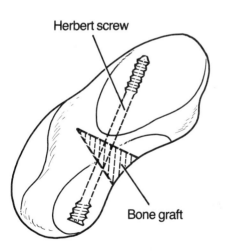

Herbert screw

Bone graft

**Fig. 7.9**   Reconstruction of a collapsed scaphoid by a wedge corticocancellous graft and screw

adjacent bones and significant pain or weakness of grip, bone grafting of the scaphoid is indicated. This may take the form of a Russe bone graft, using two cortical blocks laid into a trench on the volar aspect of the scaphoid (Fig. 7.10). If the scaphoid is angulated and foreshortened, a volar wedge corticocancellous graft is required. Arthritis limited to the scaphoid articulation may be treated by a Silastic scaphoid replacement. If the degenerative changes in the wrist are more extensive, it may be necessary to consider wrist arthrodesis, replacement or limited carpal fusion. The long-term benefit of intercarpal fusion and Silastic replacements is uncertain at present.

## FRACTURES OF THE LUNATE

These fractures are uncommon and present as cracks with minimal displacement. The carpus is splinted in a Colles' plaster for 4 weeks. The majority of such fractures heal satisfactorily and full wrist mobility is regained. If the vascular supply to the lunate has been compromised, the patient may develop Kienböch's disease. It is prudent to perform radiographs on all lunate fractures at 3 and 6 months from the injury.

### Kienböch's disease

The Austrian radiologist Kienböch first described the radiological features of avascular necrosis of the lunate (Fig. 7.11). Injection studies reveal that

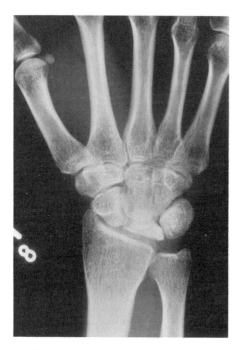

**Fig. 7.11** Kienböch's disease

approximately one-third of lunates have a precarious arterial supply, with either a single vessel or two end arteries which do not anastomose. Infrequently a radiologically visible fracture of the lunate may progress to avascular necrosis. However the majority of cases probably arise from stress microfractures developing within the lunate. These may follow wrist injuries, or relate to anomalies in surrounding structures. A portion of the lunate articulates with the radius, while the remainder overlies the triangular cartilage. The latter may provide inadequate support to the lunate in compressive loading and cause stress fractures within the bone. Softening and collapse of the lunate occurs, associated with pain and restricted wrist motion. Splintage may ease discomfort in the short term but does not arrest the bone collapse, or the development of surrounding degenerative changes. The inadequate support provided by the triangular cartilage as revealed by an apparently short ulna (negative ulnar variance) has led to clinical trials of radial shortening (or ulnar lengthening) as a means of arresting the progress of the disorder. Lunate excision with a Silastic replacement preserves wrist motion and

relieves pain if degenerative changes are limited to that area of the carpus. Revascularisation of the lunate by vascularised bone graft techniques has been attempted. The benefit in arresting lunate collapse remains to be assessed.

## DISLOCATIONS OF THE LUNATE

Disruption of the carpus may produce pressure on the median nerve in the carpal tunnel. This is particularly common with the volarly dislocated lunate. A sprained wrist, with persistent severe pain or associated carpal tunnel syndrome, requires urgent reassessment.

### The perilunate dislocation

This injury is frequently initially missed, being regarded as a wrist sprain. The carpal bones, with the exception of the lunate, dislocate dorsally, leaving the lunate in correct alignment with the radius (Fig. 7.12). The dislocation is most readily seen on the lateral radiograph, with no articulation between capitate and lunate. Closed reduction can usually be achieved, but carpal instability may persist after reduction. This will be evident on the lateral radiograph as an abnormal scapholunate angle. Stabilisation with Kirschner wires in a corrected position is advised. The instability can usually be corrected by applying longitudinal traction to the carpus as the Kirschner wires are inserted. On occasion, the proximal pole of the scaphoid remains attached to the lunate, producing a trans-scaphoid perilunate dislocation. Reduction of the dislocation is coupled with internal fixation of the scaphoid fracture to achieve carpal stability.

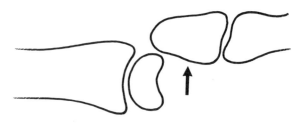

**Fig. 7.12** Perilunate dislocation of the wrist

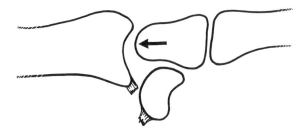

**Fig. 7.13** Lunate dislocation: the capitate is articulating with the radius and the lunate is displaced volarly, this may produce compression of the median nerve

## Lunate dislocation

The perilunate dislocation may be the first stage of the mechanism by which the lunate is dislocated. The capitate and surrounding carpal bones rebound from their dorsal position and as they reduce on the radius, dislocate the lunate volarly (Fig. 7.13). The lunate dorsal capsular attachments are disrupted, with variable damage to the volar structures.

Carpal distraction, dorsiflexion and pressure over the lunate will usually reduce the dislocation. If carpal instability remains apparent on the lateral radiograph, the carpal bones should be stabilised with Kirschner wires in correct alignment. Open reduction of the lunate is required if closed manipulation is unsuccessful. Volar capsular repair may improve carpal stability. The carpus is splinted in a plaster cast to allow the disrupted capsule and ligaments to heal. Radiographs at 3 or 6 months may reveal Kienböch's disease.

## FRACTURES OF OTHER CARPAL BONES

### The triquetrum

Flakes of bone, raised from the dorsal aspect of the triquetrum, are frequently seen after falls on the hand with forced dorsi or palmar flexion. The radiotriquetral ligament insertion is avulsed from the triquetrum. Support in a Colles-type plaster for 3–4 weeks usually allows the discomfort to settle.

### The trapezium

These fractures are uncommon. The joint surfaces articulating with the first metacarpal or scaphoid are often involved. The fracture is probably caused by hyperextension of the first ray, causing compressive loading at the joint. Displacement is usually minimal and conservative management indicated.

### The capitate

A fall on the outstretched hand, at speed, may produce this uncommon injury. The capitate fractures across the body and the proximal pole may rotate through 180°, so that the fracture surface faces the lunate. The malalignment is not always obvious on routine radiographs and lateral tomograms may be required to confirm the diagnosis. If a fracture is minimally displaced, conservative management is appropriate. If the proximal pole is rotated, open reduction and stabilisation with Kirschner wires is required. Impaired circulation to the proximal pole of the capitate may cause subsequent bone softening, collapse and degenerative arthritis.

### The hamate

Fractures to the body of the hamate are rare and arise from severe crush injuries to the ulnar border

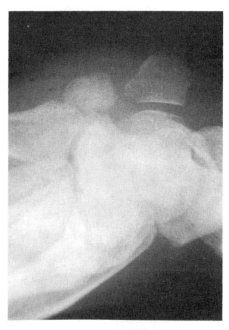

**Fig. 7.14** Fracture of the hook of the hamate

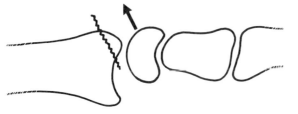

**Fig. 7.15**   Dorsal rim fracture of the radius

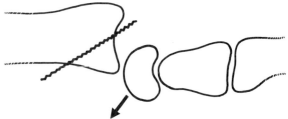

**Fig. 7.16**   Volar rim fracture of the radius

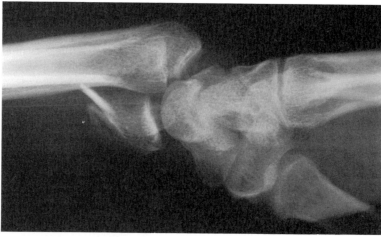

a

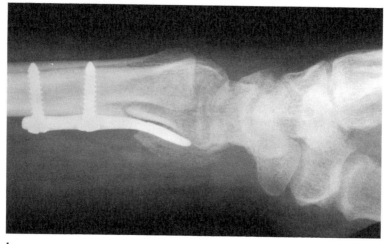

b

**Fig. 7.17**   Volar rim fracture with joint subluxation (**a**) treated with a buttress plate (**b**) and early mobilisation

of the hand, or compressive loading of the fifth ray. Injury to the hook of the hamate is also uncommon but is of interest. Untreated, the condition causes prolonged disability, yet appropriate treatment relieves symptoms completely. The patient is usually enthusiastic and successful at a sport that requires racquet, club or bat. If two hands are used on the sporting equipment, it is the more proximal of the two that is involved. The patient complains of a sharp pain over the hypothenar eminence after a vigorous swing of club or racquet. Discomfort may be more prominent on the dorsal aspect of the carpus towards the ulnar side. Pain persists on vigorous use and restricts function. Mild ulnar nerve sensory symptoms may be apparent. Pressure on the hook of the hamate may be painful. Routine radiographs are unremarkable. Serial X-rays in 10° increments from the true lateral will skyline the hook of the hamate and reveal the fracture non-union (Fig. 7.14).

The carpal tunnel view will reveal fractures near the hamate tip, but does not give a satisfactory view of the junction between the hook and the body of the hamate. Excision of the hook of the hamate relieves discomfort and permits return to full activity.

## FRACTURES OF THE RADIAL RIM

### Dorsal (Fig. 7.15)

This fracture may be associated with radiocarpal dislocation. Reduction is usually achieved without difficulty. There is a tendency for recurrent dorsal subluxation of the carpus in the healing phase. If the dorsal bone fragments are sufficiently large, internal fixation with screws and Kirschner wires will achieve radiocarpal stability. Early mobilisation of the wrist is then appropriate with the best chance of full mobility.

### Volar (Fig. 7.16)

Barton in 1838 described both dorsal and volar rim fractures of the radius, but his name is now associated with the latter. There is a disruption of the radial articular surface. Treated conservatively, there is a tendency for increasing articular incongruity with volar subluxation of the carpus. A volar buttress plate (Fig. 7.17) maintains reduction of the articular fracture, blocks volar subluxation of the carpus and permits early mobilisation of the wrist. This form of treatment is also indicated for an oblique Smith's fracture. If treated conservatively the entire wrist joint may slip volarly.

# 8. Nerve injury and repair

*Principal author:   P. J. Smith*

The cellular anatomy of the peripheral nervous system renders it vulnerable to injury. The centrally located cell bodies maintain the viability of an enormous peripheral axon process whose length may exceed a metre in comparison to a cell body measured in microns. The axon terminates distally at a sensory mechanoreceptor or motor end-plate and the function of these structures depends upon the anatomical integrity of the axon. Injury at any point along the length of the axon process produces biochemical and ultrastructural changes within the nerve cell body and these are more pronounced if proximal. If severe, nerve cell death may result. In proximal injuries if the nerve cell body survives, it attempts to regenerate a new peripheral axon process. This is an enormous task in metabolic terms and proceeds slowly. However, the resulting loss of axonal tissue may exceed the neurone's capacity for repair.

Nerve cells do not exist in isolation but are grouped together in bundles lying in a connective tissue stroma to form peripheral nerves. Proliferation of the connective tissue elements occurs at the site of nerve injury as in other tissues. However, in nerves regeneration is essential if there is to be a satisfactory functional outcome. A conflict may therefore exist between the regenerative and reparative processes. Regeneration is often required over a considerable distance and there is a time lapse between its commencement and eventual recovery of function. If no clinical signs of recovery are apparent, the surgeon must consider intervention before the peripheral mechanoreceptor and effector sites become irreversibly altered. However, the information derived from clinical examination becomes apparent too slowly to indicate those cases which require re-exploration to achieve the best results.

## Assessment of clinical recovery

In judging the progress of nerve regeneration, reliance is placed upon the advancing Tinel sign. This is difficult to detect until approximately 2 or 3 months after injury, due to the rate of axonal regeneration occurring at the repair site. The technique of eliciting this sign is discussed in Chapter 20. Shortly after the advancing Tinel sign reaches the fingertips it disappears. Tingling develops spontaneously, or in response to gentle stroking. Protective sensation is established when the patient withdraws from painful or hot stimuli. Discriminating sensation may then re-establish itself in which the patient is capable of differentiating between textures. Once this has been established, assessment of the postinjury peripheral innervation density may be made by a multitude of tests. Many are time consuming, difficult to perform with precision and require the complete co-operation of an intelligent patient. The results are difficult to interpret. No satisfactory method of objective sensory evaluation as yet exists and there is little scientific evidence available upon which decisions can be based. Anomalous innervation may suggest motor recovery where none has actually occurred. Lack of objectivity in the documentation of results renders their assessment and comparison between techniques difficult.

## ANATOMY AND PHYSIOLOGY

At present, there is no universally accepted surgical nomenclature for the various constituents of a peripheral nerve, although a long-accepted anatomical terminology has been based on microscopic findings. The use of the electron microscope has clarified the anatomical situation.

The fundamental unit of any peripheral nerve is the axon process (Fig. 8.1). Sensory axons conduct impulses from peripheral receptors towards nerve cell bodies which lie in the dorsal root ganglia. Motor axons conduct impulses from the anterior horn cells to motor end-plates distally. Conduction in axons may occur in both directions but transmission between neurones across synapses is normally in one direction only. The maintenance of axonal function depends upon a constant flow of axoplasm ('axon transport') produced by the nerve cell body. Axoplasm flow is a bidirectional activity bringing nutrients to the distal

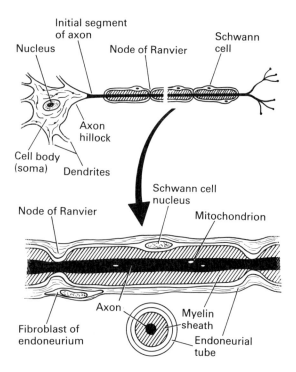

**Fig. 8.1** The fundamental unit of any peripheral nerve is the axon process which runs from the nerve cell body to peripheral neuromuscular receptor sites or from peripheral mechanoreceptors to a centrally placed nerve cell body

nerve as well as returning metabolites. The axon is surrounded by a single layer of Schwann cells. The cytoplasm of the Schwann cell wall (a trilaminar unit membrane) comprises a multilayered lipoprotein sandwich and is referred to as myelin. This acts as an insulating body. At points of contact between adjacent Schwann cells, there are gaps which allow contact between the bare axonal process and the surrounding extracellular fluid. Depolarisation can only occur at these uninsulated areas and thus nerve conduction involves electrical jumps from one uninsulated area to the next. This form of conduction is called saltatory conduction and the bare areas are known as the 'nodes of Ranvier'. It is the most rapid method of conduction and is only possible in lamellated or myelinated fibres.

One or more axons may lie within an endoneurial tube. This is a connective tissue tubule, the walls of which are formed by networks of delicate collagen fibrils and homogeneous ground substance. The endoneurial tubule and its contents comprise a nerve fibre. Such nerve fibres pursue a sinuous course within the nerve. Mild stretching of the nerve merely straightens these fibres. Fibre branching also occurs. Groups of fibres are collected together and surrounded by a dense and strong sheath of connective tissue — the perineurium. This unit is a nerve *fascicle* and each fascicle contains a variable number of fibres and thus they are of differing diameters. Groups of fascicles are collected within a sheath of loose connective tissue called the inner epineurium and the outer surface of the nerve is surrounded by a slightly denser collection of the same material, the outer epineurium (Fig. 8.2).

The fibres within a mixed peripheral nerve can be classified into three groups on the basis of diameter and conduction rate. The largest (1 $\mu$m to 20 $\mu$m in diameter) and the most rapidly conducting are the A fibres. These are myelinated and are subdivided into four groups, one of which, the A beta fibre, is responsible for transmitting moving light touch sensibility. The fibres of group B are found in the autonomic nervous system. C fibres are small diameter fibres which are slowly conducting and transmit impulses concerned with the appreciation of pain. Such sensibility is also transmitted by the A delta fibres (see Table 8.1).

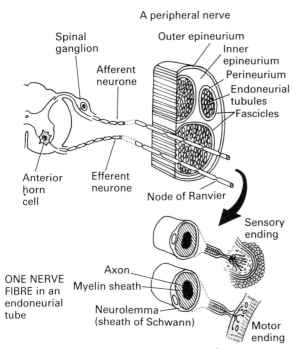

**Fig. 8.2** The peripheral nerve unit. Nerve fibres are grouped together to form fascicles. These may be well defined at certain sites in peripheral nerves

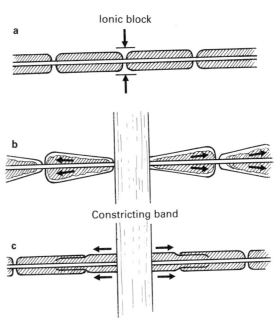

**Fig. 8.3** Neuropraxia. **a** The effect of a local physiological block, such as a pharmacological agent. **b** Mechanical compression producing bulging of the myelin and back flow. **c** Myelin intussusception

**Table 8.1** Nerve fibres

| Group A | 15/100 ms | Large Myelinated |
| Group B | 3/14 ms | |
| Group C | 0.5/2 ms | Small Unmyelinated |

| Number | Origin | Letter equivalent |
| --- | --- | --- |
| I a | Muscle spindle, annulospiral ending | A α |
| b | Golgi tendon organ | A α |
| II | Muscle spindle, flower-spray ending; touch, pressure | A β and γ |
| III | Pain and temperature receptors | A δ |
| IV | Pain and other receptors | d.r. C |

## TYPES OF INJURY

Nerve injuries have been classified into various grades and these are discussed below. However the surgeon must decide — will the lesion recover spontaneously or does the structural damage to the nerve require repair?

*Neuropraxia* (first degree injury) may be caused by pressure and produces a localised physiological block. There may be ultrastructural alterations detectable only by electron microscopy such as myelin intussusception (Fig. 8.3). These blockages can be transient and rapid spontaneous recovery may be expected with return of full function.

*Axonotmesis* (second degree injury) leads to peripheral axon death. A series of changes occurs which are histologically described as Wallerian degeneration. The endoneurial tubules however remain intact and regenerating axons will inevitably pass down their appropriate tubules, if regeneration occurs. Lesions such as these should be capable of a good recovery in the long term.

*Neurotmesis* (third, fourth and fifth degree injuries) is associated with disruption of the gross internal architecture of the nerve. In third degree injuries, the endoneurial tubules are disrupted but fascicular continuity remains. Fascicular disruption may occur (fourth degree injury) or there may be total neural disruption resulting in a complete division (fifth degree injury). There is little therapeutic relevance in differentiating between third, fourth and fifth degree injuries. These degrees of neurotmesis indicate the state of a nerve that has been either completely divided or subjected to such serious internal disorganisation that spontaneous regeneration is impossible. Neurotmesis may be caused by laceration, traction injury, injection of noxious drugs or ischaemia. From the clinician's point of view, it is important to realise that neurotmesis and axonotmesis are clinically indistinguishable in the early phases, but electrical testing may help to ascertain which of these lesions will recover spontaneously, as early surgical intervention is indicated for the remainder.

The neurone's response is governed by the severity and level of the injury. Provided the cell does not die, hypertrophy of the nerve cell body occurs during the first week in preparation for axon regeneration. The intracellular RNA fragments within 24 hours of injury (chromatolysis) (Fig. 8.4).

At the site of injury, the divided nerve stumps swell as axoplasmic flow continues for a short while. Proximal to the site of injury, the axon degenerates to a varying extent. Schwann cell proliferation commences in 48–72 hours and axon sprouting has begun by the fourth day. Fibroblastic proliferation is the most prominent feature at this stage arising from the connective tissue components of the nerve. Minimal tension at the repair interface may encourage the moulding and linear orientation of collagen, but excessive tension will prejudice regeneration. Three weeks

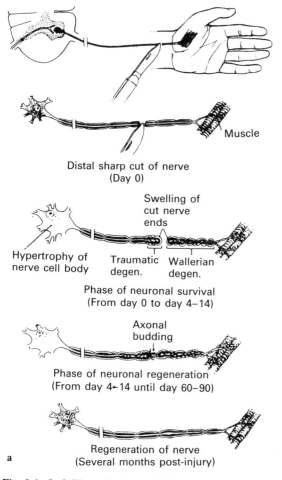

Muscle

Distal sharp cut of nerve
(Day 0)

Swelling of
cut nerve
ends

Hypertrophy of    Traumatic    Wallerian
nerve cell body    degen.    degen.

Phase of neuronal survival
(From day 0 to day 4–14)

Axonal
budding

Phase of neuronal regeneration
(From day 4–14 until day 60–90)

Regeneration of nerve
(Several months post-injury)

a

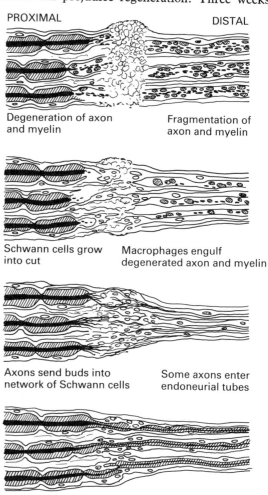

PROXIMAL                    DISTAL

Degeneration of axon          Fragmentation of
and myelin                    axon and myelin

Schwann cells grow        Macrophages engulf
into cut                  degenerated axon and myelin

Axons send buds into      Some axons enter
network of Schwann cells  endoneurial tubes

b

Axons continue to push along endoneurial tubes of distal stump, are enfolded by Schwann cells and form new myelin

**Fig. 8.4 Left** Illustration from Grabb and Smith, showing the effect of injury on the nerve cell body. **Right** The progressive changes that occur at the site of injury in a peripheral nerve

after injury, axon regeneration predominates, but these regenerating axons may be trapped in the proliferating fibroblastic tissue at the nerve interface, thus forming a neuroma.

In the distal stump, oedema immediately follows injury. The whole of the distal axon undergoes Wallerian degeneration. It fragments within 2–3 days of injury and by the second week no histological trace of the axon is left. This may be due to the accumulation of metabolites causing a breakdown of lysosomes. Myelin sheath disruption occurs and the Schwann cells phagocytose the fragmented myelin. Schwann cell proliferation produces cords of cells filling the collapsing endoneurial tubules. At the distal nerve stump, the Schwann cells and fibroblasts proliferate, producing a swelling which contains a mass of scar tissue containing no neural elements. By convention it is termed a glioma. The endoneurial tubules display their elastic properties by instant recoil after nerve division. Prolonged delay, prior to repair, undoubtedly contributes to chronic shortening and narrowing of the endoneurial tubules leading to a reduction in fascicular size. The degree of re-extension possible at a later date is unknown.

Changes following nerve division occur in the peripheral effector sites at the neuromuscular junctions, in the muscle itself, and at the sensory mechanoreceptor sites. The distal endoneurial tubules and motor end-plates are relatively normal for the first 3 months following injury. As time passes, the motor end-plates become increasingly distorted due to connective tissue proliferation. There is progressive shrinkage of muscle fibres, but these are capable of reinnervation for up to 3 years after denervation. During this time muscle atrophy is associated with proliferation of connective tissue within the muscle. As time passes, the degree of expected functional recovery diminishes. After 3 years muscle fibre disorganisation is established to such a degree that rennervation at this stage is unlikely to be followed by any functional recovery.

Within 3 days of injury changes may be noted in Meissner corpuscles, and within 2 weeks of injury nerve terminals can no longer be demonstrated within these corpuscles. Progressive shrinkage of the sensory corpuscles occurs and the regenerating axon may have increasing difficulty in penetration. Sensory recovery is dependent upon reinnervation of pre-existing corpuscles rather than on the development of new ones.

There are four phases of regeneration:

1. The phase of delay. During this period protein synthesis is occurring in the cell bodies. The duration of this quiescent stage depends on the severity of the injury and the distance from the nerve cell body. During the phase of delay, there are no detectable changes in the patient's clinical condition.

2. Axon penetration of the nerve interface (the contact surface between the repaired nerve ends). Axon sprouting occurs from the proximal nerve end and must penetrate the fibrous tissue present at the nerve interface. The sprouting commences just proximal to the area of retrograde myelin degeneration. Many sprouts are formed and the number of small axons attempting to cross the scar tissue at the interface greatly exceeds the number of axons present in the nerve proximally. The presence of scarring at the nerve interface or the presence of a large gap will diminish the likelihood of axons entering the distal endoneurial tubules. They are already collapsed but this is reversible at this stage. Nonetheless, the smaller fibres may be more successful in penetrating the endoneurial tubules. This may explain why there appears to be a recovery of pain and temperature sensation prior to the re-establishment of moving light touch. In the long term, many patients are left with protective sensation but no discriminating ability.

3. Distal axon regeneration. Once the nerve interface has been penetrated and the distal endoneurial tubules contain growing axons, their rate of advancement depends on the level of nerve injury. Proximally, the axons advance more rapidly but their progress is distally reduced. The rate of advancement may be altered by external factors such as the chemical milieu. It is known that steroids slow this rate and (T3) tri-iodotyrosine and Nerve Growth Factor may increase it. In general axon advancement occurs at an approximate rate of 1 mm per day distal to the repair site. It is during this phase of distal axon growth that the Tinel sign is most useful. There is normally

a latent period of 3–4 weeks before this is detectable. As the axons advance, myelination proceeds in a centrifugal manner. The regenerating axons reconnect with their end-organs and the axon diameter subsequently enlarges. However, even when satisfactory reinnervation occurs in this manner, absolute measurements of nerve conduction velocity show that there is a permanent reduction to perhaps 20–60% of normal.

4. The phase of functional recovery. Function returns to a variable extent after end-organ re-innervation. Sensory re-education may improve the patient's ability to interpret sensations through fewer innervated receptors.

It can be seen that nerve regeneration is a complex process. The ultimate functional recovery is governed by numerous factors.

1. The number of surviving neurones capable of producing axonal regeneration.

2. Problems at the nerve interface. The gap may be too large as a result of inadequate surgical apposition. There may be an abundance of scar tissue preventing axon penetration. Inaccurate approximation of the nerve may misdirect axon sprouts. Collapse of the distal endoneurial tubules may be such as to prevent the entry of regenerating axons. Loss of nerve substance may result in dissimilar fascicular patterns at the nerve interface enhancing axon sprout loss. This is due to the interfascicular plexus arrangement which occurs throughout the length of the nerve.

3. End-organ disruption may mean that function will not recover despite satisfactory reinnervation across the interface.

The surgeon can only influence certain aspects of the whole process. Accurate approximation of the nerve ends is necessary to achieve the best results. Gentle handling, the use of fine instruments and good haemostasis all contribute to creating the best environment for subsequent nerve regeneration. Early repair of divided nerves is desirable before it becomes difficult to approximate the nerve ends. This allows reinnervation to proceed before permanent endoneurial tubule collapse occurs and irreversible changes develop in the end-organs.

## CLINICAL DIAGNOSIS OF NERVE INJURY

Division of a mixed peripheral nerve is immediately followed by cessation of sweating within its cutaneous territory. The skin appears dry and tactile adherence diminishes. This is most easily displayed by the plastic pen test (see Ch. 20). Response to pin prick is a less reliable sign. If divided nerve ends are in good approximation, pin prick sensitivity and moving light touch may be temporarily preserved. As pin prick testing is both uncomfortable and unreliable it is best avoided. Tactile adherence is always absent in complete nerve division and this is immediately and easily detectable. With the passage of time, the area of reduced sensitivity diminishes due to overlap from adjacent territories. Atrophy of the subcutaneous fatty tissue in the affected area leads to spindle-shaped dry fingers.

Division of motor fibres leads to immediate paralysis. Careful clinical testing will reveal lack of function. However, at the time of initial injury, pain may prevent full patient co-operation. Nevertheless it is important to ascertain and document the opposition and abduction function of the thenar muscles after median nerve division, using the tests described in Chapter 20. Without establishing such a baseline, the surgeon may overlook the presence of dual or anomalous innervation and attribute later recovery of function to intrinsic reinnervation, when in fact, none has occurred.

## NERVE REPAIR

Fine instrumentation and delicate surgical technique make accurate approximation of nerve ends possible. The operating microscope allows the surgeon to visualise and thus control his own refined movements; its role in peripheral nerve repair is established. However, the choice of repair technique remains debatable.

A choice between epineurial and interfascicular repair is rarely necessary; both are indicated in different circumstances and at different levels within the nerve. The principle involved is the accurate approximation of neural tissues. As the structure of the nerve varies — from the plexiform fascicular pattern associated with areas of mobility to the more uniform cables seen in less mobile areas — the technique required for repair will also vary. The achievement of accurate fascicular apposition is governed by both the site of injury and the timing of repair.

## The timing and technique of nerve repair

If the mechanism of injury is a sharp laceration, nerve shortening to remove devitalised tissue is not required and repair can be undertaken without undue flexion of adjacent joints. Primary repair allows regenerating axons to cross only one suture line (as opposed to grafting).

When nerve repair is attempted early, the nerve ends have not undergone any secondary changes. There is, however, an inevitable retraction of the divided nerve ends due to the internal elastic properties of the fibres within the nerve. The epineurium appears to retract and the fascicles bulge from the divided nerve ends like toothpaste from a tube. The epineurium is soft and flimsy

and it is difficult to pick it up and approximate the two nerve ends. Pearse forceps are ideal for handling the epineurium. Usually it is not possible to re-approximate the divided ends of, for example, a median nerve at the wrist using two 10/0 nylon sutures alone when the wrist is in a neutral position. The nerve ends should be approximated temporarily using larger sutures (8/0 nylon which absorbs the tension until the repair has been completed with 10/0 sutures). The tension sutures are then removed. Tension at the repair site is reduced by flexing the wrist. If an epineurial repair is undertaken, careful approximation of the epineurium around the circumference of the nerve is required. Some trimming of the fascicles may be necessary to avoid fascicular pouting through the epineurial repair (Fig. 8.5a). Where the nerve structure is such that fascicles are arranged in clear groups with a significant amount of intervening connective tissue, fascicular repair may be undertaken. In such cases, the epineurium is generally shortened and two or three sutures are

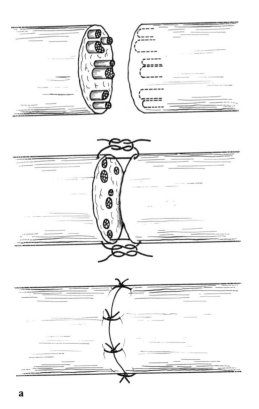

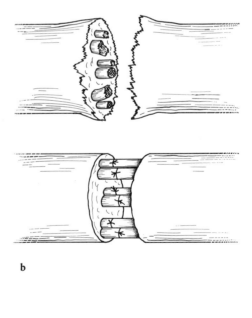

Fig. 8.5  a Primary or secondary epineurial repair.
b Primary interfascicular repair

a

carefully placed to approximate respective fascicular groups (Fig. 8.5b). A combination of the two techniques can be used involving sutures which penetrate the epineurium, pick up underlying fascicular bundles, and approximate them to their fellows. It is thought that excessive epineurial stripping may promote a marked connective tissue response, resulting in excessive scar tissue formation.

Delay presents the surgeon with tissues which have been altered by the response to injury. The nerve ends are adherent to surrounding structures. It may be difficult to define the nerve end from the surrounding fibrous tissue. Proximally, the nerve end is swollen forming a neuroma consisting of dense fibrous tissue and enmeshed and intertwined nerve fascicles. The epineurium surrounding the nerve is grossly thickened. Distally, the swollen nerve stump consists of fibrous tissue alone (glioma). Once freed, the thickened nerve ends are more rigid and easier to handle than their counterparts in the acute situation. Serial transverse section of the nerve stumps is necessary until healthy fascicles are visualised. This may produce nerve shortening and possible fascicular mismatching. Approximation of shortened nerve ends may require an excessive amount of joint flexion. The protection of the nerve repair may require prolonged immobilisation in such a posture, producing a conflict between joint func-

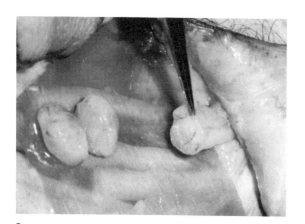

a

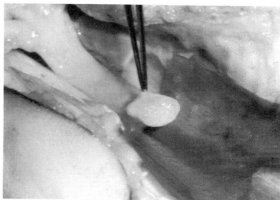

b

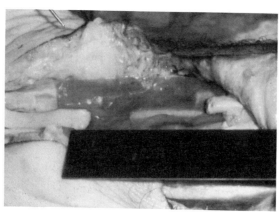

c

**Fig. 8.6** **a** A patient referred for grafting of his median nerve. Resection of the contact point between the two nerve ends showing the proximal nerve stump with fascicular pouting. **b** The distal nerve stump. **c** Measurement of the distance between the two nerve stumps. Approximately 15% extra length is inserted when taking the nerve graft

tion and nerve repair. It is inadvisable to flex a joint more than 30° to achieve approximation of nerve ends. In such circumstances, it is preferable to bridge the gap using a nerve graft. Nerve grafting may even prove necessary in cases of attempted primary repair.

In secondary repairs, it may prove possible to approximate the nerve ends. An epineurial repair can be undertaken or an interfascicular repair as previously described. Although the insertion of the sutures is easier in a secondary repair, nerve shortening may necessitate a graft.

*Nerve grafts* may be taken from various donor sites. The diameter and length of the graft required and the subsequent donor site morbidity

will determine the correct choice of donor nerve. Sural nerves have little donor site morbidity, can be vascularised if required (Figs. 8.6, 8.7) and are appropriate cable grafts in plexus or large nerve repairs (e.g. median at the wrist). The medial cutaneous nerve of the forearm provides a smaller nerve more suitable for digital nerve grafting. However, the resultant area of anaesthesia on the medial side of the arm is troublesome to many patients. The lateral cutaneous nerve of the forearm is often small and in several branches and occasionally represents the only termination of the superficial radial nerve. These nerves may be difficult to locate. A small nerve graft may be obtained from the lateral sural cutaneous nerve

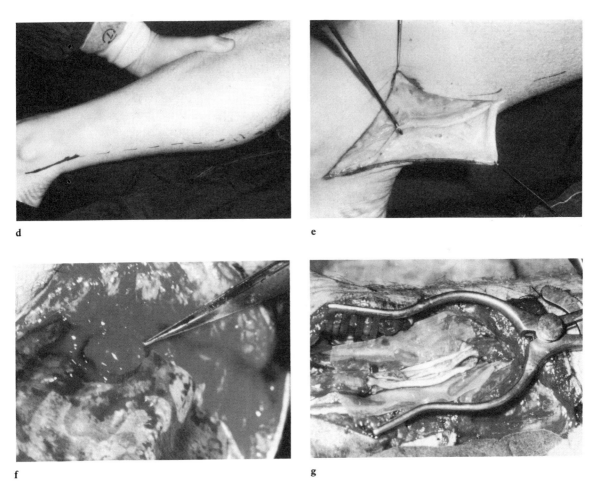

d                                    e

f                                    g

**Fig. 8.6  d** Site for sural nerve harvesting. **e** Location of the sural nerve graft and the short saphenous vein. **f** Release of the tourniquet prior to insertion of the grafts shows bleeding from the proximal nerve stump. Bleeding points must be controlled by bipolar coagulation or a haematoma may develop. **g** Insertion of the cable grafts, between the two nerve stumps

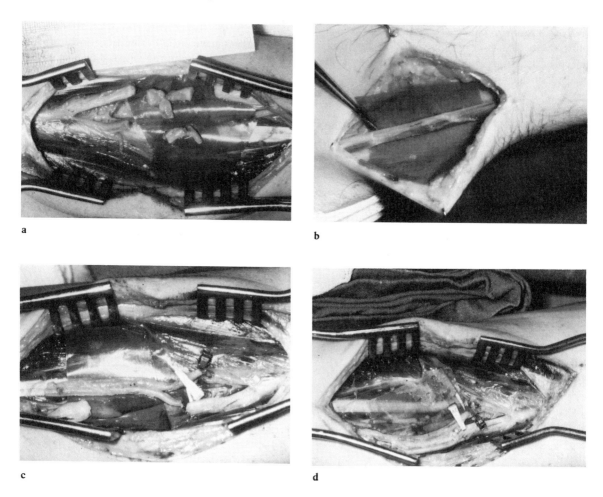

**Fig. 8.7** A case similar to that in Figure 8.6, with a poorly vascularised bed. **a** Resection of the damaged segment of nerve. **b** Sural nerve graft and short saphenous vein are taken together. **c** Insertion of a vascularised nerve graft. **d** Vascular repair has been undertaken and the tourniquet is about to be released

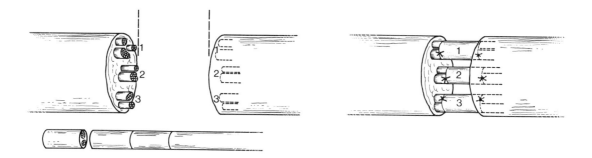

**Fig. 8.8**   Interfascicular nerve grafting

(cutaneous branch of the popliteal nerve) with less morbidity. It would seem logical to reverse nerve grafts in an attempt to prevent loss of regenerating axons through branches of the graft. They are inserted approximately 15% longer than the gap to allow for subsequent shortening. A well-vascularised bed is essential and small diameter grafts may give better results. Haemostasis must be obtained to prevent undue fibrosis. It has been suggested that when using cable grafts in a large nerve with many fascicles, the grafts are sutured to fascicular groups in a staggered fashion to ensure optimal apposition (Fig. 8.8).

The nerve repair must be protected until its tensile strength is adequate. Experimental studies suggest that this takes 4 weeks. However, if joint flexion has been required to achieve neural approximation, protection may be required for a longer interval. Metal markers may be used to allow subsequent assessment of the integrity of the nerve repair by radiography.

## CLINICAL SIGNS OF NERVE RECOVERY

Immediately following nerve repair some patients will describe the return of 'sensation'. This is a temporary phenomenon with reversion to the pre-operative state within the next few days. These comments are often dismissed, but evidence is accumulating that this is a real phenomenon.

Wallerian degeneration follows. The Schwann sheath cells act as phagocytes, removing the debris left by axonal disruption. There are no detectable clinical changes during this phase. Axonal regeneration follows with penetration of the nerve interface. Distal migration of these regenerating axons may be localised by the advancing Tinel sign which is the earliest detectable clinical evidence of nerve recovery. Due to the rate of distal axonal migration, the advancing Tinel sign is difficult to detect until approximately 2 or 3 months after injury. The technique of eliciting this sign is discussed in Chapter 20. When the axons reach the fingertips and reinnervate sensory end-organs, the Tinel sign disappears. The relative proportion of advancing axons to those caught up in the scar tissue or whose direction has been lost at the nerve repair site can be determined by comparing the advancing Tinel to the static Tinel at the scar site. Good progress is indicated by a prominent advancing Tinel and a diminished or absent static Tinel. The rate of advancement of the Tinel sign can be measured by noting its distance from the scar site at each outpatient visit.

An advancing margin of sensation may be detected following the advancing Tinel sign both temporally and geographically. Shortly after the Tinel sign reaches the fingertips it disappears. Tingling develops spontaneously in the fingertips or in response to gentle stroking. This represents a relinkage of the peripheral mechanoreceptors with the regenerating ABeta fibres. A form of moving light touch response then becomes established in the area — sensation being described as distant or as if feeling through a glove or through thickened skin. At the advancing margin of sensation there is a heightened response to pin prick (hyperpathia) followed by a diminished response. It should be noted that some form of moving light touch response does appear before the return of protective sensation (response to pain and temperature).

Temperature sensitivity begins to return. All denervated and reinnervating areas are cold sensitive from the time of injury. This diminishes very slowly but leaves the patient with some degree of permanent cold intolerance even if only minor. Hypersensitivity to cold objects and spontaneous pain in cold weather may occur. It is believed to be related to neural sensitivity and not to ischaemia. Warm sensitivity slowly returns — initially the response is greatly delayed and quantitatively diminished but later becomes immediate and virtually normal in quality. Protective sensation is re-established when the patient withdraws from painful or hot stimuli.

Discriminating sensation becomes established after the return of protective sensation to an area. This is an indication of the extent of recontact between the regenerating A beta fibres and the peripheral mechanoreceptors. Little is to be gained by testing for these capabilities until the regenerating A beta fibres have reached the fingertips and re-established contact with the peripheral mechanoreceptors. The Tinel must have advanced to the point of disappearance. Vibration sense testing using a tuning fork (C256) at the fingertip will detect re-establishment of A beta fibre contact. Dellon's technique using the vibrating tine (prong) on the fingertip is more sensitive than conventional use of the base. Once vibration sense has been re-established, specific tests of peripheral innervation density may be attempted. Static two-point discrimination has been the standard test for many years. Dellon has shown that moving two-point discrimination will return prior to static two-point discrimination as it is a more sensitive test. The ridging test may also be used (See Ch. 20). Many of these tests are time consuming, difficult to perform with precision, and the results are difficult to interpret. No satisfactory method of objective sensory evaluation as yet exists. An attempt to quantify sensory recovery has been made by the Medical Research Council (Table 8.2). The reappearance of sweating heralds the final phase of nerve recovery and little improvement in discriminating sensation can be expected once sweating has achieved normal levels in the automonous territory. Sweating is diminished only in those patients who have achieved a poor recovery in sensation following nerve repair.

Table 8.2   MRC classification of nerve recovery

Motor recovery

| | |
|---|---|
| M0 | No contraction. |
| M1 | Return of perceptible contraction in the proximal muscles. |
| M2 | Return of perceptible contraction in both proximal and distal muscles. |
| M3 | Return of function in both proximal and distal muscles of such degree that all *important* muscles are sufficiently powerful to act against resistance. |
| M4 | Return of function as in Stage 3 with the addition that all synergic and independent movements are possible. |
| M5 | Complete recovery. |

Sensory recovery

| | |
|---|---|
| S0 | Absence of sensibility in the autonomous area. |
| S1 | Recovery of deep cutaneous pain sensibility within the *autonomous area* of the nerve. |
| S2 | Return of some degree of superficial cutaneous pain and tactile sensibility within the autonomous area of the nerve. |
| S3 | Return of superficial cutaneous pain and tactile sensibility throughout the autonomous area with disappearance of any previous over-reaction. |
| S3+ | Return of sensibility as in Stage 3 with the addition that there is some recovery of two-point discrimination within the autonomous area. |
| S4 | Complete recovery. |

For those patients who achieve discriminating sensation, sweating slowly returns to pre-injury levels but this takes some considerable time.

On the motor side the earliest sign of regeneration is reactivation of the first muscle distal to the nerve repair site. The distance to this muscle is measured and an estimate can be made of the expected time-lapse to reinnervation. Should the muscle resume activity when expected, the prognosis is good.

However, delays may occur even in the presence of regenerating advancing axons due to anatomical variations in the level of motor branching. At first, muscle activity is detected by minimal contraction. Later antigravity activity is possible. At this stage postural deformities may spontaneously correct, especially in the young. The adduction of the thumb consequent upon thenar muscle denervation corrects with reinnervation of the abductor pollicis brevis. Alternatively the reactivation of muscle groups may produce postural deformities for the first time. In high ulnar nerve lesions, clawing is absent. After nerve repair, reinnervation of the profundi produces temporary clawing of the digits in the recovery phase.

The reinnervation of muscles intrinsic to the hand has in the past been overestimated in adults. Careful documentation of opposition and abduction is rarely performed pre-operatively. Without establishing this baseline many patients will be noted as having thenar muscle reinnervation when they have anomalous innervation. The opponens muscle may be dually innervated. Median nerve division may thus lead to immediate weakness of opposition which is interpreted as paralysis. Hypertrophy of the ulnar innervated muscle fibres will lead to a return of opposition within 6–8 weeks of injury. This may be mistakenly interpreted as thenar muscle reinnervation. Following denervation of *abductor pollicis brevis* abduction may rapidly return upon removal of the plaster due to 'trick' movements (Jones). The long flexor and extensors of the thumb acting in conjunction with abductor pollicis longus produce a see-saw movement of weak abduction. These movements are integrated by the brain so that abduction rapidly appears normal. However, if tested it is extremely weak. Abduction of the thumb is partly a positioning movement but, in addition, strong abduction is required to balance adduction, thus stabilizing the thumb and allowing flexor pollicis longus to contribute power to grip strength. In the absence of this stabilizing force, objects such as a tennis racquet cannot be gripped firmly — the thumb collapses into adduction and the power of flexor pollicis longus is lost. True reinnervation may occur after documented loss of abduction and opposition, particularly in children. It takes 4 months or more and muscle strength will return to powerful levels, although less than those before denervation. The time-scale is important in assessing which of these events is occurring. Trick movements will establish themselves within a few days of removal of the plaster (4–5 weeks post-injury). Hypertrophy of dual innervated muscles will take longer (6–8 weeks). Successful reinnervation takes longer still (4 months or more) but probably produces most power.

Similar problems are encountered in ulnar nerve injuries. The first dorsal interosseous is often innervated by the median nerve explaining why it may function well in the absence of any function in the remaining interossei. Trick movements may give the impression of active contraction of *abductor digiti minimi* producing finger abduction. This is due to contraction of flexor carpi ulnaris pulling on abductor digiti minimi through the pisiform. Extensor digiti minimi also contributes. If the wrist is held flat on the table while testing, this apparent active contraction will disappear.

Intrinsic reinnervation is thus frequently poorly documented in publications relating to nerve repair. Absolute evidence of reinnervation may be obtained only by EMG studies. It should be realised that minimal intrinsic tone is required to prevent clawing, thus detailed testing may reveal no intrinsic power yet sufficient resting tone may exist to overcome the claw deformity.

## PROGNOSIS FOLLOWING NERVE INJURY

The surgeon has no influence over many important prognostic factors such as the age of the patient, the mechanism and level of injury. The pre-existing state of the nerve and its surrounding bed is already determined should the patient be referred for secondary surgery. The surgeon's influence on the outcome following nerve injury can only be affected by the timing and the technique of the surgery he employs.

Primary repair appears to produce more satisfactory results than secondary repair and should preferably be undertaken in clean-cut injuries. However, in dirty and severely traumatised wounds, secondary or delayed primary repair should be performed. If secondary surgery is to be undertaken, then the results that can be expected are proportional to the interval between injury and repair. A prolonged delay may lead to irreversible motor end-plate and sensory receptor damage so that nerve repair may not produce satisfactory results. The shorter the interval between injury and repair, the better the prognosis. Good general wound care and careful surgical technique may avoid the occurrence of delayed wound healing, tissue necrosis and secondary infection, all of which are deleterious to the results of nerve repair.

One of the most important factors that the surgeon may influence is the avoidance of tension at the repair site. Direct approximation of the divided nerve ends produces better functional results than nerve grafting. However, the deleterious effects of undue tension must be balanced against those of a double nerve interface. Such judgements are difficult. If grafting is necessary, it is unwise to undertake it in a wound which is contaminated. If the graft fails, the patient must undergo a further surgical procedure to repair the injured nerve and a donor site has been needlessly sacrificed. When nerve grafting is indicated it should therefore be undertaken as the secondary procedure in the majority of circumstances. Prognosis may be influenced by the length of time that the repair is protected. The nerve repair should be protected for a period of 4 weeks but there is little evidence at present to suggest that more prolonged protection will lead to improved results.

In secondary referrals, the bed in which the nerve lies may be unsatisfactory. Fibrous tissue forms a poor bed and nerve grafts fail to function when embedded in such tissue. A well-vascularised soft tissue covering is required. Flap cover should be provided as the results of nerve grafting in well-vascularised beds are significantly better.

The considerable improvement in the results of

peripheral nerve repair in recent years has been due to advances in surgical technique. Magnification, and the use of fine instruments and suture materials have diminished the secondary surgical trauma inflicted during a repair. Although the surgeon cannot influence the major prognostic factors such as age of the patient, level and mechanism of injury, his contribution in terms of refined surgical technique should not be underestimated as it may have a significant influence on the prognosis.

## FAILED NERVE REPAIRS

In assessing the results of nerve repairs in a patient who is referred soon after primary management, the hand surgeon must consider the likely quality of the original repair. If an unsatisfactory repair has been performed in a primary care situation the hand surgeon should await wound healing and undertake re-exploration as early as possible, refashioning the repair to ensure the best possible outcome. Alternatively, the surgeon may feel that the quality of the initial repair, performed elsewhere, was satisfactory. After such a repair, the rate of recovery as monitored by the advancing Tinel sign may be slow leading eventually to a poor and inadequate functional outcome.

Patients who present later may have neuroma, pain syndromes or dysaesthesia. Poor return of function after repair may be associated with a weak or absent advancing Tinel sign indicating a problem at the nerve repair site. However, there may be a marked Tinel sign at the repair site associated with a palpable neuroma. Such a situation is an indication for re-exploration with resection of the neuroma and direct repair of the nerve ends if possible. This is a difficult clinical decision as the benefits of surgery are not always predictable. Grafting will be necessary if the resulting gap is too large. It should be realised, however, that due to variations in branching the time taken for reinnervation may vary by as much as 3 to 5 months from the expected interval. Therefore it is usual to wait for some 8 months following median, ulnar or radial nerve repair in the forearm before deciding on the adequacy of functional return and for 5 months for median and ulnar

nerves at the wrist. After this period of time, if function is inadequate, re-exploration may be considered. Poor ultimate function may be associated with a satisfactory distal migration of the Tinel sign if the sensory receptors and motor end-plates and muscles have undergone irreversible changes.

Many factors must be taken into consideration when nerve repair has resulted in an inadequate functional outcome. The patient's attitude to his deficiencies may be such that he is capable of coping with his everyday activities and work and does not wish to undergo surgical treatment. Age and personality will influence the outcome. A patient who has achieved an M3, S3 quality of repair following nerve injury at the wrist has a less than 50% chance of improving this by secondary surgery. If the nerve is found to have dehisced at the repair site or a neuroma is present, resection of the neuroma and the scar tissue around the distal nerve stump is essential. The nerve ends are resected until apparently healthy fascicles are visible. Although these may look healthy to the unaided eye, microscopic examination may reveal that as much as 30% of the axon content of the nerve is missing. It is thus a useful exercise to resect a small portion of the proximal nerve end and submit it for subsequent histology as the presence of a high percentage of empty endoneurial tubules will indicate a poor potential prognosis. Rarely it is possible to directly approximate the two healthy nerve ends without the need for undue flexion of adjacent joints. The presence of a fusiform neuroma-incontinuity associated with a poor functional recovery requires exploration of the neuroma. The nerve fascicles must be teased from the neuroma under magnification. Electrical fascicular recordings may be useful if available but resection of such neuromas should not be undertaken unless the surgeon is certain that the existing functional result is unsatisfactory for the patient and there is no prospect of spontaneous improvement.

If the return of function is inadequate and further nerve surgery is unlikely to yield improved results, consideration may be given to the use of neurovascular island flaps to restore sensation to important areas and tendon transfers to redistribute the remaining functional parts (see Ch.

10). Neurovascular island flaps are rarely used nowadays for nerve injuries, as protective sensation is usually re-established following nerve repair. If nerve injury is associated with soft tissue loss, free innervated pulp transfers may be undertaken. These comprise a toe-pulp and its feeding vessels and nerves which are transferred by microvascular anastomosis. The use of such techniques avoids the scarred donor area which occurs in a neurovascular island flap.

*Pain syndromes* may develop, producing an unsatisfactory result after nerve repair. These are most commonly due to a neuroma or a reflex sympathetic dystrophy. Painful neuromas are uncommon if the proximal nerve stump is in a quiet area cushioned by subcutaneous tissues. All nerves produce a neuroma upon division but only a few are painful. Troublesome neuromas are most commonly found in distal sensory nerves (for example the radial) and the treatment of these problems proves difficult. It is best to avoid the situation by leaving divided nerve ends in a quiet well-padded area where they are unlikely to be tethered to surrounding structures.

In the patient who presents with an established troublesome neuroma, it may be useful initially to try conservative measures such as a desensitisation programme. This involves repeated massage of gradually increasing intensity and tapping over the involved area. Transcutaneous nerve stimulation may prove effective if commenced at an early stage. Patients who fail to respond to such conservative measures require simple resection of the nerve end and its placement in a quiet area. Although many patients will respond to this form of treatment, a troublesome minority will continue to have symptoms and for such patients, a variety of surgical manoeuvres has been developed. Proximal crushing and ligation of the nerve trunk, epineurial stump closure upon resection, coagulation of the proximal nerve end, and steroid injections into the nerve end have all been attempted. The nerve may be capped with silicone or buried into bone in an attempt to inhibit axon sprout regeneration. The nerve may be split and the two halves sutured together. The wide variety of manoeuvres that is available to treat this problem serves only to confirm the fact that none of them is dramatically effective. Occasionally, a patient will return complaining of discomfort over the brachial plexus at the site where a nerve block has been used. The patient will recall that attempts at producing the nerve block were difficult or perhaps even unsuccessful. There is an area of tenderness associated with a Tinel's sign and burning discomfort. Shooting pains and paraesthesia may occur in the arm in the majority of patients; these symptoms of *plexus neuritis* will usually settle over several months. During this period, the neuritis may be a source of great discomfort to the patient and occasionally may produce a full sympathetic dystrophy. This syndrome is thought to be related to either direct nerve damage at the time of injection or as a result of perineurial haematoma.

## REFLEX SYMPATHETIC DYSTROPHY

This syndrome may follow hand trauma and is often seen after nerve injuries. Patients are affected by a burning pain which is aggravated by physical and emotional stimuli. Disproportionate pain after injury or poor progress in regaining motion should always raise the question of a possible sympathetic dystrophy. Early diagnosis is of importance, for early treatment is more likely to lead to a rapid resolution of symptoms. The patient complains of pain in the limb and will protect it, resisting any attempts at contact. On examination, the hand is swollen, flushed and sweaty. At a later stage, the limb becomes less painful and the skin dries, becoming vasoconstricted and possibly cyanotic. Pain, oedema and disuse lead to stiffness and osteoporosis. It is thought that the majority of such cases develop within the first 24 hours of surgery or injury and most of the remainder develop within the next few days. Diagnosis is often delayed with the clinician attributing the patient's symptoms to psychological overlay or to a low pain threshold. Sympathetic blockade is the most effective form of treatment supplemented by intensive physiotherapy to mobilise and encourage use of the hand. Physiotherapy is most effective when applied immediately following sympathetic blockade. Guanethidine blocks are preferred to stellate ganglion blockade because they are more easily tolerated by the patient and are equally effective. Early diagnosis and swift treatment offer the best prospect of satisfactory resolution (See Ch. 2).

## SUMMARY

The results of nerve repair have improved over the last 50 years, but complete motor and sensory recovery are, at present, an unrealised dream. Technical advances (refined instrumentation, microsutures and the operating microscope) have contributed to these improvements. There has also been an appreciation of the importance of early repair. In the care of a competent hand surgeon, no less than an M3 S3+ result would now be expected and a lesser result would prove disappointing. A plateau in the quality of results has become apparent and this is unlikely to improve through further technical advances. A biological frontier has been reached in which the manipulation of the processes occurring at the nerve interface may contribute more to improved results than any other factor.

# 9. Brachial plexus injuries

*Principal author:*  *F. D. Burke*

TRACTION INJURIES OF THE BRACHIAL PLEXUS

The most common injury to the brachial plexus (Fig. 9.1) is the adult traction injury. Ninety per cent are sustained in road traffic accidents, 80% of these involving motorcyclists. The majority fall into the 16–23-year-old age-group and are predominantly male manual workers. The inci-

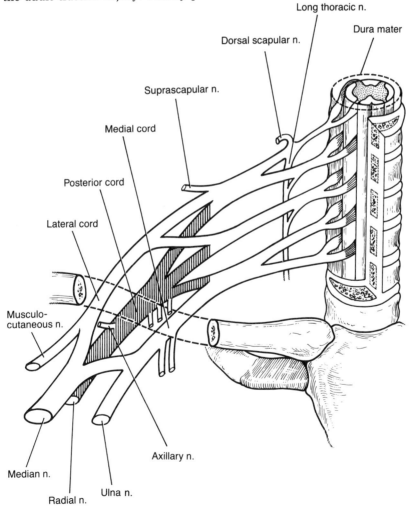

**Fig. 9.1**  The brachial plexus

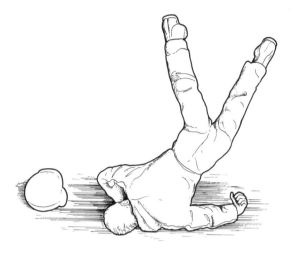

Fig. 9.2 The mechanism of injury

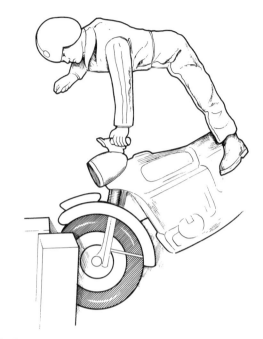

Fig. 9.3 An alternative mechanism of injury

dence of the condition is probably rising as motorcycle sales increase. The mechanism of injury to the brachial plexus is uncertain. The most commonly accepted view is that the patient is thrown from his motorcycle and, as he lands, his head is pushed towards one shoulder (Fig. 9.2). At the same time the opposite shoulder is depressed and the two movements result in traction being applied to the brachial plexus. Not all patients, however, present with bruising of the cheek or shoulder on the affected side. An alternative view is that the patient is thrown up from his bicycle and fails to let go of the handlebars. He sustains a direct traction injury to the plexus (Fig. 9.3).

There are three main varieties of injury to the plexus (Fig. 9.4), although mixtures of these types may occur with different injuries at different root levels:

A Root avulsion: the nerve roots have been ruptured from the spinal cord. No spontaneous improvement is to be anticipated and the injury is not amenable to surgical repair.
B Rupture of the brachial plexus distal to the intervertebral foramina. Spontaneous improvement is unlikely but the disruption is accessible to surgical repair.
C Traction injury to the brachial plexus which

is less severe and, although the nerve is damaged, the overall continuity of the structure is preserved. This produces a neuropraxia or benign axonotmesis and spontaneous improvement over weeks or months may be anticipated.

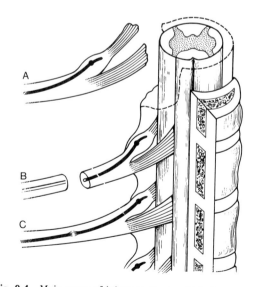

Fig. 9.4 Main types of injury to the brachial plexus

It is important that all patients presenting with brachial plexus injuries are assessed at an early stage. The management of each type is different and if nerve repair is felt to be required, the best results occur if surgery is performed within 6–12 weeks of the injury (according to Narakas). There is a tendency to await spontaneous improvement of brachial plexus injuries and this should be avoided. Early classification is of benefit in all three groups, allowing the appropriate treatment to be provided. To employ a 'wait and see' policy is to deprive the nerve repair group of the opportunity of early surgery. The root avulsion group can drift on for many months, unable to return to employment, awaiting a recovery that is unlikely to occur. A patient's interests are better served by early assessment, early advice as to the likely outcome and the appropriate rehabilitation programme. Job retraining may be necessary, and .all patients should be returned to playing as active a role in society as their ultimate disability will permit.

Months of inactivity and uncertainty at best delay, and probably reduce, the chances of the patient returning to his maximum potential. Brachial plexus injuries produce disability in three ways:

1. Sensibility is lost.
2. Muscles are weakened or paralysed.
3. Pain.

Approximately 10% of patients with plexus injuries have serious problems with pain in the first few months following injury, but half of these will settle within the first 2 years. The patients who have suffered a root avulsion tend to present with chronic pain. Many patients acknowledge that they can be distracted from their pain either by work or by any pastime which absorbs their attention. Prolonged periods of inactivity following a plexus injury increase, rather than diminish, the amount of pain experienced by a patient.

## The assessment of brachial plexus injuries

Assessment involves the drawing together of several tests and examinations to produce an overall picture. Few single investigations permit one to classify a patient into any one of the three groups with certainty. Patients frequently sustain plexus damage in association with multiple injuries. Long bone fractures in the upper limb will make early neurological assessment difficult. The patient may have head or chest injuries and the diagnosis of a plexus injury may be delayed for several days.

### History

If injury has occurred as a result of a road traffic accident it is worthwhile obtaining an assessment of the speed of impact at the time of the accident. If a head-on collision has occurred the aggregate speed of the vehicles is relevant. Low-velocity injury tends to be associated with neuropraxia or benign axonotmesis with a spontaneous recovery anticipated. High-velocity injuries are more likely to produce complete disruptions of the plexus. These disruptions may be distal, or at root level.

### Examination

Full neurological examination is required as soon as possible after the injury to form the baseline from which any subsequent improvement may be measured. All muscle groups related to the upper limb should be tested and it is convenient to use an Assessment Chart of the type popularised by Narakas (Fig. 9.5). Examination will give a general impression of the *root values of the paralysed muscles*. Particular attention should be paid to those muscles innervated by nerves which leave the plexus at a proximal level (the rhomboids, upper portion of pectoralis major and latissimus dorsi). If these muscles are functioning normally and yet other muscles of similar root value are paralysed, then it is likely that the damage to the plexus is sufficiently distal to be accessible to surgical repair. It is prudent to check the *reflexes in the lower limbs*. The presence of lower limb hyperreflexia suggests a root avulsion at cord level, causing upper motor neurone signs in the legs. *Horner's syndrome*, with ptosis, enophthalmos, anhidrosis and miosis, strongly suggests a root avulsion of the first thoracic nerve. Uncommonly, a Horner's syndrome may improve spontaneously several weeks after the accident. This is probably due to haematoma around the stellate ganglion, or

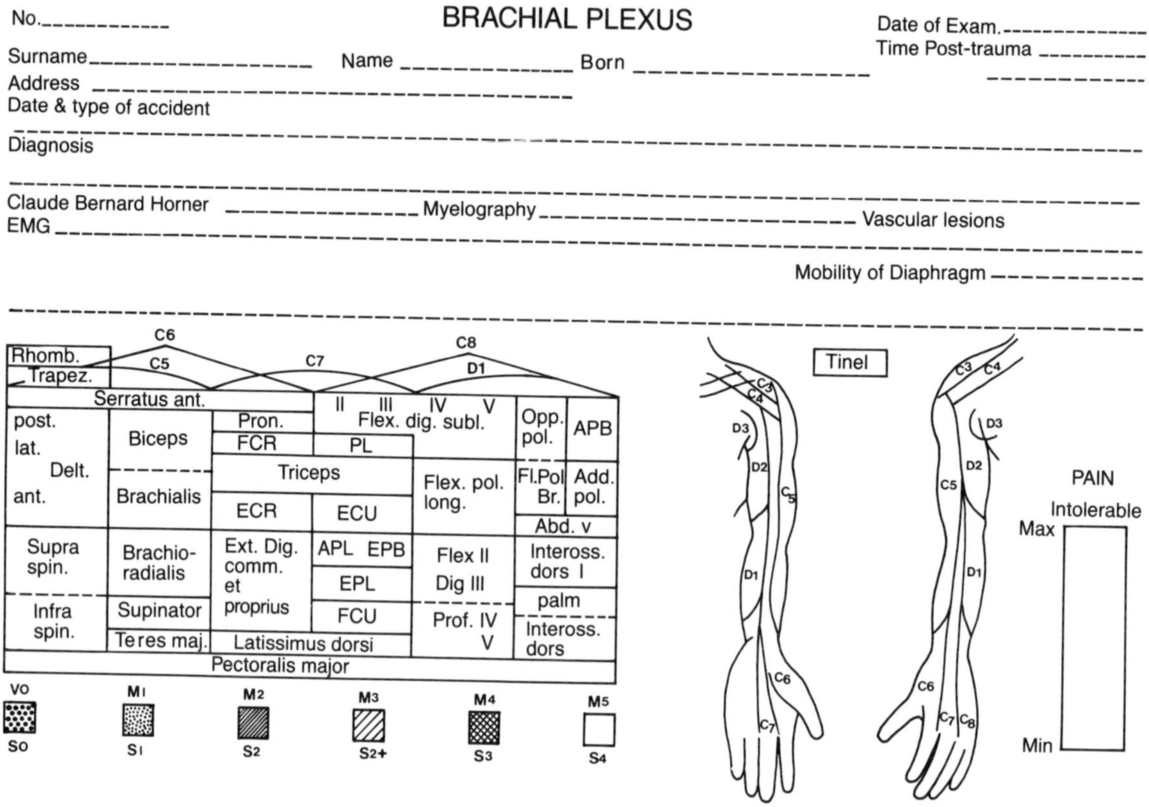

## BRACHIAL PLEXUS

No._____

Surname_____   Name _____ Born _____

Address _____

Date & type of accident

Diagnosis

Claude Bernard Horner _____ Myelography_____
EMG_____ Vascular lesions

Date of Exam._____
Time Post-trauma _____
_____

Mobility of Diaphragm _____

| | | | | | |
|---|---|---|---|---|---|
| Rhomb. Trapez. | | | | | |
| Serratus ant. | | | | | |
| post. lat. | Biceps | Pron. FCR | II III IV V Flex. dig. subl. PL | Opp. pol. | APB |
| Delt. ant. | Brachialis | Triceps ECR ECU | Flex. pol. long. | Fl.Pol Br. | Add. pol. Abd. v |
| Supra spin. | Brachio-radialis | Ext. Dig. comm. et proprius | APL EPB EPL FCU | Flex II Dig III Prof. IV V | Inteross. dors I palm Inteross. dors |
| Infra spin. | Supinator Teres maj. | Latissimus dorsi | | | |
| Pectoralis major | | | | | |

C6 C5 C7 C8 D1

VO  MI  M2  M3  M4  M5
SO  SI  S2  S2+  S3  S4

Tinel

PAIN

Intolerable
Max

Min

**Fig. 9.5** A brachial plexus assessment chart

to local bruising. *Tinel's sign* is a useful test in the assessment of brachial plexus injury, and may indicate the level of the nerve damage. It is important to percuss along the line of the nerve from distal to proximal. There are two features to elicit — the level at which tingling (and often discomfort) radiates down towards the hand and the strength of the 'signal'. Localisation on early assessment may well indicate the site of nerve injury and may be used to monitor spontaneous recovery or progress following nerve repair. A strong Tinel that fails to progress distally on serial examination suggests plexus rupture has occurred at that level. There is probably a loose correlation between the strength of the signal and the percentage of axons growing back down the nerve. Light percussion producing marked tingling distally suggests that many axons have crossed the nerve repair site. Neurological assessment should

be performed at weekly intervals in the first month and less frequently afterwards.

*Investigations*

There are several investigations designed to reveal whether the damage to the plexus is *preganglionic* or *postganglionic*. The principle underlying all these investigations is that root avulsions from the spinal cord leave the dorsal root ganglion in continuity with the distal portion of the nerve. The nuclei of the cells continue to nourish the sensory axons distally. Investigations, which reveal this apparent viability of the sensory nerve in the absence of sensibility, indicate a poor prognosis, as the damage to the nerve is so proximal that surgical repair is impractical. The *histamine triple response* is composed of a central capillary dilatation, a weal, and a surrounding flare. The flare depends on the presence of an intact nerve distal to the nucleus and if present in insensitive skin, suggests that damage has occurred proximal to the dorsal root ganglion. The value of this test is limited by the variability of the sensory dermatomes, but nevertheless the test may be of benefit.

**Nerve conduction studies may be performed.** The presence of sensory action potentials in nerves supplying insensate skin may indicate that damage has occurred proximal to the dorsal root ganglion. Degeneration of peripheral fibres following post-ganglionic rupture is a gradual process. Sensory action potentials may persist for 2–3 weeks following rupture and the test is unreliable in the earliest weeks following injury. Lesions at two levels of the brachial plexus (10% in Narakas' series in 1978) will appear on the above tests as distal plexus injuries, even though the more proximal of the lesions may be a root avulsion.

**Electromyography.** May be of value at two stages in brachial plexus injuries. In the early phase of assessment, electrodes may be inserted into the deep posterior cervical muscles. Normal activity indicates that the segmental nerve supplying that area has not been damaged and a root avulsion has not occurred. These segmental nerves are the most proximal branches of the plexus arising from the nerve roots as they pass through the intervertebral foramen. An electromyograph revealing denervation in these muscles suggests a root avulsion is present. Localisation to a specific nerve root may be difficult, but root avulsions of two or three levels will be more obvious. In the recovery phase, EMGs may be of value as a means of showing whether early re-innervation is occurring. EMG sampling of the more proximal paralysed muscles may be performed several weeks after injury, prior to exploration. The first signs of spontaneous recovery may be revealed. As with many investigations, the information obtained must be interpreted in association with other tests and serial clinical examinations.

Evoked responses may be recorded from the plexus and spinal cord following stimulation of a peripheral nerve. This technique is still being assessed, and it remains to be seen whether it will provide any information that is not available from careful clinical examination and routine electromyography.

**Radiology.** *The site of the adjacent fractures* may help to localise the nerve injury. Fractures of the transverse processes of the lower cervical vertebrae suggest that the lesion may be proximal. Clavicular and upper humeral fractures may indicate a more distal plexus lesion. *Screening of the diaphragm* will reveal whether phrenic nerve function has been affected. As the phrenic nerve is one of the most proximal branches arising from the upper portion of the plexus, the information may well be of use in deciding whether an exploration is indicated.

**Myelography.** Is a valuable test in plexus injury evaluation. Root avulsions distort the root sleeve visible in a normal *cervical myelogram*. Myeloceles suggest that root avulsion has occurred. The accuracy of the test is around 80%. However, deformity of the root sleeve does not always indicate that a root avulsion is present. On occasion a root avulsion may not significantly alter a myelogram. The test is usually performed 3–4 weeks after injury when oedema of the surrounding area has settled.

**Nuclear magnetic resonance.** Offers the prospect of better visualisation of nerve roots and may render the myelogram redundant.

## Management of brachial plexus injuries

### Group I: neuropraxia or benign axonotmesis

Spontaneous improvement is anticipated. This group will tend to be low-velocity injuries with patchy loss and signs of motor and sensory recovery in the more proximal muscles. An advancing Tinel's sign may be found. EMGs may confirm early reinnervation. The patient's progress needs to be closely monitored and physiotherapy provided to maintain a passive range of motion in involved joints. Dynamic or static splints may be required in the short term.

### Group II: distal plexus disruptions

No spontaneous improvement is anticipated. Nerve damage is accessible to surgical repair. These patients tend to have been involved in high-velocity accidents, and if the Tinel's sign is present it is static and does not move down the

**Table 9.1**  Brachial plexus injury: summary

| Assessment: | | | |
|---|---|---|---|
| | Low velocity<br>Advancing Tinel's sign<br>Patchy loss<br>Proximal recovery<br>EMG — early<br>reinnervation | — Neuropraxia<br>or benign<br>axonotmesis | — Physiotherapy<br>Temporary<br>joint bracing |
| | High velocity<br>Static Tinel's sign<br>No spontaneous<br>improvement<br>Proximal muscles spared<br>No myeloceles<br>Abnormal histamine triple<br>response<br>Normal EMG — deep<br>posterior cervical muscles | — Distal plexus<br>rupture | — Exploration<br>Cable grafting<br>Physiotherapy<br>Joint bracing<br>Sensory re-<br>education |
| | | | Pain clinic<br>(early)<br><br>Tendon transfer<br>(late) |
| | High velocity<br>Weak or no Tinel's sign<br>No spontaneous<br>improvement<br>Proximal muscles not<br>spared<br>Sensory loss extending into<br>neck<br>UMN signs in lower limbs<br>Phrenic dysfunction<br>Horner's syndrome<br>Histamine triple response<br>Abnormal EMGs —<br>Deep posterior cervical<br>muscles<br>Myeloceles | — Root avulsion | — Flail arm<br>splint<br>Job<br>retraining |

*Principle:* early assessment and active treatment

limb. They require *exploration and nerve repair* at an early stage and certainly *within 12 weeks* of the injury. Although direct nerve suture may on occasions be performed, *grafting* of the damaged segment is more usually required. The sural nerve is most frequently used for the graft. Exploration is performed above and below the clavicle to avoid the risk of missing a second lesion to the plexus. The damaged portions are identified and trimmed back to healthy nerve tissue. Sural nerve grafts are then sutured into the defect avoiding tension and using 8/0 or 10/0 nylon sutures. (Fig. 9.6). The operating microscope is used. The arm is restricted in a collar and cuff under clothes for approximately 4 weeks and then mobilised. Rein-

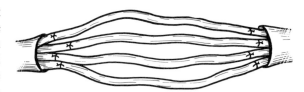

**Fig. 9.6**  Grafting to the plexus

nervation is slow. C5/6 grafts may take 18–36 months to recover shoulder and elbow function. Lower roots, with longer distances to cover, will take even longer. Physiotherapy is required to maintain the passive range of motion of the involved joints and a flail arm splint may help to preserve body image during the recovery phase.

Which plexus injuries benefit most from surgical repair? Children do better than adults, even if repair has been delayed beyond 12 weeks. Lesions to the upper portion of the brachial plexus (Erb's paralysis: C5/6) produce the most gratifying results. The patient presents with an inability to control the shoulder or flex the elbow. Sensibility is reduced in thumb and index finger, but function in the hand and wrist is otherwise excellent. The patient is, however, unable to place his hand in space and is greatly incapacitated. Recovery of shoulder control and biceps function returns the patient to virtually normal function. Lesions limited to the lower portion of the plexus (Klumpke's paralysis C8 and T1) are less common and the results of nerve grafting disappointing. The patient has poor control of wrist and hand, but normal function at shoulder and elbow. Reinnervation after repair is prolonged and intrinsic function is rarely enough to permit handwriting and fine manipulative skills.

**Mixed lesions**, partly at root level and partly more distally, may merit exploration. Grafts of those parts accessible to repair may benefit the patient, but the overall result is undermined by the presence of root avulsions.

**Total plexus lesions.** C5 to T1 without root avulsion. The role of nerve grafting here remains uncertain. Both sural nerves may be harvested and used to graft the upper roots. The ulnar nerve (and artery) may be taken from the involved arm and used as a (vascularised) graft to the median nerve. The aim of surgery is to achieve shoulder and elbow control with some recovery in function on the median side of the hand. It is too early to say whether the results of such surgery will prove to be of functional value to the patient.

**Assessment of results.** To an extent it is irrelevant whether a patient gets Power 2 or 3 back in a muscle group. Success is dependent on whether such return of power permits the patient to use the limb in a more effective manner. It is on the functional gain in the limb that success must be gauged. A good C8/T1 recovery still leaves the patient greatly handicapped. Power 4 return to the intrinsics enables the patient to write, but with great difficulty, and he remains unable to perform many fine manipulative skills.

*Group III: root avulsions*

No spontaneous recovery is anticipated and the damage is not amenable to surgical repair. These patients should be informed at an early stage that the prospects of recovery are poor and that plans should be made on the expectation of no or little improvement. The patient is offered a flail arm splint (Fig. 9.7). This is more likely to be used in the longer term if the patient is admitted to an occupational therapy workshop for fitting and intensive training. The patient's occupation must be assessed and, if necessary, retraining provided in an attempt to return him to as active a role in society as his injury permits. A positive approach, presenting realistic objectives to the patient, is preferred to prolonged inactivity and uncertainty.

*Alternative surgical options in brachial plexus injury*

These options are usually considered when the

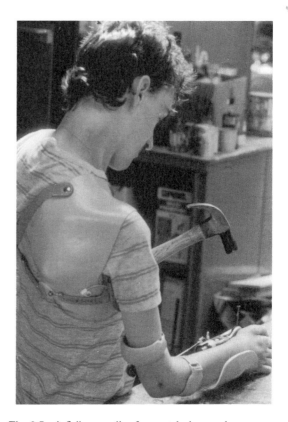

**Fig. 9.7** A flail arm splint for a total plexus palsy

neurological state in the upper limb has stabilised and no further improvement is anticipated.

*Arthrodesis of the shoulder.* This is of value when the glenohumeral musculature (supra- and infraspinatus and deltoid) remain paralysed and the majority of the scapula/thoracic group (pectorals, trapezius, serratus anterior, rhomboids) are functioning. Scapula/thoracic motion is approximately 30% of the normal shoulder range. Arthrodesis of the glenohumeral joint gives these patients excellent power and stability through this limited range.

*Tendon transfers to achieve elbow flexion.* This is a crucial area in upper root brachial plexus injuries:

*1. Clark's transfer.* A portion of pectoralis major is mobilised towards the clavicle, preserving the neurovascular supply. The muscle is swung into the upper arm and is joined to the biceps tendon. The shoulder should be of either normal power or stabilised by an arthrodesis, permitting the transferred muscle to act upon the elbow effectively.

*2. Steindler transfer.* This transfer involves moving the forearm flexor origin approximately 5 cm proximally on the humerus. There is a tendency to pronate the forearm during flexion.

*3. Triceps to biceps transfer.* The triceps is required for two main functions in the upper limb:

a. Stabilising the elbow when working above shoulder height.

b. Pushing up when rising out of a low chair. The transfer may be considered in upper root plexus lesions if there is no likelihood of improvement in shoulder mobility, but should not be used in the presence of good shoulder function. The procedure is also contraindicated if there are lower limb problems that require the patient to use walking aids or if there is difficulty rising from the sitting position.

*4. Latissimus dorsi transfer.* The muscle is mobilised on its neurovascular pedicle in the axilla, released at both ends and transferred into the upper arm. The proximal end is sutured to the clavicle, the distal end to the biceps tendon.

*Tendon transfers in the wrist and hand.* Tendon transfers will depend on available motors and the variety of motor loss. Arthrodesis of the wrist is rarely indicated. It is preferable to maintain a mobile wrist with the benefit of the tenodesis effect (wrist extension potentiating the power of the finger flexors and vice versa).

## OTHER PLEXUS LESIONS

Birth injuries to the brachial plexus are uncommon. They are caused by traction injuries during delivery and they may involve the upper roots, lower roots or total plexus, depending on the direction and force applied. The majority are not ruptures, but are benign axonotmeses and make an excellent spontaneous recovery. If plexus rupture has occurred, nerve grafts may produce gratifying results, even if the repair is performed several years after injury. Lacerations to the brachial plexus are usually accessible to nerve repair or graft. If early exploration is performed, a nerve graft may not be required.

Although primary tumours of the brachial plexus do occur (neurilemmoma, neurofibroma), the majority of tumours are secondary deposits or extensions of primary tumours of the lung (Pancoast's tumour). The commonest secondary tumour is from a carcinoma of the breast. Mastectomy may have been performed 2 or 3 years previously, with postoperative radiotherapy. The differential diagnosis between radiotherapy neuritis and recurrence of tumour is difficult to make. Biopsy of the plexus itself may be required to make a firm diagnosis.

Radiation neuritis of the brachial plexus is fortunately an uncommon condition. Loss of power and sensibility is frequently patchy and slowly progressive. The symptoms may become apparent 2 or more years after radiotherapy. External neurolysis rarely produces significant improvement, even vascularised wrap-around flaps (to improve the vascular bed surrounding the plexus) have failed to halt the deterioration.

# 10. Replantation and revascularisation

*Principal authors:   D. A. McGrouther, P. J. Smith*

In 1963 the successful replantation of an amputated arm in a 12-year-old boy heralded the age of clinical replantation surgery. At that time, the scope of the technique was limited by the size of blood vessels which could be reliably anastomosed. More recent developments in optical technology, microsurgical instruments, sutures and needles, have made it possible for surgeons to anastomose small vessels and nerves. Digital replantation in man has now become routine in many centres such that this service is widely available. Success must now be judged on the degree of functional restoration rather than by survival of the part alone, since this should now be a matter of course in properly selected cases.

Replantation may be defined as the surgical re-attachment of traumatically severed tissue where the amputation has been complete. Revascularisation is the restoration of blood flow to a part which has been incompletely amputated. There is no concise term to describe the amputated part and for simplicity the term 'amputate' (from the German 'Amputat') will be used.

Microvascular surgery is dependent upon highly developed technical skills. Specific training in the laboratory is necessary for surgeons undertaking this work. However, the actual technical procedure of replantation is only the initial event in the overall treatment plan for these patients. The majority of patients require secondary surgery, particularly to the tendons, to achieve the optimal functional result. Prolonged rehabilitation is required after primary and secondary procedures.

The need for experienced patient assessment, the labour-intensive nature of the operation and the requirement for effective postoperative monitoring make regional centres for replantation necessary. As these patients require referral to a centre with the minimum of delay, it is therefore necessary for every hand surgeon to have a working knowledge of the principles involved in the first aid treatment of such cases.

## FIRST AID TREATMENT — ADVICE FOR THE EMERGENCY ROOM

At the outset it is vital to avoid delay and to avoid damage to the amputate and stump. The results of replantation are best when operation is undertaken as soon as possible. This is hardly surprising when one considers the normal limits of tourniquet time. When the injury is at a digital level the duration of ischaemia is less critical and rare successes have been reported 24 hours after injury. The ischaemia time which is permissible can be prolonged by cooling the amputate, but even so the results deteriorate considerably after 12 hours of cold ischaemia. In more proximal injuries toxins are released from anoxic muscle when the circulation is restored and can lead to severe complications: myoglobulinaemia, renal failure, and even death. Replantation of such large parts should therefore be performed within 5–6 hours. Allowing some external venous bleeding after arterial repair may flush out metabolites if there has been a long delay.

The replantation surgeon should be contacted by telephone (even in situations where there has been some delay). It is essential to ensure that the patient is fit for transfer and not suffering from other major injuries which naturally should take precedence over replantation. The transfer should be expeditious and this may require the use of a helicopter.

167

The amputate should be placed in a saline-moistened swab inside a dry polythene bag and sealed by knotting it. Polythene bags are sterilized by the manufacturing process and the interior remains so until the bag is opened. The polythene bag is then placed on melting ice in a larger polythene bag or a plastic container. The ideal storage temperature is 4° C. However, there are many potential errors in this cooling process which may damage the tissue. If the amputate is immersed in saline or other physiological fluids it will become macerated; this may damage the exposed vessel ends. Direct contact with ice or too low a temperature may freeze the tissue with considerable damage on rethawing. An insulated container (for example, a vacuum flask or transplantation container) should not be used as cooling of the amputate may be excessive.

There is no substitute for a person-to-person referral and detailed discussion with the replantation surgeon. Delegation of the cooling task to others may result in irreversible damage of the part (Fig. 10.1). The referring surgeon must take great care in the maintenance of the condition of the amputate as well as ascertaining that the patient is fit for transfer.

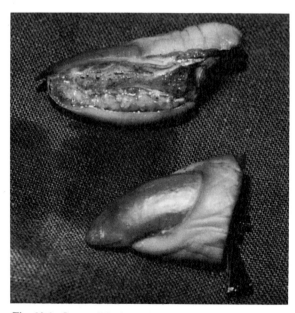

**Fig. 10.1** Irreversible damage to amputated parts. These small fingertips were replantable, but unfortunately they were mistakenly immersed in formal saline

## ASSESSMENT OF A PATIENT — THE DECISION TO REPLANT

The decision whether to undertake replantation must be made by a surgeon experienced in microsurgery in consultation with the patient. The patient's hopes must not be unduly raised at the referral centre; the patient should realise that he is being transferred for *consideration* of replantation. Having sustained a painful and distressing injury, the patient will not be in the best position to judge his future with or without the amputated part. The replantation surgeon, however, should be able to judge the outcome based on experience and knowledge of the literature. The questions which the surgeon must ask in making a decision are:

1. Is it *wise*.
2. Is it *possible* from a technical point of view?
3. Is it *desirable* functionally?

A provisional decision may then be made whereupon the surgeon must ascertain:

4. What are the patient's wishes?

### 1. Wise

The presence of other injuries and the patient's general health must be considered, as must the patient's age. Whereas replantation should be attempted in children, teenagers and young adults, the indications are few over the age of 60 because of the long rehabilitation period necessary. Vessel disease is also more likely in the elderly.

### 2. Technically possible?

The possibility of replantation is governed by two factors: the technical feasibility of vessel repair or grafting and the integrity of the distal microcirculation. The nature of the tissue damage must be considered. In clean-cut amputations the vascular injury is localised and minimal bone shortening can allow end-to-end anastomosis of the vessels. In crushing or rotational injuries the vascular injury is quite extensive proximally and long vein grafts are often required (Fig. 10.4). Saw cuts remove tissue, the amount of which depends upon the width of the blade. There is also a varying extent of crush and avulsion extending beyond the wound.

The distal microcirculation may be disrupted primarily as a result of the mechanism of injury. Secondary damage may occur with prolonged ischaemia producing cellular disruption. This produces the 'no reflow' phenomenon (despite successful technical vessel anastomosis there is no venous return from the replanted part).

A distal amputation with gross crushing of the amputated part and disruption of the capillary bed will inevitably result in failure to re-establish a distal circulation. Attempts at replantation in such cases are fruitless. In other circumstances, replantation may be technically feasible although this may only be ascertained on exploration. The real question is whether or not it is functionally desirable.

### 3. Functionally desirable?

The functional benefit of replantation should be assessed by predicting hand function with or without the replanted parts. Replantation must be compared with amputation and not normality. In considering the functional result of replantation predictions should be made of:

a. Sensation.
b. Mobility.
c. The incorporation of the replanted part into the overall function of the hand.

   *a. Sensation.* If the digital nerves are cleanly cut in the amputation process and it is possible to repair them primarily, good sensory results can be anticipated. Such results will match those seen in isolated digital nerve repairs. However, extensive tissue damage requires secondary grafting. Poor results may be anticipated if the graft lies on a relatively avascular bed.

   *b. Mobility.* Mobility may be predicted from the level of individual digital injury.

   *c. Functional incorporation.* An assessment should be made as to whether the replanted parts are likely to be incorporated into the overall function of the hand. The more digits that have been lost the stronger the indication for reconstruction. Amputation of the thumb or the whole hand is an absolute indication and should be attempted even

in the worst injuries. Loss of digits on the radial side of the hand requires replantation to maintain key and pinch grip. Reduced mobility of the radial digits will usually still permit satisfactory key and pinch grip, although power grip will be impaired. On the ulnar aspect a stiff ring and little finger will detract from grip strength without significant impairment of fine manipulative skills. The functional desirability of replantation can be gauged by whether the replanted part is likely to be incorporated into total hand function or detract from it.

### 4. The patient's wishes

Having decided what is possible and desirable the patient should be informed of the predicted outcome of replantation in terms of mobility and function. The patient's wishes should then be considered in relation to work and recreational activities. Some patients will decline replantation, usually for economic reasons, preferring a speedy return to work. Others may request an attempt at replantation despite the surgeon's predictions.

## GENERAL PREPARATIONS FOR OPERATION

It is necessary to reserve a theatre for several hours for this procedure. The patient must be resuscitated with adequate attention paid to blood volume replacement and maintenance of body temperature.

Anaesthesia is usually by regional nerve block to avoid the necessity for prolonged operation under inhalational anaesthesia. Supraclavicular block is desirable and can be topped up if a cannula is left in situ. It is possible to obtain anaesthesia for 12–14 hours with long-acting local anaesthetics before a top-up is required. Throughout the operation the anaesthetist must pay particular attention to the maintenance of the peripheral circulation. Control of the body temperature is most important and is achieved by regulation of the theatre temperature. The patient may also be warmed with a heated mattress and space blanket.

Ideally, two surgical teams should prepare the stump and the amputate simultaneously, operating with Loupe spectacle magnification or operating

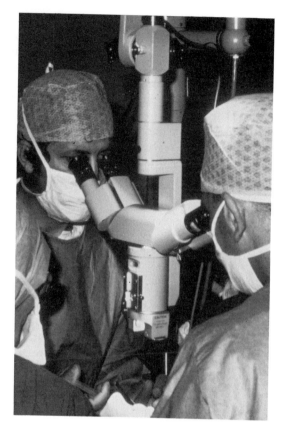

**Fig. 10.2**  Operating microscope

microscopes (Fig. 10.2). Opinions differ on the use of a pneumatic tourniquet, but this facilitates stump preparation. An adequate débridement is performed together with identification of all pertinent structures. Nerves, arteries and veins should be labelled with stitches or microvascular clips in a systematic manner (e.g. white silk for arteries, black for veins). Any necessary trimming of tendons and skin edges is performed at this stage, but the nerves, arteries and veins are usually trimmed under the microscope after bone fixation. The amputate is prepared in a similar fashion. Bone shortening is performed distally to preserve maximum stump length lest replantation fails. The amputate is placed on cool sterile packs during dissection and particular care is taken to avoid desiccation of both amputate and proximal stump.

## OPERATION TECHNIQUE

The order of repair of the individual structures in replantation is open to debate, although bone fixation must be undertaken first to achieve skeletal stability. Where there has been a considerable delay, arterial repair should be performed next, but in general the sequence is:

1. Bone fixation.
2. Repair of the dorsal structures — extensor tendons, veins and skin.
3. Repair of the volar structures — flexor tendons, arteries and nerves.

### Bone fixation

Bone shortening should be undertaken. Even in a clean-cut injury, post-traumatic oedema will produce relative shortening of all soft tissues and approximately 0.5–1 cm of shortening is required. In a blunt injury greater shortening is indicated to allow trimming of the damaged soft tissues.

Rigid internal fixation permits early passive joint motion (Fig. 10.7b). Sufficiently rigid fixation may be achieved by intra-osseous wiring with an oblique Kirschner wire or by plates and screws. A single longitudinal Kirschner wire or crossed Kirschner wires do not give rigid fixation and may immobilise adjacent joints. Obliquely placed crossed Kirschner wires may also damage vessels, cheese-wire through the lateral skin or may obstruct the motion of tendons. These techniques are therefore inferior to intra-osseous wiring. At metacarpal level, and more proximally, plates should be used. Bone union is delayed in such severe injuries.

If the level of amputation is near a joint, there is a dilemma as to whether to excise the short bone segment and arthrodese the joint or to preserve the part and undertake an osteosynthesis in the hope of preserving joint function proximally and distally. The decision will depend on the exact level of injury and prospects for recovery of joint motion in each case.

### Tendon repair

The techniques of tendon repair are those used for simple division, except that trimming of the ends may be necessary in a blunt injury. All tendons are repaired, but limited movement may be anticipated distal to the replantation site as all healing structures are involved in one wound. An adherent tendon repair however acts as a functional tenodesis at the injury site and will at least add power to the proximal joints.

## Nerves

In the clean-cut injury, nerve repair should be performed at the time of replantation. With a blunt injury, nerve grafting should be undertaken as a secondary procedure. These procedures should be performed under the magnification of an operating microscope.

## Microvascular repair of arteries and veins

To restore circulation, repair of at least one artery and one vein is necessary for each digit (Fig. 10.3). Ideally more vessels should be repaired. The ratio of veins to arteries is controversial. Two veins to one artery is common practice. Because of small vessel size the magnification of an operating microscope is necessary with instrumentation as used for free tissue transplantation. The techniques of small vessel surgery allow a patency rate of 100% in 1 mm vessels in experimental situations. Therefore the failures of replantation surgery should not be due to primary anastomotic failure, but to other factors, e.g. long segment vessel damage, delay or operative inexperience.

A relatively clean cut amputation will require minimal bone shortening and trimming of vessel ends to allow end-to-end suture. If amputation has been caused by blunt injury, reversed vein grafts should be used electively (Fig. 10.3c). Small veins, suitable for interposition in the digital arteries, can be harvested from the volar aspect of the wrist. These are dilated in situ with heparinised blood. Larger forearm veins are suitable for reconstruction of radial or ulnar arteries or long loops for attaching multiple fingers to 'jump vein grafts'.

The major problem in a blunt injury is to ascertain the extent of vessel damage. Some indication

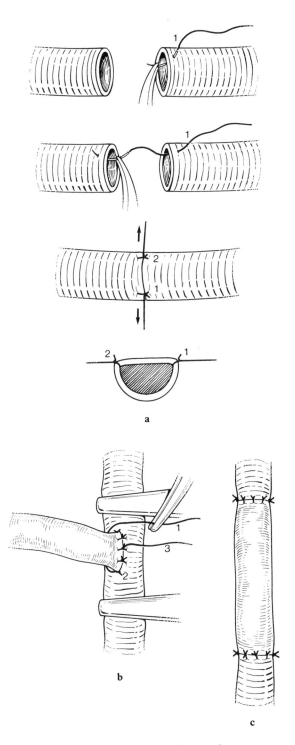

**Fig. 10.3** The basic technique for microvascular surgery. **a** End-to-end anastomosis. **b** End-to-side anastomosis. **c** Vein grafting

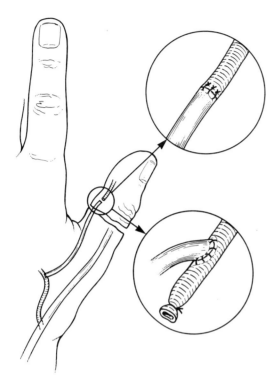

**Fig. 10.4**    A jump vein graft

is given by the history and by examination of the stump and amputate. Linear bruising along the amputate (the Chinese red streak) is a bad prognostic sign. Avulsion is the most frequent cause of long segment vessel injury. In a blunt injury the vessel is stretched between fixed points so that damage extends at least as far as the first major branch in each direction. Judgement of the length of damaged vessel is difficult. Such vessels should be trimmed under the microscope until pulsatile blood flow is obtained from a clean-cut vessel end.

If there is doubt about the proximal vessel this may be by-passed altogether. In the thumb, for example, it is possible to use a 'jump vein graft' (Fig. 10.4) from the radial artery just distal to the anatomical snuff-box to by-pass the damaged proximal vessel. This may be sutured end to side to the distal artery, by-passing a potentially damaged artery in the amputate. Alternatives to vein grafts for thumb replantation are transfers of neurovascular bundles from the index or middle fingers. Venous pedicle transfers may also be

dissected from the dorsum of the index finger and routed to the thumb.

## Skin closure

Tight skin closure must be avoided and it is better to leave wounds open and apply split skin grafts to the raw areas. Split skin grafts may even be applied over vein grafts. Skin graft take may be reduced by exudation from the raw surface of the replanted part. However, the skin protects the vein grafts by avoiding desiccation and flow should be maintained. On occasion, the skin graft acts only as a temporary dressing. Rarely, flap cover of the replantation site is possible using local skin flaps to cover skin deficiencies.

## REPLANTATION AT DIFFERENT LEVELS OF INJURY

It is possible to predict the functional outcome by assessing the level of injury (Fig. 10.5). This allows the surgeon to define clearly what function he is aiming to restore and this functional prediction can be of value in deciding whether or not to proceed with the replantation procedure. In terms of achieving viability, the level of injury of the vessel is the most important factor, but in relation to later motor function, the level of injury of the skeleton and musculotendinous structures is more relevant. Reinnervation is generally satisfactory in restoring sensation, but recovery of intrinsic muscle function is exceptional.

### Level 1 — through the distal phalanx

Vascularisation is difficult at the level of the distal phalanx, but an excellent functional result can be anticipated (Fig. 10.6). One longitudinal Kirschner wire provides adequate bone fixation. Technically it may be possible to repair only one artery, but no veins. Adequate perfusion can be maintained by encouraging external bleeding from the veins which are volarly situated at this level. Leeches (Fig. 10.6e) are particularly valuable as they will ingest some blood and the anticoagulant they inject will promote bleeding for up to 12 hours. Some surgeons use heparin postoperatively as an

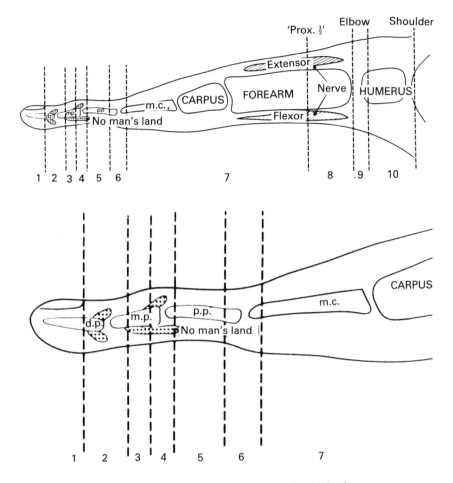

**Fig. 10.5** A classification of amputation by level

adjunct in these distal replantations. Alternatively, it may be possible to perform an anastomosis of one artery and to join the remaining distal artery to a draining vein. No other method of fingertip reconstruction is available which so adequately restores length and a sensate pulp. Return of nail growth may be virtually normal.

### Level 2 — through the distal interphalangeal joint

Vascularisation is marginally easier than at Level 1 as it may be possible to find dorsal draining veins. The distal joint is destroyed, but the action of flexor digitorum superficialis should maintain normal function at the proximal interphalangeal

joint, and a very useful functional digit can be restored (Fig. 10.7).

### Level 3 — through the middle phalanx

The extensor tendon central slip is intact and must be preserved (Fig. 10.8). The flexor tendons are repaired in the hope of preserving a range of motion at the proximal interphalangeal joint.

Repair of the flexor tendons at this level is unlikely to yield distal mobility. The aim must be to achieve maximal proximal interphalangeal motion. Kirschner wire fixation of the distal joint will concentrate all rehabilitation forces on the proximal joint.

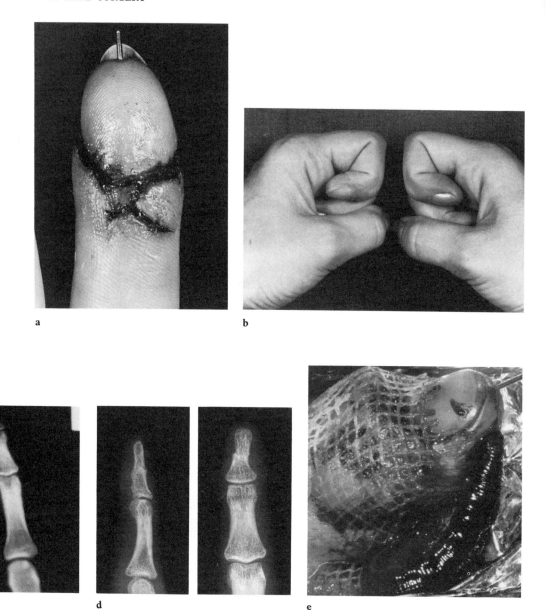

**Fig. 10.6**   Level 1, replantation. **a–d** Although technically difficult, distal replantation provides the best reconstruction of the fingertip. **e** The application of a leech to a distal replantation of the thumb. This encourages external bleeding if the venous return is inadequate

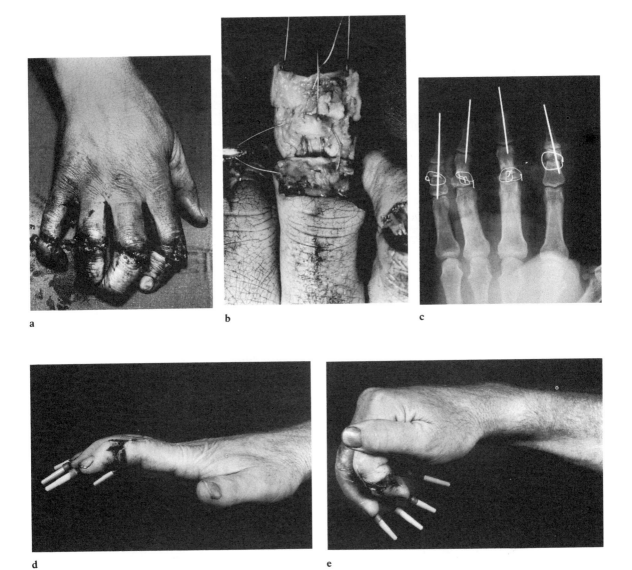

**Fig. 10.7**  **a** Incomplete amputations at different levels in the digits. **b, c** The technique of bone fixation is noted. **d, e** Immobilisation of the distal joints by Kirschner wires allows the maximum effort of rehabilitation to be concentrated on the proximal interphalangeal joints

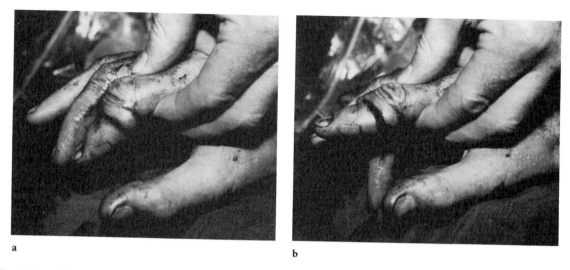

a                                    b

**Fig. 10.8   a, b** Level 3, incomplete amputation. An intact central slip is demonstrated, although all other structures and the digit have been damaged. This finger was not replanted as the patient was 71 years old

## Level 4 — through the proximal interphalangeal joint

If there is destruction of the proximal interphalangeal joint the finger will be stiff (Fig. 10.9). At the time of replantation it will be necessary to undertake a primary arthrodesis or arthroplasty or accept a fibrous ankylosis. A realistic view must be taken of this injury as it is likely that poor tendon function will render the distal joint immobile. Both interphalangeal joints will therefore be

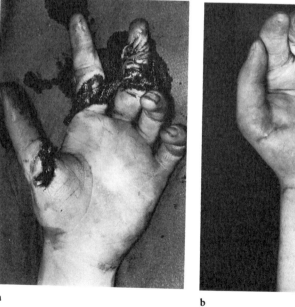

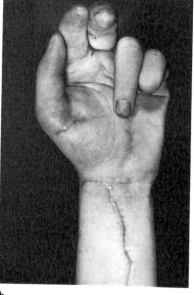

a                                    b

**Fig. 10.9   a** A Level 4 injury in the middle finger through the proximal interphalangeal joint and a Level 5 injury through the proximal phalanx in the index. **b** These fingers have only metacarpophalangeal flexion, but contribute greatly to overall hand function

stiff. Tendon repair does, however, contribute to the power of metacarpophalangeal flexion. In single finger injury replantation may be unrewarding, as the finger will have a different arc of motion from its neighbours. Multiple digital injuries at this level should be replanted, as several such fingers, although only capable of metacarpophalangeal flexion, will provide useful power. A stiff hyposensitive digit may be a success in isolation when it is the only digit against which the thumb can oppose, but is a failure in good company when other digits function well and it does not.

Joint reconstruction is possible, usually at a later stage, by Swanson interpositional arthroplasty, or by vascularised joint transfer from a toe or adjacent damaged finger.

The combination of injury to the joint and flexors and extensors however mitigate against a good result.

## Level 5 — through the proximal phalanx

The bony injury is complicated by a flexor tendon injury in no man's land and an injury of the extensor apparatus in an area where it has three separate slips and the prognosis for future func-

tion is poor (Fig. 10.9). Rigid internal fixation of the fracture should be undertaken with early passive movement to maintain joint range. Primary flexor tendon repairs in such complicated injuries have poor results and it may be better to consider staged tendon reconstruction. The aim is to achieve some motion of both the metacarpophalangeal and proximal interphalangeal joints either by primary or secondary tendon reconstruction.

## Level 6 — through the metacarpophalangeal joint area

This is a particularly unfavourable level in view of the destruction of the joint, but worthwhile results can be achieved by primary metacarpophalangeal joint arthrodesis with shortening, particularly in a marginal finger on the radial side (Fig. 10.10). One flexor tendon alone should be repaired and a concentrated effort must be made to restore proximal interphalangeal joint motion. The aim is to keep one mobile joint in the digit; because of the damage to the interosseous tendons the chance of adequate distal interphalangeal joint motion is reduced. Alternatively, joint reconstruction may be undertaken, especially in injuries to the ulnar digits.

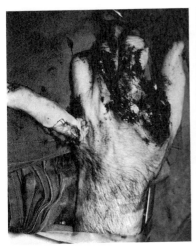 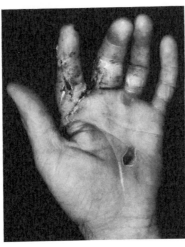 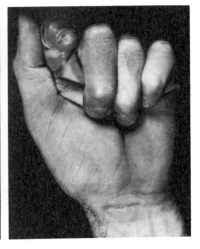

a                                    b                                    c

**Fig. 10.10** **a** Amputation through the metacarpophalangeal joint with an associated dorsal injury to the middle finger. This level is often considered unfavourable, but the patient requested replantation, and there was a dorsal injury of the middle finger. **b** The early result. **c** The late function contributed significantly to the patient's function

## Level 7

From the mouth of the flexor tendon sheaths in the palm to the proximal third of the forearm the reconstructive problem has common features (Figs. 10.11 and 10.12). There is injury to the bone or joints together with injuries of the extrinsic extensor and flexor tendons. The proximal muscle units are, however, innervated and the problem is principally one of achieving satisfactory skeletal stability together with multiple tendon repairs.

Intrinsic palsy from direct damage to the intrinsic muscles or from ulnar and median nerve injuries is inevitable. Very good functional results can be obtained, although secondary tendon surgery may be necessary for intrinsic paralysis.

## Level 8

Above the level of innervation of the forearm muscles the quality of recovery depends on the

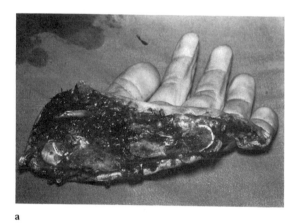

a

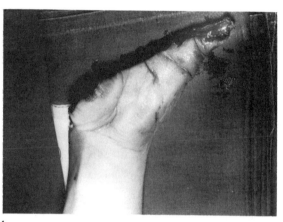

b

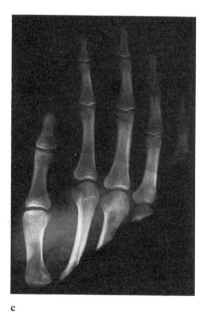

c

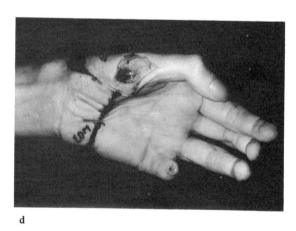

d

**Fig. 10.11   a–c** Level 7 injury through the middle of the hand. Replantation was successful and restored extrinsic tendon function (**d**). Later tendon transfers were necessary to restore intrinsic function

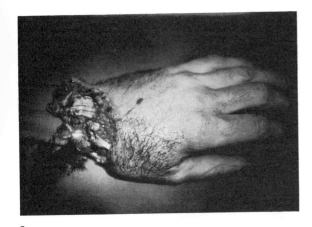

a

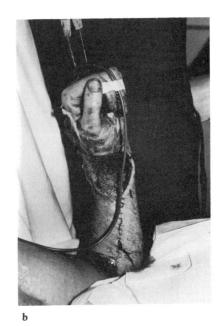

b

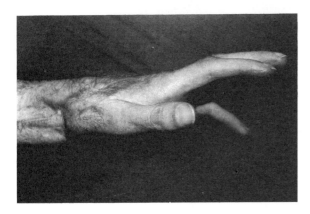

c

**Fig. 10.12   a, b** Amputation at the level of the wrist. **c** The patient returned to heavy work 1 year after injury

reinnervation of the forearm muscle masses (Fig. 10.13). Adequate bone shortening is justified to allow primary nerve apposition. Replantation at such high levels is unlikely to be functionally rewarding, except in children.

In relation to adjacent digit injuries, undesirable results are:

1. Adjacent fingers with different arcs of movement.
2. Different stump lengths (battlement type of hand).

Co-ordinated function is thus made difficult and these factors should be taken into account when making the decision for or against replantation. A favourable result may be anticipated:

a. Distal to no man's land (see Ch. 5).
b. Proximal to no man's land up to the level of the innervation of the forearm muscles.

Unfavourable results should be anticipated:

a. In no man's land (due to stiffness).
b. Proximal to the innervation of the forearm muscles (due to their poor reinnervation).

These unfavourable results relate to the limitations of current techniques. Clearly there is scope for improvement by directing attention to new techniques of preventing tendon adhesions, of maintaining mobility in the digit and of preserving joint function. Such technical innovations may in time alter the indications for replantation.

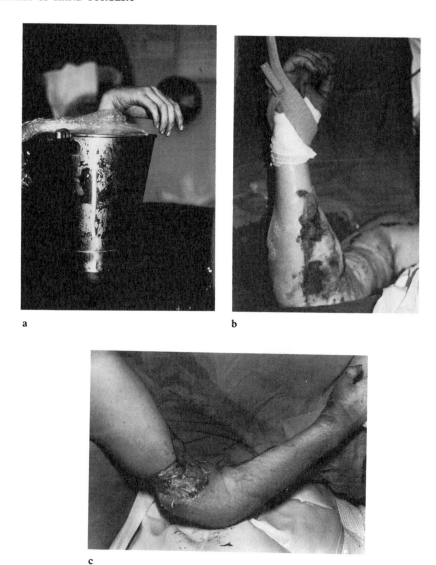

a                                         b

c

**Fig. 10.13    a, b** Amputation above the level of innervation of the forearm muscles. **c** Return of function is limited

## REVASCULARISATION

The restoration of circulation may require reconstruction of arteries and/or veins depending on the
nature of the injury. Whenever the circulation is
doubtful, early referral to a hand surgeon with
microvascular expertise is always wise. Recognition of circulatory impairment can be a major
problem. The clinical interpretation of changes in
skin circulation can be extremely difficult. A
finger which is pink may have a normal circulation

or mild venous congestion. The white finger has
no, or very low, arterial inflow due to arterial spasm
or thrombosis. A blue finger may indicate congestion or venous back-flow. Tissue turgor is of great
significance and may be demonstrated by the pulp
compression test. The restoration of circulation
may require reconstruction of the arteries or veins,
depending upon the nature of the injury.

Revascularisation may be simple with damage
limited to neurovascular structures, but it
becomes progressively more complicated as more

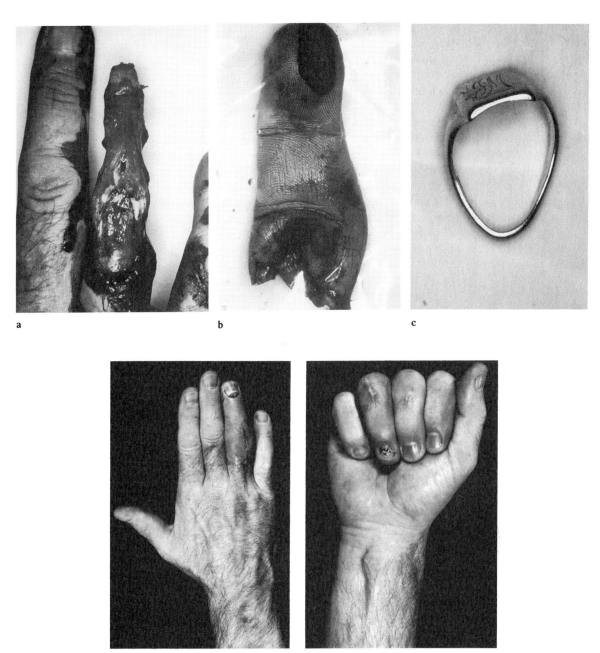

**Fig. 10.14**   **a–c** A ring avulsion injury. This was replanted using vein grafts. **d, e** The late function was excellent

tissues are divided. At one end of the spectrum the prospects are excellent and at the other end the functional outcome is equivalent to replantation. Ring avulsion injuries may require revascularisation (Fig. 10.14). They comprise a spectrum of injuries of simple contusion at one end to complete skin avulsion requiring replantation at the other.

The operative approach is similar to replantation. Fractures are fixed as described above. End-to-end vessel repair may be possible in clean-cut injuries or vein grafts may be necessary. Intermediate grades of ring avulsion may require revascularisation by vein grafts to restore venous flow if there is venous congestion. Alternatively, vein grafts to both arteries and veins may be necessary if there is no circulation at all.

If a number of digits are damaged and not all suitable for salvage, the use of a finger as a donor of tissue should be considered. Such a finger may provide tissue for grafting or free vascularised transfer of bone or joint for an adjacent digit. For this reason damaged digits should be retained as a tissue source for secondary reconstruction. Banked fingers such as these may be used for thumb reconstruction.

## POSTOPERATIVE CARE FOLLOWING REPLANTATION AND REVASCULARISATION

The limb should be elevated on a pillow in a warm environment. Cold may cause arterial spasm which may then lead on to thrombosis. Temperature control of the room is advised together with the use of space blankets and attention to body fluid balance. Dressings should be loose or, where practical, no dressing applied at all.

Meticulous postoperative observation is necessary to detect circulatory problems at the earliest stage. A routine chart should be kept of nursing observations of the replanted part, for colour and turgor. Considerable experience and skill are necessary to interpret the adequacy of the circulation postoperatively. For this reason, technical aids may be employed to permit a more objective assessment. Devices are available to monitor temperature, transcutaneous $Po_2$ or pulsatile capillary blood flow. Although systems of this type require time and effort to set up and are not wholly reliable, they may provide the earliest warning of circulatory problems. Corrective measures are instituted at the first sign of vascular insufficiency. This may require positional readjustment, release of any constricting dressings, surgical re-exploration with revision of anastomoses or the insertion of vein grafts. A theatre should be permanently available during the postoperative phase. Doubt about circulation merits return to the operating theatre at the earliest possible stage. Many pharmacological aids have been investigated, but there is no universal agreement on their efficacy. Low molecular weight dextran 1 unit/24 hours for 5 days is generally administered. Aspirin and Persantin may be used for their antiplatelet adhesion action.

Hand therapy is commenced with passive motion on the fifth day and active motion at 21 days. The commencement of mobilisation requires vascular stability. Should the part change colour, becoming more pale or more blue, a further period of rest may be necessary. Skin grafts require 5 days to take and further immobilisation is unlikely to be beneficial. The start of mobilisation is always a compromise between the fear of disturbing circulation and the prediction of stiffness. The aim of mobilisation is to maintain some relative motion between the individual structures which are contained in the one healing wound.

Secondary procedures may be necessary to maximise potential function. Unstable skin cover may require replacement. Fracture non-union may require later bone fixation or joint arthrodesis. Staged tendon reconstruction may be beneficial where good passive distal joint motion is achieved by rehabilitation. Nerve grafting imports sensation, but motor function should not be anticipated. The replantation is often merely the first step in a staged reconstruction of functional parts.

# 11. Infection

*Principal author: F. D. Burke*

## INTRODUCTION

If hand infections are well treated, one may expect rapid and complete resolution of the problem. Poor treatment, however, leads to delayed, and sometimes incomplete resolution with permanent incapacity, due to stiffness of the fingers and reduced grip.

Delayed or inadequate primary treatment of hand injuries remains a frequent cause of hand infections. Penetrating injuries of the hand are common and retention of a foreign body should always be considered. Hand infections are more common among deprived social groups, due to poor hygiene and malnutrition. Sepsis is frequent among drug addicts, because of the conditions under which injections are administered. Late presentation and poor patient compliance further complicate the management of this group. Diabetes mellitus, steroid or immunosuppressive therapy and blood dyscrasias increase vulnerability to infection in general and hand infections under these circumstances are both more frequent and serious. Any condition that reduces the blood supply to the tissues of the hand (vasculitis due to rheumatoid arthritis, Raynaud's disease or scleroderma) affects the host's ability to respond to bacterial invasion.

The principles underlying the management of infections in the hand are as follows:

Early diagnosis is essential. If the infection is at an early stage and there is no localisation of pus, non-operative management is appropriate. The hand should be rested on a splint in the optimal position for immobilisation and the arm elevated. Antibiotic therapy is commenced. Inpatient treatment or daily outpatient review will be required in these cases.

Surgical intervention is indicated if prompt resolution of signs and symptoms does not occur. Patients presenting with a throbbing pain in the hand of sufficient intensity to cause loss of sleep, nearly always have a significant infection requiring incision and drainage of pus. The procedure is best performed under general anaesthesia. Local anaesthesia causes further distension of the surrounding tissues and is inappropriate for all but the smallest collections of pus. There is no role for ethyl chloride spray as an anaesthetic in the management of hand infections. A pneumatic tourniquet should be used which provides satisfactory haemostasis during surgery. Application of an Esmarch's bandage to the infected part would risk spreading the infection, and elevation of the limb prior to inflation of the cuff is all that is required. Incisions must be sufficiently extensive to permit full drainage of infected material. The incision is performed over the area of maximal tenderness. On occasion the position of nerves, blood vessels, flexor tendons and sheath may modify the site of incision. Although the skin incision is made with a knife, deep dissection is best performed by spreading fine pointed scissors. Pus is released and the walls of the cavity are copiously irrigated and cleaned with saline gauze. Following surgical decompression, dressings are required to ensure continued drainage, absorb exudate and to rest the hand. The wound edges are held apart with a small paraffin gauze wick and a sterile gauze dressing applied. The wick is used to promote drainage of the cavity and to allow healing to occur from deeper to superficial layers. It is important that the wicks are not packed into any cavity too tightly, as drainage will be impeded. If a raw surface is present, the part is dressed with a sheet of paraffin gauze. This readily permits the passage of discharge from the tissues to the overlying dressing gauze yet does not adhere firmly to the underlying tissues. Discharge from the tissues will not pass through several layers of paraffin gauze, and if the gauze is folded upon itself, it will be unable to perform its function satisfactorily. If the hand is oedematous, it should be rested on a volar slab in the optimal position and the arm placed in a high sling. A 5-day course of the appropriate antibiotic may expedite resolution. As the inflammation and oedema settle the hand is mobilised with physiotherapy.

## INFECTIONS ARISING FROM DELAYED OR INADEQUATE PRIMARY CARE OF HAND INJURIES

Many hand infections are caused in this way. The patient may present late or a small penetrating wound may result in an unsuspected infection of pulp, web space or palm. More regrettably, a patient may attend and receive inadequate primary treatment. This is most frequently due to retained foreign material in the wound. Organic material is most likely to cause infection, glass or metal usually cause fewer difficulties.

## ANTIBIOTIC THERAPY

The majority of hand infections, both primary and secondary, are caused by *Staphylococcus aureus*. It is the organism most frequently isolated from carbuncles, pulp or palmar space infections or sepsis in the flexor tendon sheath. Approximately 80% of isolates in the UK are penicillin resistant and for these an isoxazolyl penicillin (eg flucloxacillin (Floxapen, Beechams, UK) or oxacillin (USA)) is the antibiotic of choice. Alternative therapies for patients allergic to penicillin include erythromycin and clindamycin. Oral cephalosporins are frequently used because they offer a broader spectrum of activity which includes Gram-negative organisms. However, this activity is rarely required and cephalosporins are no more effective than isoxazolyl penicillin in the treatment of staphylococcal infection. Also there are disadvantages in the use of cephalosporins. They are more expensive than the penicillins and they appear to encourage colonisation of wounds by Gram-negative organisms such as coliforms and pseudomonads. If infection involves bone or joint, flucloxacillin therapy may advantageously be combined with fusidic acid. The latter achieves excellent levels in bone and joint fluid. Treatment may need to be contined for several weeks. Fusidic acid should always be given with another antibiotic to prevent the development of fusidic acid resistance.

## TETANUS PROPHYLAXIS

*Clostridium tetani* is widely distributed throughout the environment. It is found in human and animal faeces and many spores are present in soil. A course of immunisation should be started in infancy and supplemented with routine booster doses of toxoid. The need for tetanus prophylaxis following injury depends on the extent of the injury, the degree of contamination of the wound and the patient's immunisation record. Clean lacerations in patients who have had a full immunisation course and recent toxoid boosters only require surgical toilet. A toxoid booster is required if one has not been given in the previous 5 years. If patients have not previously received an immunisation course, a toxoid injection is given as the first of a series of three, to establish immunity. Patients who have contaminated infected wounds with devitalised tissue require human tetanus immunoglobulin in addition to a toxoid booster. The immunoglobulin confers passive immunity for a month. Penicillin therapy may be used to control clostridial contamination of the wound. Meticulous removal of foreign and devitalised tissue from the wound remains an essential part of tetanus prophylaxis.

## PRIMARY HAND INFECTIONS

### Paronychia

The infection involves the soft tissues adjacent to the nail. It may extend proximally to involve the eponychium (the nail-fold adjacent to the proximal matrix) (Fig. 11.1). The most frequent cause is a minor penetrating injury. The patient complains of pain and swelling in the nail-fold, adjacent to

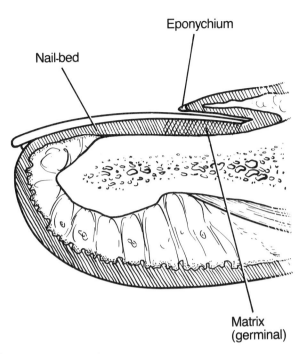

Fig. 11.1 The nail-bed

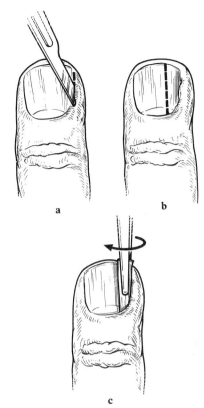

Fig. 11.2 a Incision of a paronychia. b Removal of the lateral quarter of the nail. c Removal of the nail

the nail. If the infection is limited to this area, an incision can be made adjacent to the border of the nail (Fig. 11.2a). Pus is released and the area cleaned with saline-soaked swabs. The wound edges are held apart with a small paraffin gauze wick and a sterile gauze dressing applied. On occasion the swelling in the lateral border of the nail is so great that inadequate drainage results from this procedure. It is then appropriate to remove the lateral quarter of the nail (Fig. 11.2b). If the infection has extended proximally to the eponychium, it should be gently raised from the dorsal surface of the nail and the area cleaned with saline-soaked swabs. A single thin paraffin gauze sheet may then be placed between the eponychium and the nail. If pus has tracked beneath the nail at the level of the eponychium, removal of the nail is indicated (Fig. 11.2c).

An alternative management is to treat all paronychias by nail removal. This is performed by inserting one blade of a thin haemostat under the nail close to the margin. The haemostat is closed and rotated, thus removing the entire nail without damage to the nail-bed. Although this procedure may be perceived by some to be excessive, the technique is easy to perform, safe, and almost universally successful in draining the paronychia. In addition, it does not involve incision of the tissues which may spread infection, or heal with unsatisfactory scarring. Abnormal nail growth is exceptional.

A minority of acute paronychias are due to infection by the herpes simplex virus. These infections frequently involve dental, medical or paramedical staff. Pain is intense, with swelling and erythema. There is a characteristic vesicular eruption and the virus may be grown from the vesicular fluid. Incision and drainage is not indicated and the condition is self-limiting.

### Chronic paronychia

This condition is common in people whose job entails frequent immersion of the hands in water.

It is often caused by *Candida* and is treated by the application of antifungal creams. *Candida* infections are difficult to eradicate if the skin remains macerated by continuing immersion. The hand should be kept dry to control infection. Surgery is rarely indicated.

### Carbuncle

Carbuncles occur on the dorsal aspect of the hands and probably originate from an infected hair follicle. They are frequently found in patients whose general health is poor. They may be caused by penetrating injuries in the presence of poor personal hygiene. Incision and drainage are required.

### Pulp space infection

Pulp space infections arise most commonly from penetrating injuries to the fingertip. The finger-pulp is composed of many small fat-filled compartments separated by strong fibrous septa passing from skin to distal phalanx (see Fig. 11.1). If an infection develops in the distal pulp, the tension in the involved compartment increases rapidly. The tissue distension causes pain and unless decompression is performed there is a risk of progressive fat necrosis, skin necrosis or osteomyelitis of the distal phalanx (Fig. 11.3). The patients present early with rapidly increasing pain in the pulp associated with moderate swelling and local tenderness. The area of maximal tenderness

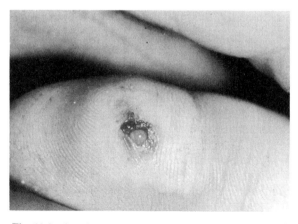

**Fig. 11.3**   A pulp space infection

is identified and incision and drainage performed at that point, taking care to avoid digital nerves and vessels. If significant amounts of fat or skin are lost to the pulp, long-term disability will be experienced by the patient. Fine manipulative skills are reduced by alteration in the conforming properties of the pulp or tenderness in the scar.

### Infections of the flexor tendon sheath

Sepsis in the flexor tendon sheath is uncommon but it represents one of the most serious types of infection which may occur in the hand. Delayed diagnosis or inadequate treatment will result in long-term disability, with stiffness of the involved finger. Reduced movement of the finger may occur even if adequate treatment is provided promptly. The injury most frequently follows an apparently trivial laceration to the volar aspect of the finger. The cruciate portions of the flexor tendon sheath are very superficial at the levels of the proximal and distal interphangeal joint creases. If the laceration occurs when the finger is held in a flexed position, the flexor tendons compress the cruciate pulleys against the skin. Superficial lacerations may thus breach the flexor tendon sheath. Patients present with increasing pain in the finger, which is held in a semi-flexed position. Careful inspection may reveal evidence of a partly healed superficial laceration at the interphalangeal joint crease. There is moderate swelling along the entire length of the finger (Fig. 11.4), with diffuse tenderness over the flexor tendon sheath. Active or passive movement of the proximal interphalangeal or distal interphalangeal joints is exquisitely painful. The flexor tendon sheath is a relatively non-distensible structure and increasing pressure within the sheath jeopardises the tendon blood supply and may proceed to tendon necrosis. Urgent surgical decompression of the flexor tendon sheath is required. This is best performed by opening the sheath at the level of the distal interphalangeal joint, and proximally at the level of the A1 pulley. The sheath is irrigated by passing fine catheters up the sheath and perfusing the area with Ringer's solution. Irrigation may be continued into the postoperative period, retaining the fine catheter in the flexor tendon sheath for 48 hours. Alternatively it may

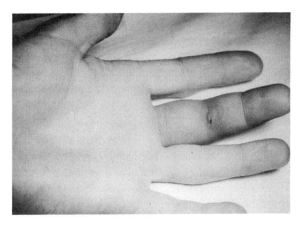

**Fig. 11.4** Flexor tendon sheath infection of the middle finger with healing laceration over proximal interphalangeal joint

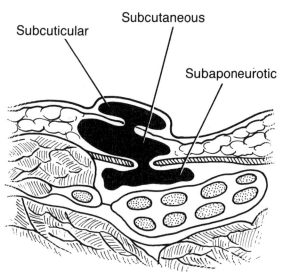

**Fig. 11.5** Collar stud abscesses and tissue planes

be discontinued at the end of the operation and the skin loosely sutured. The hand is rested upon a volar slab and parenterally administered antibiotics prescribed. As soon as it is apparent that the inflammation is resolving, intensive physiotherapy to mobilise the hand must be considered.

### Interdigital infection

This often arises through a superficial infection developing in dry or cracked web space skin. The infection may remain in the web space area, diverging the fingers, or spread via the lumbrical canal to the deep palmar area. Incision and drainage of pus limited to the web space itself are best performed through the web. The more sensitive volar aspect of the palm is undisturbed and a longtitudinal scar at the base of the web settles well without contracture. If the infection has extended more proximally into the deep palmar area, drainage through the web space may prove inadequate and an incision will be required on the palmar surface itself.

### Palmar space infection

These infections can be due to direct penetration, or to spread from more distal sites. Flexor sheath infections may spread proximally to palm (midpalmar space) or wrist. Web space infections may also spread proximally to the palm along the

lumbrical canal. The loculation in this situation is somewhat different to the proximal spread of the flexor sheath infection and has been described as the deep palmar space. Classical descriptions of the palmar spaces in previous texts are not readily demonstrated in clinical practice. Swelling on the palmar aspect of the hand may be minimal, but dorsal swelling is common. The patient is toxic and complains of pain in the palm on firm pressure. Such infections are uncommon and require exploration under tourniquet by a surgeon with a profound knowledge of the anatomy of the hand.

If the infection is well established, it may spread through the palmar fascia to the subcutaneous area and perhaps more superficially to form a subcuticular abscess. These collections of pus, connected by small defects in the fascial planes, produce 'collar stud' abscesses (Fig. 11.5). It is important when draining an abscess to ensure that there is no deep connection which has been overlooked.

### Streptococcal cellulitis

The causative organism is *Streptococcus pyogenes* (the Lancefield Group A beta haemolytic streptococcus). This is one of the few hand infections that does not require early incision and drainage. The infection is not localised. The patient is sometimes toxic and may be moribund. There is often severe discomfort and marked swelling of the hand. Ascending lymphangitis to elbow and axilla is usually present. The patient should be admitted to hospital and the hand rested on a volar slab in the optimal position. The arm is elevated and parenteral benzyl penicillin is given. Pyrexia and discomfort usually abate within 24 hours. If the patient fails to respond, then a careful search for pus is required.

## Septic arthritis

This almost invariably occurs following a penetrating injury. There is swelling around the joint and frequently an effusion. Movement of the joint is usually extremely uncomfortable, but this is not invariably so. Early exploration of the joint is required, usually from the dorsolateral aspect. Swabs are taken for bacteriology and the joint is irrigated with copious amounts of saline solution. The wound is loosely sutured with incomplete closure of the joint capsule to permit drainage into

the dressing. The hand is rested on a volar slab. *Staph. aureus* is the usual causative organism and flucloxacillin and fusidic acid are prescribed. Damage to the articular cartilage may be avoided by early surgical intervention, control of infection with antibiotics and avoidance of prolonged immobilisation.

One of the commoner varieties of septic arthritis of the hand is the 'bite' injury (usually to the fourth or fifth metacarpophalangeal joints) (Fig. 11.6a). The patient is involved in a brawl and strikes his opponent on the face. His clenched knuckle strikes the upper incisor of his opponent and this penetrates the skin, extensor tendon and dorsal joint capsule. As the finger extends, the puncture wound to the skin retreats proximal to the metacarpophalangeal joint. The extensor tendon also moves proximally (Fig. 11.6b). The patient commonly ignores the laceration (Fig. 11.6c) and even if he does attend the casualty department, will frequently conceal the mechanism of injury. The hand is usually examined with the fingers extended and the depth of involvement

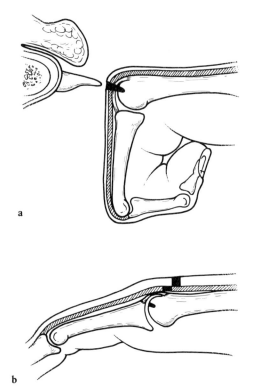

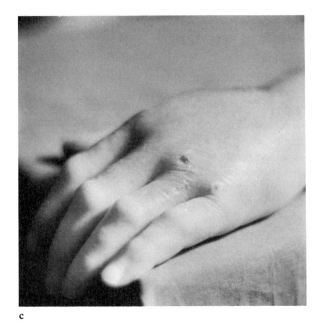

**Fig. 11.6** The human bite: mechanism of injury (**a, b**) and the presentation (**c**)

will be missed unless the significance of the site of injury is appreciated and the fingers flexed to reveal damage to both tendon and capsule. The human mouth contains several hundred different species of bacteria. These are present in saliva and gingival scrapings to a concentration of $10^9$–$10^{10}$ per ml. Human bite infections are therefore usually polymicrobial, with anaerobic organisms predominating. Early exploration is required with irrigation of the metacarpophalangeal joint. If the patient is seen at an early stage, the tissue edges may be trimmed and the skin loosely sutured. Delayed suturing may be considered. The hand is rested on a volar slab. The pus should be submitted for microbiological examination, including Gram stain, as a guide to therapy. The appropriate antibiotic therapy is penicillin (Penidural depot injection guarantees patient compliance) with metronidazole for increased activity against anaerobic organisms.

## Animal bites

The majority are dog or cat bites. The limbs are most frequently involved. There may be abrasions, puncture wounds or deep lacerations contaminated with organisms from the animal's mouth. Horses cause considerable crushing to the tissues. Rodent bites are particularly deep and may involve bone or joint. Primary management should include adequate wound toilet with careful cleansing and débridement. Prophylactic antibiotics should be considered in all cases. Because of the likely group of infecting organisms penicillin V (phenoxymethylpenicillin) is an appropriate choice.

In cases presenting with established infection, a swab or pus specimen should be sent for laboratory examination. A Gram-stained smear of the specimen may yield helpful immediate guidance for antibiotic therapy. The wound is débrided, packed and dressed. Secondary closure is indicated when the infecting organism has been isolated and an appropriate antibiotic prescribed. The mouth flora of animals is similar to that of man with oral streptococci and mixed anaerobes present in profusion. There is, however, an organism present in the mouths of dogs and cats which very frequently causes bite infections:

*Pasteurella multocida* is a Gram-negative bacillus which causes septicaemic/meningitic illness in cats and dogs. Spreading infection of this type in man may involve bone or joint, or even cause septicaemia, pneumonia and meningitis. *Pasteurella multocida* is penicillin sensitive and the route of administration chosen depends on the severity of the infection.

## Erysipeloid

This is most frequently seen in butchers, abattoir workers or fish handlers. The organism is *Erysipelothrix rhusiopathiae*. The skin is inflamed and oedematous (*peau d'orange*). The organism is sensitive to penicillin.

## Orf

This is a large pox virus which causes ulceration around the mouth of sheep. The virus may enter an abrasion on the forearm or hand of a vet, abattoir worker or shepherd. A firm painless nodule develops. The dome of the nodule separates to reveal an ulcerated base which heals in 2 or 3 weeks. The diagnosis is made on the characteristic appearance of the painless lesion and a history of exposure to sheep. Confirmation of the diagnosis can be made by electronmicroscopic examination of material from the lesion. The condition does not respond to antibiotics, but it is self limiting. A secondary transient generalised rash may occur after 10–14 days.

## Interdigital sinus

A discharging sinus in a web space characteristically affects hairdressers and is a pilonidal sinus (Fig. 11.7). If the sinus is small it may settle on removal of the hair, but if involvement is more extensive, excision of the tract will be required.

## Pyogenic granuloma

These granulomas arise from exuberant granulation tissue following a laceration. They are merely a dramatic overabundance of granulations and may produce a pedunculated vascular swelling (Fig. 11.8). Small granulomas may be treated by

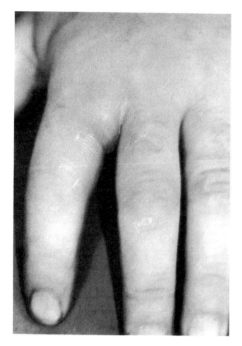

**Fig. 11.7**  An interdigital sinus

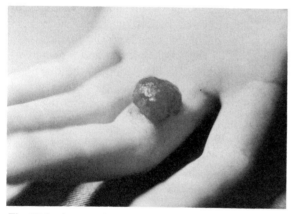

**Fig. 11.8**  A pyogenic granuloma

the application of a silver nitrate stick, but larger ones will require excision and skin closure or the application of a skin graft. The differential diagnosis from malignant melanoma may be difficult and histology of the specimen should always be obtained.

## High-pressure injection injuries

These injuries are caused by the accidental injec-

tion into the tissues of material from spray guns or hydraulic systems. The fluid is usually in an oil base. Modern spray guns work at pressures in excess of 20 700 kPa (3000 lbf/m²), which is sufficient for the fluid to penetrate the intact skin and diffuse widely in the tissues. The index finger or thumb is frequently involved as the patient attempts to clear the blocked nozzle of a spray gun (Fig. 11.9). Initially the patient feels some discomfort in the fingertip, but there is frequently little evidence of the extent of the damage. Careful examination may reveal a small entry wound. The diagnosis is frequently missed by both patient and casualty officer. Pain relentlessly increases over the succeeding hours. A radiograph may reveal air or radiopaque material (particularly lead-based paints) within the soft tissues (Fig. 11.10). Most commonly the flexor tendon sheath remains intact, but this is not always the case. Treatment involves early exploration, with attempts to remove as much of the foreign material as possible. Extension into flexor tendon sheaths or joint may occur. All necrotic fat should be removed. The oil-based

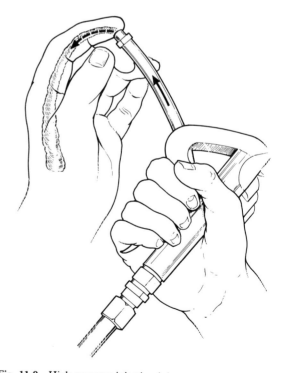

**Fig. 11.9**  High-pressure injection injury

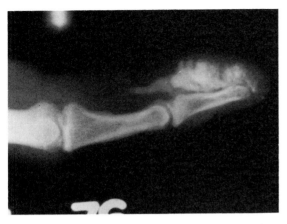

Fig. 11.10 Lead-based paint in the soft tissues of the finger

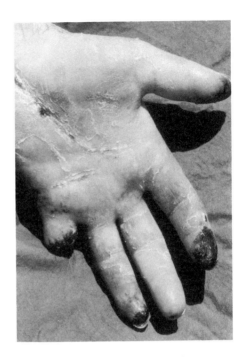

Fig. 11.11 Distal infarction of a drug addict's hand

material is mopped out on gauzes. Exploration is frequently required from fingertip to midpalmar level, or even more proximally. The wound is loosely sutured or delayed closure with skin grafts may be necessary. It is rarely possible to remove all the injected material and chronic inflammation, often with the development of persistent sinuses, may occur. Loss of fat to the pulp reduces fine manipulative skills and direct nerve involvement may reduce sensibility to the fingertip. Some loss of motion in the finger is almost invariable. Early exploration reduces long-term morbidity. However, even in those cases where early exploration is performed, the finger may be stiff and insensate. Further reconstruction may be necessary and toe-pulp transfers are of particular value. Amputation is frequently necessary in those cases when there has been long delay in diagnosis or exploration.

### The care of the drug addict's hand

Drug addicts administering agents by injection pose problems on several levels. Recognition is the first difficulty because many addicts present with a hand problem but conceal its cause. The patient's appearance is not always informative, ranging from the destitute to the debonair. Skin sepsis, absent superficial veins or punctate scars on the forearm or the dorsum of the hand should arouse suspicion. More florid infection (lymphangitis, thrombophlebitis or even necrotising fasciitis) may be present. In addition to the infection, there

may be vascular insufficiency. This may be the predominant aspect of the symptoms and usually presents as pain. Arterial spasm following direct injection of barbiturates, or thrombosis and embolism of clot, may produce ischaemia or infarction of more distal parts (Fig. 11.11). Management of infective lesions is along conventional lines, although failure of resolution may indicate unsuspected deep sepsis or vascular insufficiency. The management of vascular insufficiency is difficult and unsatisfactory. Guanethidine and stellate ganglion blocks are of limited benefit. If massive oedema develops, surgical fasciotomy is of value on occasion. Direct arterial surgery has little to offer. Pain relief is difficult to achieve if caused by ischaemia and there is the added complication that such patients may be addicted to morphine-like drugs, therefore they no longer obtain pain relief from analgesics, despite massive doses. Local anaesthetic blocks may be a last resort in a situation of despair. Compliance cannot be anticipated unless the patient foresees an immediate short-term gain. Where pain relief cannot be secured, the patients remain restless and difficult to manage. For these reasons, the aim of treatment must be to achieve wound healing by the simplest, swiftest means. Staged reconstructive surgery is contraindicated.

The third level on which this group of patients should be considered is in relation to the hazards they pose to hospital staff and other patients. The addict group have a high incidence of potentially lethal viral illnesses (serum hepatitis and AIDS). A barrier nursing approach may be quite impossible, due to poor compliance, which may be carried to the level of physical violence to staff or other patients. In addition, there is a security risk in relation to drugs, syringes and any items of potential value.

# 12. Burns

*Principal author: D. A. McGrouther*

A burn injury of the hand threatens its structure and function in a variety of ways. There is primary cellular damage from the thermal change. Loss of the protective barrier of the skin surface allows the entry of infection, which increases local tissue destruction and may spread to become systemic. The inflammatory response to the burn injury, although designed by nature to provide protection, permeates all adjacent tissues. Oedema fluid distends the skin envelope, producing the characteristic posture (p. 18) and predisposing to fibrosis and contractures. Pain may be intense as a result of the rich innervation and, if inadequately controlled, will deter the patient from motion and therefore contribute to postural deformities. Measures must be adopted to counteract all of these responses in addition to ensuring adequacy of skin cover.

Burns may be classified into three levels. The most *superficial burns* will heal with little or no permanent sequelae. When the damage extends deeper into the dermis (*deep dermal burn*) the wound will heal from the residual skin adnexal structures, but the destruction to the dermis is such that the scar will become hypertrophic and lead to contractures. The overlying unstable epithelium may prove unsatisfactory and skin resurfacing is often necessary. *Full thickness burns* destroy the dermis as a whole, the wound granulates and healing is only possible by marginal ingrowth of epithelium. A burn which remains unhealed at 3 weeks can be considered full thickness. Healing from the margins is a slow process which progresses little from month to month. Surgical intervention is required for all but the smallest full thickness burns if satisfactory wound healing is to be achieved.

## CAUSES OF HAND BURNS

### Scalds

The hand and upper limb are areas which are frequently involved in scalds by tea or boiling water. Children are particularly vulnerable. Scalds usually produce a superficial burn with erythema and blistering, although deeper areas are encountered where contact with the hot fluid is prolonged, such as when a child falls into a bath of boiling water. Steam scalds in adults are frequently caused by industrial accidents.

### Hot fat burns

Hot cooking fat causes deep burns as the fat remains in contact with the skin surface and cools slowly. Small splashes are often superficial, but larger burns are usually deep.

### Flame burns

These burns vary in depth depending on the length of exposure, but they are almost always deep in parts. The skin surface may be covered with soot or debris making assessment of depth difficult. There may also be tattooing of the skin with foreign material when the burn is the result of an explosion.

### Electrical burns

There are several mechanisms of injury in an electrical burn. The primary damage is caused by passage of current through the tissues, but there may be additional injury due to contact with heated metal or flash burns. Electrical transformers contain oil and may produce an additional mechanism of burning from the heated oil. Bar fire burns in children are not typical electrical burns, but are localised deep burns, usually on the palmar surface of the hand as a result of grasping the heated element of a domestic fire. These injuries are still seen frequently, despite fireguard regulations. These are disastrous injuries requiring repeated operations to relieve contractures during growth. The fingers remain permanently scarred.

The amount of damage in electrical burns depends on the current which passes through the tissues. A burn generally occurs at both the entry and exit sites and there is a varying amount of damage in the intermediate tissues. High voltage injuries (defined as more than 1000 volts) produce considerable coagulation of tissue with gross swelling and circulatory disturbance. Fasciotomy should be undertaken in such injuries as the current is conducted by vessels, nerves and muscles and there will be considerable swelling of the limb. Deep damage to the limb is always greater than would be anticipated by external inspection. Electrical injuries due to domestic supply (50 MHz) are particularly likely to result in immediate death from cardiac asystole or fibrillation and may therefore not reach the hand surgeon. Damage is less extensive than in the case of high-voltage injuries.

## Chemical burns

Chemical burns of the hand are not uncommon and may be due to a variety of acid or caustic substances. Specific information on antidotes may be available from the place of work. Dilution with large volumes of water is the mainstay of treatment, but specific chemical neutralisation may be necessary in addition. Hydrofluoric acid burns produce progressive tissue necrosis and require neutralisation by the local injection of calcium chloride. Erythema may develop hours after exposure to some chemical substances and it may be difficult to distinguish between a burning type of injury and an eczematous reaction.

## ASSESSMENT OF BURNS

Before attention is directed specifically towards the hand, it is essential to establish the total burned surface area and to institute fluid replacement if this is in excess of 15% in an adult patient and 10% in a child. Other injuries, resuscitation and treatment of smoke inhalation take priority over consideration of the hands, but the programme of total patient management must include care of the hands.

The hand burn must be assessed as to area, depth and the adequacy of circulation. Area and depth are estimated simultaneously by the appearance of the burned part. Loss of pin-prick sensation can be helpful in identifying areas of deeper burn, especially on the palmar surface. The depth of the burn injury is the most important single factor in predicting the outcome. It is therefore important to estimate depth at the outset, as this will influence the co-ordinated treatment plan. Erythema and blistering suggest a superficial burn confined to the upper dermis. White coagulated collagen is a sign of a deep burn. The intermediate deep dermal burn is more difficult to recognise. Any intensely red, weeping surface with white areas can be considered to extend in depth to the deeper layers of the dermis and may be full thickness. The skin on the palm of the hand is much thicker than that on the dorsum and when the hand sustains a generalised injury, as in scalding, the depth of the injury will generally be greater on the dorsal surface. Any burn sufficiently deep to penetrate the palmar skin constitutes a severe injury resulting in gross oedema and likely circulatory disturbance (Fig. 12.1).

## ASSESSMENT OF CIRCULATION

Circulatory disturbance is most likely with deep burns, particularly deep palmar burns and circumferential burns of the digits or proximal limb. The adequacy of the peripheral circulation can be difficult to estimate in extensive burns, particularly when the patient becomes shocked. If there is a circumferential burn of sufficient depth to form an 'eschar' or layer of coagulated tissue it is always safer to perform a surgical release of the eschar (Fig. 12.2). This procedure should be undertaken in a sterile environment to avoid the introduction of infection. Haemostasis is necessary

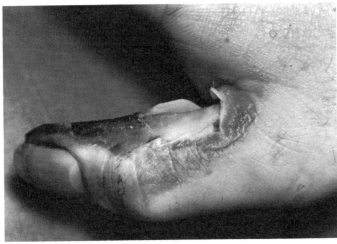

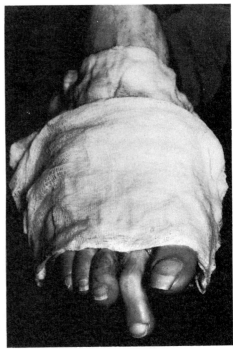

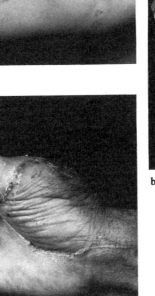

**Fig. 12.1 a** A deep contact burn of the thumb with loss of circulation. Amputation was performed. **b** Harvesting of the second toe. **c** Thumb reconstruction by second toe transfer

as blood loss can be considerable from large subcutaneous veins. A longitudinal incision is made in the burned tissue, generally over the dorsal surface. In the digits, a dorsolateral incision is usual. The tissues spring apart leaving a gap which is dressed with Jelonet, gauze and crepe bandages.

## TREATMENT OF THE BURN INJURY

Treatment of the burn injury is principally directed towards:

1. Control of pain.
2. Control of infection.
3. Control of oedema.
4. Restoration of mobility.
5. Avoidance of postural deformity.
6. Restoration of skin cover.

### Control of pain

Superficial burns are the most painful and adequate analgesia is required at the outset. Pain will be greatly relieved when the surface is covered

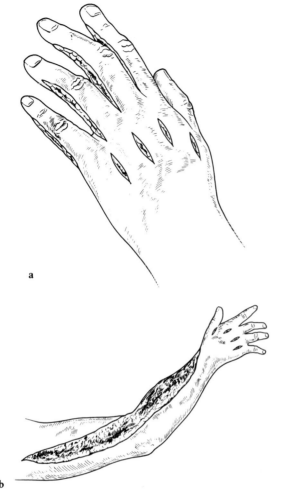

**a**

**b**

**Fig. 12.2**   Escharotomy. A longitudinal incision is made in
the forearm. Lateral or dorsolateral incisions are used in
the fingers. Additional incisions on the dorsum of the hand
allow release of the fascia over the interosseous muscles

(see below). Intravenous morphine in small doses
is relatively safe in the patient whose general
medical history is unknown. However, this is not
often required when the burns are confined to the
hands.

## Control of infection

Organisms on the skin surface proliferate and
produce clinical infection, generally between the
second and fifth day after burning. Exposure of
the burned surface to the air to allow the forma-

tion of a dry eschar is one means of controlling
infection, but it is undesirable in the hand, as
crusting limits motion and the margins of the
eschar tend to become infected. The best method
of preventing infection while maintaining motion
is to place the hand in a polythene bag with an
antibacterial agent (Fig. 12.3). Polythene dispos-
able examination gloves are an alternative allowing
individual finger movements. The bactericidal

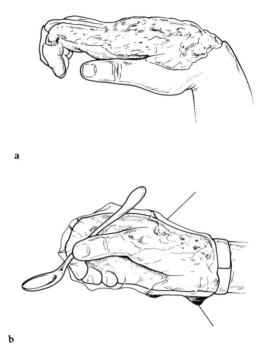

**a**

**b**

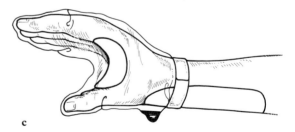

**c**

**Fig. 12.3**   **a** The oedematous burned hand assumes a
posture of extension of the metacarpophalangeal joints and
flexion of the interphalangeal joints. **b** The hand is placed
in a polythene bag containing antibiotic. Function of the
hand is encouraged within the bag. **c** Between exercise
periods and at night a splint is applied over the bag to
dorsiflex the wrist and abduct the thumb

effect of silver sulphadiazine (Flamazine) in this situation lasts 48 hours, but generally the polythene covers require changing once or twice daily for large amounts of exudate will collect, especially in the early phase. The skin of the hand becomes considerably macerated during this treatment. Assessment of depth must therefore be undertaken before treatment commences, for interpretation of the appearance will subsequently become difficult if Flamazine has been used, due to adherence of a deposit.

### Prevention of swelling

Fluid leaks from damaged capillaries. In addition, the inflammatory reaction to the burned tissue produces oedema, not only of the immediately adjacent tissues, but of the entire hand. An oedematous hand tends to assume a posture of wrist flexion, metacarpophalangeal extension and proximal interphalangeal flexion. The precise reasons for the adoption of this posture are not certain, but it is likely that pain and swelling combine to deter the patient from motion and the action of gravity allows the wrist to flex. A number of factors contribute to the claw position of the digits (see Ch. 2). Distension of the skin envelope tends to flex the proximal interphalangeal joints as the dorsal skin is more distensible than the inelastic palmar skin. Oedema is best prevented by elevation of the hand and early mobilisation. The hand should be elevated in a corrective splint (Fig. 12.3c) between exercise periods, which are supervised by a physiotherapist. An ambulant patient must be encouraged to maintain the hand aloft. Restrictive dressings must be avoided. A full thickness burn may produce an eschar with constriction and progressive distal oedema. This may provoke a vicious circle with a deteriorating distal circulation. Early escharotomy may prevent swelling, avoiding muscle ischaemia leading to ischaemic contractures or even limb infarction.

### Restoration of mobility

The patient must perform frequent active movements, supervised by a physiotherapist, to ensure that all joints are achieving an adequate range of motion. In addition, the patient should be encouraged to undertake as much of his own care as possible to maintain hand motion (Fig. 12.3b). A patient in polythene bag dressings is able to feed himself. Passive exercises may be necessary in addition if the patient is not achieving an adequate range of active joint motion.

### Avoidance of postural deformity

Elevation and active mobilisation will contribute greatly towards the prevention of postural deformity. The patient should wear a wrist support splint between exercise periods to hold the wrist in dorsiflexion. Such splints should also be worn at night. The splint should be moulded immediately on admission before oedema is established. Where progressive stiffness is developing, dynamic splintage, using outrigger splints, is possible later, but these are difficult to fit in the early stages. If the burn is deep and severe, and early surgery is undertaken, it may be advisable to immobilise the interphalangeal joints in extension, by the insertion of longitudinal Kirschner wires through the distal finger-pulps. The patient's extrinsic tendons thereafter maintain a good range of metacarpophalangeal joint motion. It is rarely necessary or desirable to immobilise the metacarpophalangeal joints by Kirschner wires, although this may be indicated in severe deep burns as a salvage procedure. It is possible to use a single wire to immobilise the metacarpophalangeal joints in flexion and the interphalangeal joints in extension.

### Restoration of skin cover: surgical options

*Early tangential excision and skin grafting*

This may be considered for deep dermal burns and would be performed within 48 hours. Successive layers of the burned tissue are shaved with a split skin grafting knife until a healthy bleeding dermal bed is reached (Fig. 12.4), upon which split skin grafts are applied (Fig. 12.5). The rationale of this treatment is that deep dermal burns will heal slowly with considerable scarring. The healing process can be expedited by this method. However, it is a technique which requires considerable experience in the interpretation of

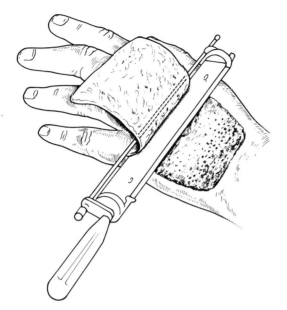

**Fig. 12.4** Treatment of the burn by early tangential excision using a split skin grafting knife. The burned skin is removed in layers until a healthy bed is found

the wound bed. The interpetation is particularly difficult when the operation is performed under tourniquet, but without tourniquet blood loss is considerable.

*Early excision and split skin grafting*

This approach is applicable to deep burns (Fig. 12.6). The rationale is to excise all devitalised tissue down to a healthy bed and apply split skin grafts, thereby avoiding the process of sloughing. If necrotic tissues are removed immediately, early skin cover allows more rapid restoration of function. The disadvantages of this technique are that it requires a co-operative patient whose general condition will tolerate early surgery. The application of this method requires the ready availability of a surgeon and anaesthetist and a considerable investment in time. The great disadvantage of early surgical excision is that movement is not possible for a 5-day period after skin graft application and stiffness is therefore temporarily increased. Should the skin grafts fail and require a second application the delay in mobilisation can be considerable.

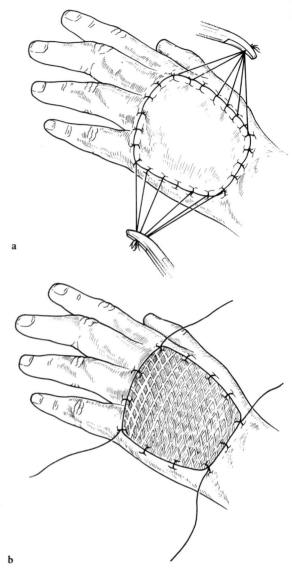

**Fig. 12.5 a** The technique of application of a split skin graft. The stitches are left long to allow them to be tied over a bolus dressing. **b** Meshed split skin prevents the collection of serous fluid beneath the graft

*Late surgical desloughing and application of split skin graft*

This method aims to speed up the desloughing process by surgical débridement. Demarcation is generally very straightforward at the fourteenth day, but if débridement is undertaken earlier the exact edge of the necrotic tissue may be less

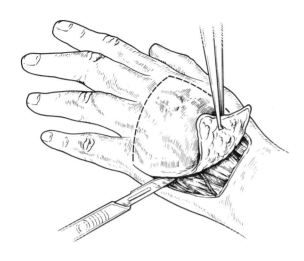

**Fig. 12.6** Treatment of the burn by early excision. This technique is applicable to deep burns and the entire thickness of the burn tissue is removed with a scalpel. Thereafter split skin grafts are applied

apparent. A variation of this method is to treat the hand by the bag method until demarcation of areas of full thickness burning is apparent. At this stage, it is possible to continue with the regimen of active mobilisation and await spontaneous desloughing, subsequently treating the granulations by the application of split skin grafts. In the intervening interval much of the hand oedema will have resolved due to the mobilisation programme.

An improvement on this method is to shave the granulation tissue down to a healthy bed with a graft knife before application of skin grafts. Granulation tissue matures to form scar tissue and this should be avoided. If a surgical débridement exposes fat it is likely that a further eschar will form if a skin graft is not applied immediately. A second débridement may be necessary. Generally the split skin grafts are applied at a later operation (delayed application) or in the ward several days later to reduce the chance of graft loss from bleeding. The grafts may be applied without dressings. Exposure to the air reduces the chance of *Pseudomonas* infection.

*Skin flap cover*

Flap cover is indicated in burns where the surgical excision uncovers bare tendon, bone or open joints. If spontaneous desloughing uncovers these structures there is likely to be considerable infection and wider débridement will be necessary.

Tissue of doubtful viability is rarely saved by the application of a flap and it is better to excise damaged tissues.

The deep surface of a pedicled skin flap has poorly vascularised fat which is unlikely to sustain or adhere to damaged tissues. Fascial flaps offer a much greater potential for importing a blood supply to contribute towards healing and eradication of infection.

Flap cover has been advised in electrical burns where the primary damage is thought to be extended by secondary infection. This is prevented by achieving early skin cover.

## MANAGEMENT OF THE HEALED BURN

Some burns will heal spontaneously and others will require skin grafting. The term 'healing of a burn' implies a finite end stage, but in its common usage this term is synonymous with epithelialisation. Except in the most superficial injuries, the burn has set in motion a series of pathophysiological events which will continue for months or years. The most superfical burns heal without any change in skin texture. Deeper burns epithelialise, but have a rather reddened appearance in those areas of the skin which will subsequently become hypertrophic (i.e. raised above the surface due to fibroblastic proliferation and deposition of collagen; Fig. 12.7a). Grafted areas also develop hypertrophy at the margins of the grafts and sometimes in the graft bed itself, particularly when the grafts are thin. The hand may therefore appear mobile and well healed at an early stage but, as the scars hypertrophy, joint contractures may develop. This is particularly true with palmar burns, especially when these burns cross flexion creases. An active programme of rehabilitation is therefore required for many months following epithelialisation. Pressure garments (elasticated gloves, Fig. 12.7b) should be worn continuously to reduce scar hypertrophy. Night splintage is necessary in addition. Physiotherapy and occupational therapy are required to maintain a full range of digital motion. It may be necessary to continue with all of these measures for up to 1 year after epithelialisation.

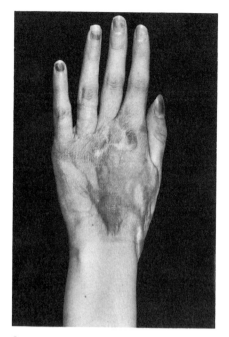
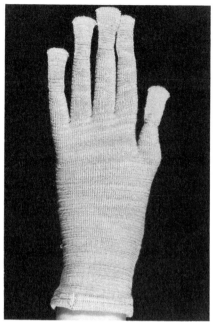

a

**Fig. 12.7** **a** The appearance of a deep dermal burn which has healed spontaneously. The scar is raised above the surface (hypertrophic). **b** Elasticated gloves apply pressure to the scarred area to encourage scar maturation. A range of sizes of gloves is readily available, but custom-made gloves are an alternative

## SECONDARY SURGERY

Secondary surgery may be necessary to release contractures and to excise unstable areas which have healed either spontaneously or following skin grafting. More elaborate reconstructive procedures may be necessary for localised deep burns such as tendon or nerve grafting and joint arthrodesis. Often it is necessary to apply skin flap cover before undertaking such staged reconstructions. Boutonnière deformity is frequent in the severely burned finger and leads to fibrous ankylosis of the proximal interphalangeal joint. Soft tissue correction is difficult because of poor skin cover. Usually the choice lies between arthrodesis or acceptance of the fibrous ankylosis.

Nail-bed deformities are difficult to improve and may require nail-bed ablation.

## RELEASE OF CONTRACTURES

Contractures are the late sequel of deeper burns on the palmar surface of the hand. Many contractures are preventable but, once established, surgical release and skin grafting may be necessary If surgical release of a digital contracture is necessary, the incision should extend from one lateral digital line to the other and the resultant skin deficit should be resurfaced by split skin grafts. Flaps and full thickness grafts are less likely to undergo subsequent contraction. However, cross-finger flaps leave a dorsal defect on the adjacent finger which may be undesirable if that digit also has a volar burn. Full thickness grafts require a well vascularized bed, but split skin grafts take well on a bed of doubtful vascularity which is frequently present.

## FROSTBITE

Frostbite affects the extremities, the fingers being more vulnerable than the thumb. The mechanism of injury differs from a thermal burn in that there is direct cellular cooling and indirect damage from vessel spasm. Initial management is by mobilis-ation in Flamazine bags. Operation is delayed for 6–7 weeks if the amount of necrotic tissue is small, but may be undertaken at 3–4 weeks where larger areas of necrotic tissue are present.

The overall plan is to prevent a loss of mobility from the pathophysiological events during the entire healing and scar maturation process.

# 13. Reconstruction of major hand injuries

*Principal authors: D. A. McGrouther, P. J. Smith*

The challenge of reconstruction of a major hand injury, with widespread damage to several tissues or loss of parts, leads the surgeon to the frontiers of knowledge and technique. In the past, injuries of this severity have often resulted in amputation or major permanent disability. The reconstructive techniques which are presently available offer the potential for functional improvement to a point where return to everyday use is now more likely.

There are two broad types of reconstructive challenge; tidy injuries where secondary repair is necessary, and mutilating injuries where tissue replacement or augmentation is required by conventional techniques or microsurgical free tissue transfer.

The patient will reach a functional plateau after primary surgery and rehabilitation. The patient's wound healing potential, age and motivation will affect the level of this plateau and the time taken to reach it. The degree of functional recovery achieved will depend upon whether the damaged structures were repaired primarily and upon subsequent complications and failures.

The patient's attitude to the result of primary surgery must be ascertained as overall hand function may be satisfactory to him despite the possibility of further improvement. However, if the surgeon can visualise a gain he must be able to communicate the potential to the patient in terms which can be readily understood. Nevertheless, the surgeon must appreciate that late reconstruction may make the process of adaptation more difficult.

Secondary reconstruction is only considered when the maximum benefit of rehabilitation has been achieved. The wounds should be healed, the circulation stable, and there should be no evidence of sympathetic dystrophy. The hand should be soft and supple prior to nerve and tendon reconstruction. However, severe injuries (crush and burns) may leave the hand stiff and contracted despite intensive rehabilitation. In such cases skin and joint surgery may be necessary to raise the functional plateau before nerve and tendon reconstruction can be considered. A staged plan of action must be conceived.

When a static phase of recovery is reached the plan for secondary reconstruction is dependent on three factors:

1. An assessment of whether or not reconstruction is necessary. The patient's position on the ladder of function must be measured and an estimation made as to whether or not it is possible to raise the patient to a higher rung of total hand function.
2. The reasons for undertaking reconstructive procedures must be defined. These are:
   a. To render existing tissues more functional.
   b. To augment function by the addition of essential, but absent, components.
3. A detailed analysis of the function of all of the remaining component parts which may be either redistributed or co-ordinated with additional tissue to improve function.

In making these assessments, the patient's occupational and recreational activities should be considered. The appearance of the hand must not be undervalued as it can almost be considered to be of functional significance in certain occupations.

Within this general assessment for reconstruction it is necessary to consider the problems likely to arise from injury to or loss of individual tissues.

## SINGLE TISSUE INJURY OR LOSS

### Skin

Injured skin is likely to develop scar *contractures*. If these cross flexion creases they may lead to flexion deformity. Contractures may arise either from healing of the wound itself or from injudicious surgical incision lines. Linear contractures arise where scars cross concavities and sheet contractures arise from healing by secondary intention or inadequate replacement following skin loss. Contractures may also develop in the bed of the skin graft or around its margins. (The management of skin contracture has been discussed in Ch. 3.)

The *durability* of any skin replacement must be considered in relation to its site. Skin grafts may be adequate in areas not subjected to heavy use (Fig. 13.1), for example, the dorsum of the hand.

Areas subjected to high pressure or shearing stresses require a tissue which matches as closely as possible the original skin cover, both in terms of mechanical properties and sensibility. It may therefore be necessary to excise grafted areas and replace these by flaps (Fig. 13.2).

*The re-introduction of sensibility to key points in the hand* should be considered when planning skin replacement. This may be done by local flaps or free tissue transfers with nerve repair (Fig. 13.3).

Spontaneous reinnervation of skin flaps is likely to produce protective sensibility in the long term, but in crucial areas, such as the thumb-tip, an innervated skin flap is preferable. Techniques of flap cover have been described in Chapter 3. Skin replacement may be required *prior to tendon or nerve reconstruction*. Skin flap cover is required with a layer of subcutaneous fat through which tendon and nerve grafts can be routed.

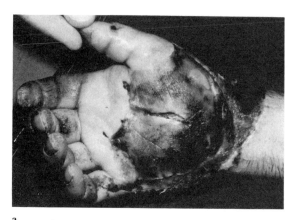

a

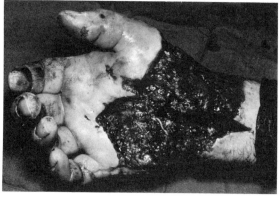

b

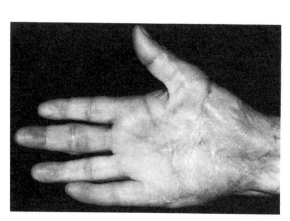

c

Fig. 13.1 Use of a split skin graft on an area not subjected to heavy usage. a Necrotic distally based flap (crush injury). b after débridement of necrotic tissue. c The area was healed by split skin grafts which proved satisfactory in the long term

## Bone

### Bone loss

Bone loss may, on occasion, be accepted where a pain-free fibrous union has developed. Proximal bone loss in a digit is likely to lead to instability and limitation of function. Bone replacement by grafts is possible in the absence of infection and if skin cover is satisfactory. Free vascularised bone transfer is an alternative technique which is not often required in the hand. Bone loss near a joint may be managed satisfactorily by excising both the fibrous union and joint and undertaking an arthrodesis. Such a resection results in further shortening of the involved ray.

### Osteomyelitis

Osteomyelitis in the hand is uncommon. Infection may be established around exposed dead bone; removal of this dead bone is required as the primary management of this problem is surgical.

### Fibrous non-union

Non-union of fractures of the hand is rare after closed injuries, but may occur in severe open wounds, particularly where there has been skin loss or infection. Non-union is also seen after replantation or inadequate attempts at fracture fixation. Non-union may result in a pain-free fibrous ankylosis, but if rigid stability is required or the non-union is painful, then excision of the fibrous tissue and bone grafting will be required. Rigid internal or external fixation is usually necessary to permit bone healing in such cases.

## Vascular structures

Secondary reconstruction of the ischaemic hand is a difficult problem. Tissue damage from vascular injury occurs at an early stage and vascular repair should always be undertaken at the primary operation. Release of longstanding contractures or joint manipulation carries the risk of damaging vascular structures, and vein grafts may be required without warning in such situations. Reconstruction of major vessel loss may be necessary prior to nerve grafting. In such situations vascularised nerve grafts may be used to achieve both aims simultaneously.

## Nerve

### Sensory and/or motor loss

If primary repair has failed or not been undertaken a secondary nerve repair may occasionally be possible. More frequently grafting will be required.

### Sensory loss where nerve repair or grafting is not feasible

Anaesthetic areas may persist despite nerve repair and it may be necessary to undertake a resurfacing procedure with an innervated flap. A neurovascular island transfer of a digital pulp to a thumb will provide a sensate area to the thumb-tip (Figs. 13.4 and 13.5). However, transfer of localisation will not take place so, if possible, the nerve should be divided and rejointed to the proximal thumb nerve. Free tissue transfers from the foot are preferred (Fig. 13.3).

### Motor loss

Loss of motor function cannot always be restored by nerve surgery and it is then necessary to consider tendon transfers.

### Pain

Pain following injury is a complex phenomenon. The pain may be due to nerve entrapment, neuroma formation or sympathetic dystrophy. Psychological factors are also relevant. Nerve entrapment is treated by release of compression (external neurolysis) with excision of surrounding scar tissue. Neuroma pain should be treated by transfer of the neuroma to a quiet area rather than by further shortening of the digit. However, there is a role for minimal bone and nerve shortening if soft tissue cover of a stump is unsatisfactory. In general, established neuroma pain is central in origin and should be managed as described in Chapter 8.

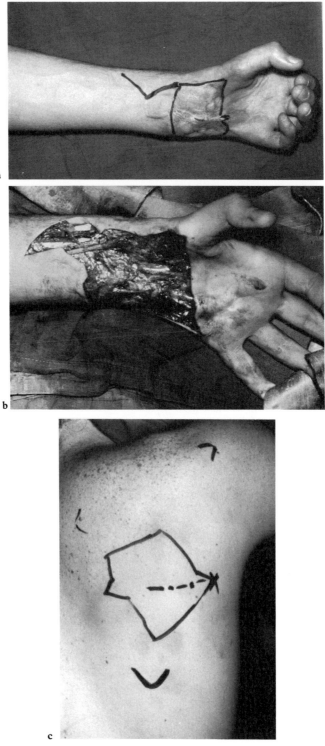

**Fig. 13.2** Use of a skin flap when skin graft cover is unstable. **a** Unstable area of scar tissue and split skin grafts. **b** The defect after excision of the grafted area. **c** Surface markings for free scapular flap. **d** The flap elevated. **e** Secondary closure of the donor defect. **f** The flap in place, microvascular anastomoses complete. **g** Result at 3 months after operation

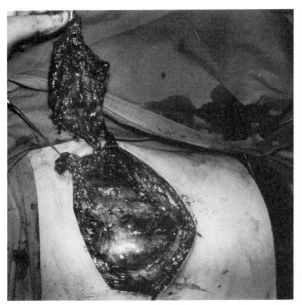

d

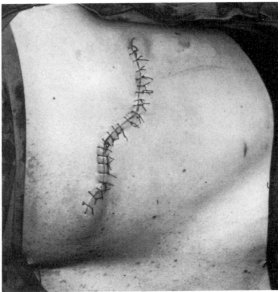

e

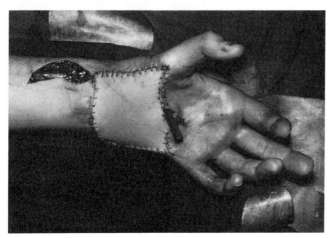

f

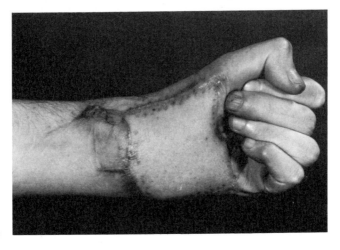

g

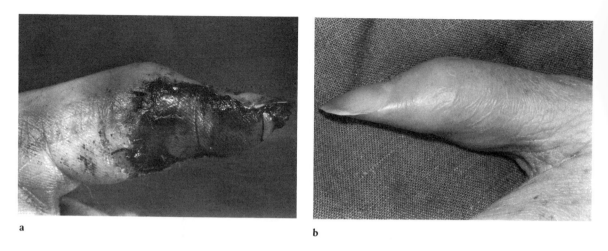

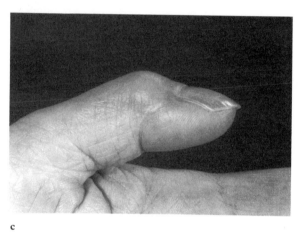

Fig. 13.3 Toe-pulp transfer. **a** Damage to the thumb-pulp from crushing. **b** After healing of the primary injury. **c** Result 1 year after transfer of a toe-pulp to the hallux

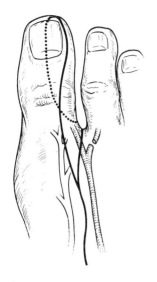

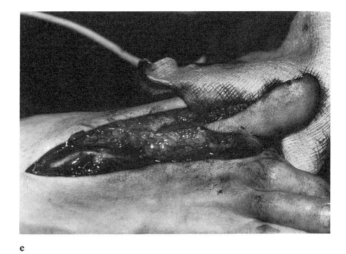

e

d

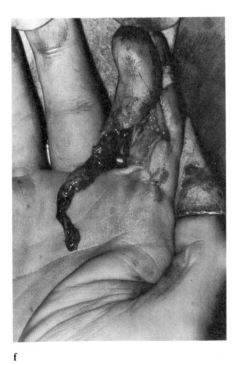

f

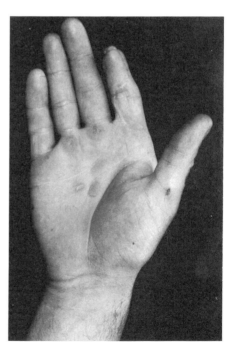

g

**Fig. 13.3   d, e** Technique of elevation of toe-pulp. **f** Application of a free toe-pulp to the index finger. The long pedicle contains veins which may be tunnelled to the dorsum of the hand. **g** The final result

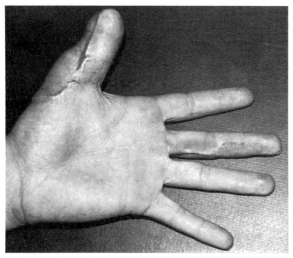

**Fig. 13.4** Neurovascular island flap transferred by the technique of Littler from the middle finger to the thumb, based on a proximal neurovascular pedicle

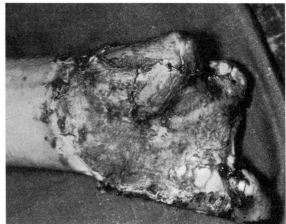

a

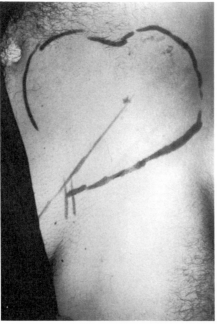

b

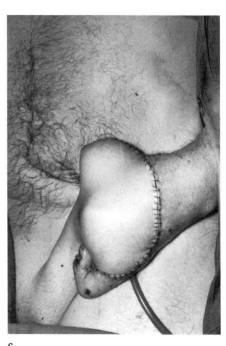

c

**Fig. 13.5** Hand resurfacing by a combined groin and hypogastric flap and thumb reconstruction by neurovascular pedicled transfer. **a** Loss of the skin of the entire hand and several digits. The little finger is flexed from a previous injury. **b** The design of a combined groin and hypogastric flap based on one pedicle. **c** The flap has been elevated, tubed and applied to both sides of the hand

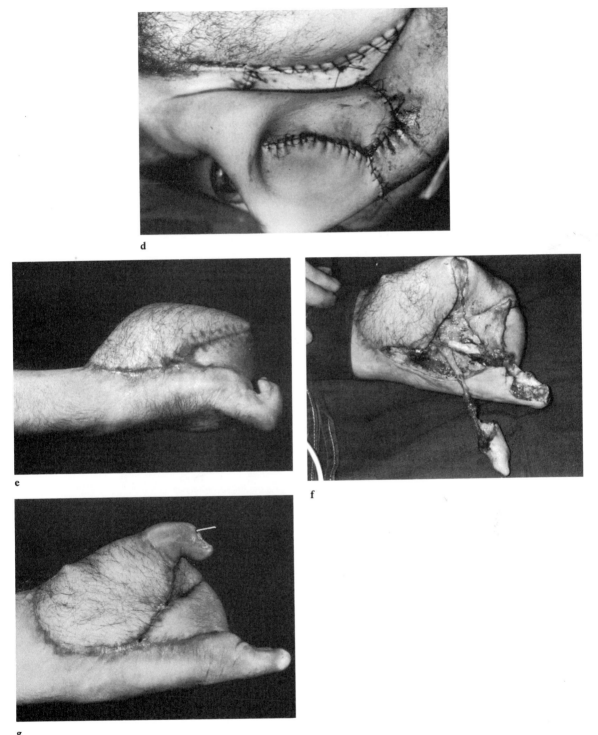

**Fig. 13.5    d** The view from above shows the groin flap cover in the dorsum of the hand, the inferior epigastric flap applied to the palmar surface and secondary closure of the donor defect. **e** Early result. **f** The hand has been defatted and the distal half of the little finger elevated on a proximal neurovascular pedicle for transfer to the thumb position. **g** Early result. This patient obtained good pinch function

## Tendon

Tendon damage may result in loss of active or passive range of joint motion. To achieve good results by secondary tendon grafting or transfer, it is necessary to have an adequate passive range. Staged procedures are generally necessary for tendon reconstruction. The outcome will be affected by secondary joint stiffness and pulley disruption (see Ch. 5). It is important to place grafts in a suitable bed which must be well vascularised. Subcutaneous fat produces a suitable gliding medium, but dense scar tissue is unsatisfactory, as firm adhesions form.

## COMPOSITE TISSUE INJURY OR LOSS

The problems of reconstruction of single tissue injury or loss are compounded when the injury or loss involves multiple tissues. Composite tissue problems include stiff joints and first web contractures.

## Joint

### Joint stiffness

Joint stiffness is a clinical sign which may have many causes. It results from injury to any of the joint components (bone, cartilage, ligaments, capsule), or to adjacent tendons and skin. The prevention of stiffness is one of the principal roles of the rehabilitation team after injury. Secondary surgical joint release may, on occasion, be required, coupled with further intensive rehabilitation and dynamic splintage to maintain the operative gain.

### Joint destruction

Joint destruction may be treated by arthrodesis or by arthroplasty. On rare occasions a silicon elastomer interpositional arthroplasty may be required for a damaged metacarpophalangeal or interphalangeal joint. A useful range of motion can be produced.

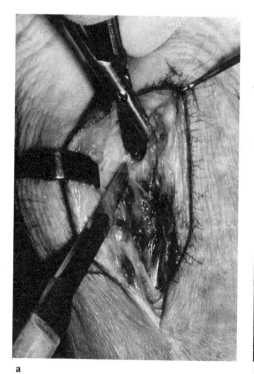 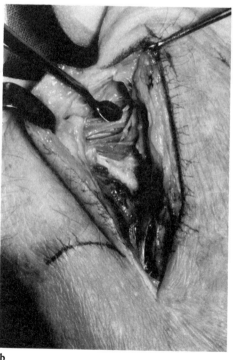

a　　　　　　　　　　　　　　　　b

**Fig. 13.6** Release of the contracted thumb web. **a** Through a dorsal approach, contracted bands of fascia are spread with the points of scissors and divided. **b** Release of contracted fascia and preservation of muscle fibres. Skin flap cover is often necessary after web release

Foucher has described the concept of a finger-bank whereby components of a severely damaged digit can be transferred on a vascular pedicle to adjacent digits. A pedicled vascularised joint transfer from a toe has a role to play in isolated joint injuries in children and young adults.

### Joint instability

Joint instability may be treated by ligament reconstruction (as in the case of ulnar collateral injury of the metacarpophalangeal joint of the thumb). If a joint is unstable, there is invariably damage to several of the structures disposed radially around the joint. There may be damage to the volar plate and extensor apparatus in addition to the collateral ligament. Correction of joint instability by soft tissue reconstruction is therefore often disappointing, frequently resulting in loss of range of motion. Arthrodesis may be required.

### Adduction contracture of the thumb web

This is a frequent complication following major injury to any part of the hand. Secondary release may be required. Release of the first web contracture comprises three separate phases:

*1. Release of contracted scar tissue.* On exploration, all contracted structures must be released; the adductor muscle, the overlying fascia and the first dorsal interosseous (Fig. 13.6). Muscle release is normally performed at the bony attachment so as to preserve any residual function. In a severe contracture it may be necessary to release the palmar and dorsal skin in addition to all of the muscular and fascial planes. In longstanding cases the capsule of the carpometacarpal joint may also require release.

*2. Skin replacement.* On occasion it may be possible to stretch the skin by serial splintage, after release of deep structures, without importation of flaps. Skin grafts are unsatisfactory as their contraction will produce an early recurrence. Many local flaps have been devised from the dorsum of the thumb or index finger or even from the palm, but none of these flaps is geometrically ideal. Distant flaps have been designed, principally from the opposite upper arm. Two flaps are required to cover palmar and dorsal surfaces. Failure to cover both raw surfaces simultaneously will result in the production of granulation tissue, which will mature to form further fibrous contracture. A free tissue transfer overcomes all these problems and, in addition, can provide satisfactory skin cover and primary wound healing over Kirschner wires.

*3. Maintenance of the released web.* Crossed Kirschner wires are required to maintain abduction of the first metacarpal. If there has been destruction of the carpometacarpal joint, it may rarely be necessary to insert a bone block to keep the thumb metacarpal in a permanently abducted position, but this should only be considered when the thenar muscles are not functional.

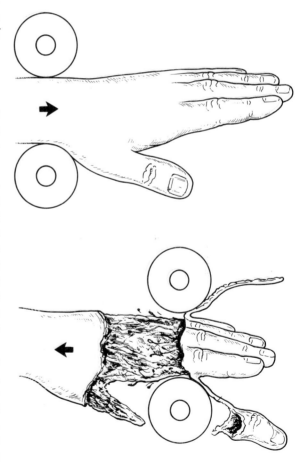

**Fig. 13.7** Mechanism of a roller injury. The hand is drawn between the rollers. The patient's tendency to withdraw the limb and the friction of the rollers combine to avulse (deglove) the skin

## MAJOR COMPOSITE TISSUE LOSS (THE MUTILATED HAND)

The hand may be said to be mutilated when there is tissue loss in association with severe injury. Primary management should be directed towards conservation of as much tissue as possible, by revascularisation if necessary. Secondary reconstruction may be considered as follows:

Dorsal loss
Volar loss
Radial loss    — thumb alone
                 thumb and index
                 thumb, index and middle
Ulnar loss    — little
                 ring and little
Distal transverse loss and proximal transverse loss
Total loss.

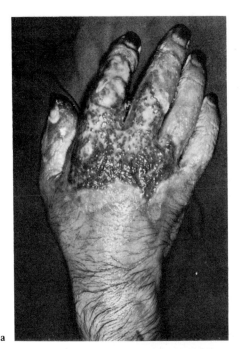

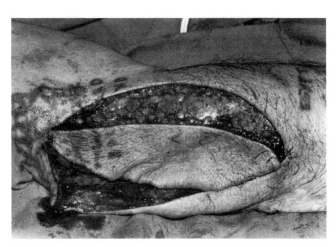

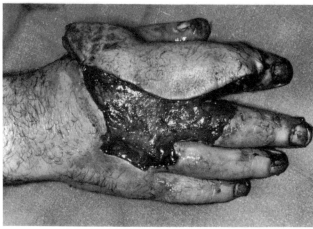

**Fig. 13.8**   Skin cover by single-stage microsurgical transfer. **a** Burn of the dorsum of the hand with exposure of the extensor apparatus of the index finger. **b** Elevation of a free lateral arm flap. **c** The lateral arm flap used to cover the extensor apparatus of the index finger. The remainder of the defect was split skin grafted

## Dorsal loss and subcutaneous tissue

Degloving of the dorsal skin may occur in a roller (Fig. 13.7) or other avulsion injury. Where skin alone is lost, grafting or flap cover may be required (see Ch. 3).

Loss of the dorsum of the hand is frequent in road traffic accidents when the hand projects through the car window and the dorsal tissues are removed by abrasion. There is usually loss of the digital and wrist extensor tendons and often the intercarpal or metacarpophalangeal joints are opened with loss of their dorsal capsules. Flap cover is necessary to cover the open joints and to provide a satisfactory tissue bed for extensor tendon reconstruction. Pedicled flap transfers,

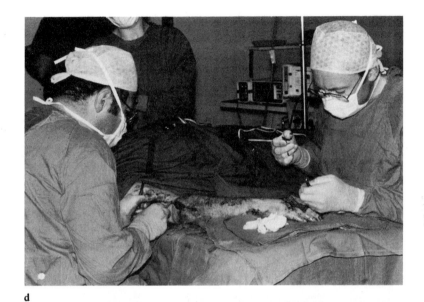

d

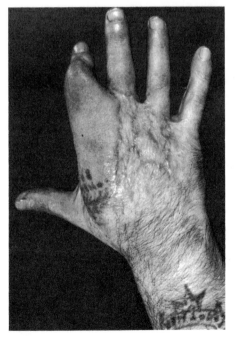

e

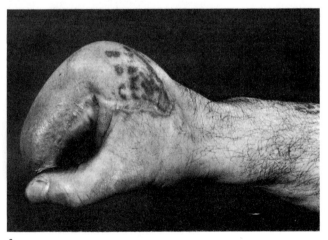

f

**Fig. 13.8   d** The use of this flap allows two surgeons to operate simultaneously with the patient under supraclavicular local anaesthetic block. **e, f** The early result before defatting the flap

such as the groin flap, are frequently used, but do not permit elevation of the hand. Immediate free tissue transfer (Fig. 13.8) allows elevation of the hand and may permit primary tendon reconstruction. This is of particular benefit as it allows primary reconstruction of the wrist extensor tendons, re-establishing the dynamic tenodesis action of the wrist.

Flap cover by single-stage microsurgical procedures offers several advantages. (Fig. 13.8). Recovery time is shortened. A permanent vascular pedicle ensures early wound healing with a reduced risk of infection and of subsequent ischaemic fibrosis. Rehabilitation may commence immediately. Although compound free flaps (e.g. DCIA, radial

flap, etc.) offer advantages of economy of tissue and the elimination of scar tissue planes between the different components, careful planning is essential to ensure the correct relationship between skin, tendon and bone. Flap design presents a difficult three-dimensional geographical puzzle. It may be better to replace skin as a free vascularised transfer and use conventional grafting techniques for reconstruction of other tissues (Fig. 13.9).

Skin flap cover may also be provided by the radial forearm flap (Fig. 13.10), although it must be realised in treating young patients that there will be forearm scars at the donor site, even if direct closure is achieved. This flap permits

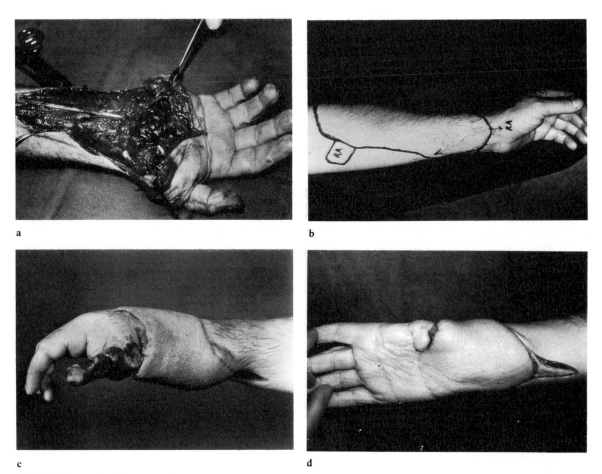

a

b

c

d

**Fig. 13.9** Acute free flap cover of an injured limb followed by later reconstruction. **a** Palmar and dorsal skin loss from a roller injury. **b** A large radial forearm flap harvested from the contralateral arm. **c** The radial flap applied to the injured hand. The vessels of the flap were used through and to bridge the vessel defect. The thumb became necrotic. **d** After amputation of the thumb

extensor tendon reconstruction at the same operation, as the palmaris longus can be incorporated in the transfer. If a distant pedicled flap is used, it is probably better to undertake the tendon reconstruction at a later stage, as there is frequently some infection around groin and other distant flaps.

## Volar loss

Loss of the palm of the hand, like dorsal loss, can also occur from roller and wringer injuries or from direct abrasion. In addition, volar tissue loss can occur from thermal and electrical burns. Volar skin replacement can be achieved by graft or flap cover. Skin grafts are satisfactory for the proximal half of the palm, but do not allow sufficient flexibility to permit folding of the distal palm. Skin flap cover is therefore preferable in this site. The radial forearm flap, groin flap or free tissue transfer provide suitable cover (Fig. 13.2).

## Radial loss

Radial loss requires thumb reconstruction. The thumb has a central importance in hand activity due to its role in pinch and grip function. Loss of the thumb from trauma is therefore a considerable disability. The best reconstruction is to replant any detached tissue and a thumb ampu-

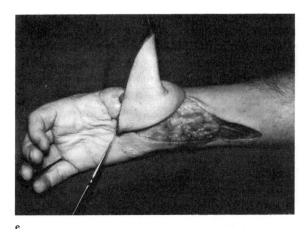

e

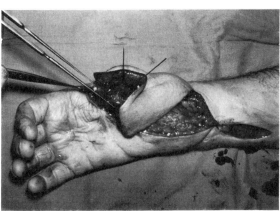

f

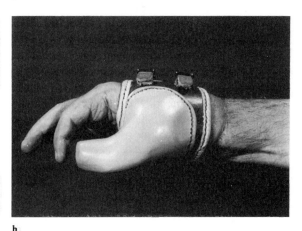

g

h

**Fig. 13.9** **e** The radial forearm flap was elevated to allow thumb reconstruction. **f** A free bone graft was fixed to the radial side of the carpus with Kirschner wires and covered by the flap. **g** The late result. **h** Excellent function was possible using an overlay prosthesis

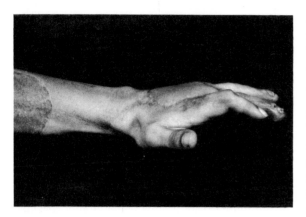

**Fig. 13.10** Radial forearm flap. A skin flap on a distally based pedicle of radial artery and venae comitantes has been transferred to the dorsum of the hand

tation at any level is therefore an absolute indication for an attempt at replantation (see Ch. 10). Terminalisation of the thumb stump will leave a shortened digit which compromises function. Some patients may choose against reconstruction, particularly in distal amputation, but in general the aim is to provide a sensate post having the same innervation as the original thumb and a similar length and range of motion. The closer the reconstruction to the original parameters the less effort will be required for patients to relearn hand function. Thumb reconstruction is, however, a prolonged process often requiring staged operations, and even if the procedure is completed in one stage there is often a delay occasioned by reinnervation. The patient must be informed of this and must be motivated to undergo the prolonged course of treatment.

*The choice of reconstructive technique depends on the level of amputation.* The level of amputation can be classified according to Mr Douglas Campbell Reid as:

1. Distal to metacarpophalangeal joint.
2. Through the metacarpophalangeal joint.
3. Proximal to metacarpophalangeal joint with preservation of thenar muscles.
4. Proximal to metacarpophalangeal joint with destruction of thenar muscles.

1. A late reconstruction would not be indicated in amputations distal to the interphalangeal joint, although primary replantation would restore pulp tissue and possibly a normal nail. Traumatic amputation through the proximal phalanx may provide sufficient length for the patient's needs, but others will require additional length or pulp replacement. An improved pulp can be achieved by free toe-pulp transfer (Fig. 13.3) and a portion of vascularised toe phalanx can be incorporated to augment length. This is only possible if there is sufficient residual skin on the stump to achieve closure. Otherwise a free vascularised toe transfer or wrap-around transfer would be necessary (Fig. 13.11).

2. After amputation through the metacarpophalangeal joint, length augmentation is generally necessary and the choice would lie between conventional and microsurgical techniques. There is no indication at this level of injury for pollicisation as the thumb intrinsic muscles are intact. A simple Z-plasty will deepen the first web and therefore produce apparent lengthening of the residual thumb stump. Techniques of thumb lengthening include metacarpal lengthening by the Matev technique (osteotomy followed by distraction using a frame; Fig. 13.12) or by the insertion of a bone graft. Extra skin can be provided by the classical technique of Gillies, described as the cocked hat flap (a distally based local flap), or a conventional pedicled flap. Other techniques of thumb lengthening include augmentation of the metacarpal by an onlay bone graft which is covered by a tubed groin flap. When the groin flap is divided the circulation of the reconstructed post will be precarious, as the flap will be deriving its flow from the wound margins. This can be considerably improved by the simultaneous application of a Littler neurovascular island flap or pulp from the middle finger. Microsurgical reconstruction techniques are by transfer of a hallux or the second toe (Fig. 13.13). The hallux produces a better functional thumb, but leaves a greater donor site deficit. The second toe is variable in size in relation to the thumb. It is generally much smaller and there are problems in achieving stability as the toe has more joints than a thumb and there are therefore insufficient tendons to achieve balance. Nevertheless, the donor site deficit is slight and a second toe provides an

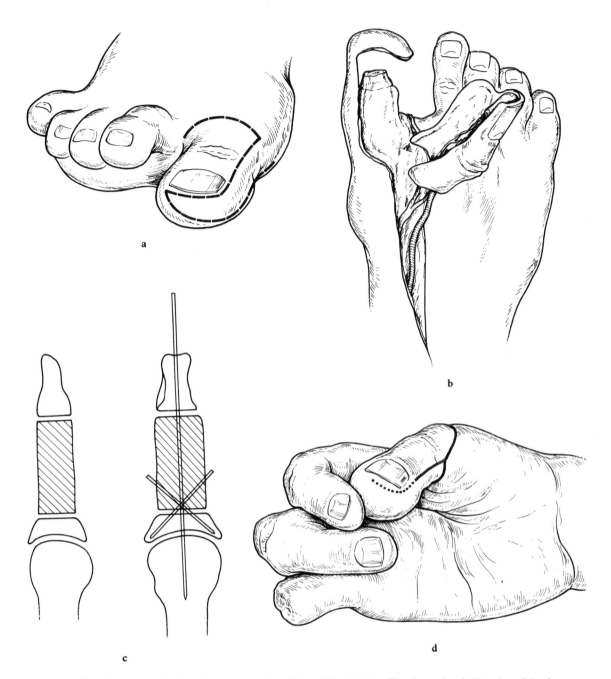

**Fig. 13.11** Thumb reconstruction by the wrap-around technique (Morrison). **a** The donor site. **b** Elevation of the flap to include the tuft of the distal phalanx. **c** Use of an interposition bone graft to achieve lengthening of the thumb. **d** The result

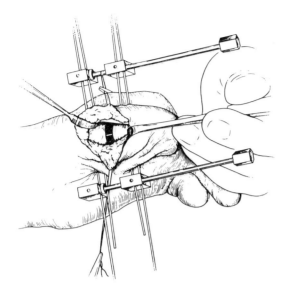

**Fig. 13.12** The Matev technique of distraction lengthening of the thumb skeleton

excellent innervated post. It is important to ensure that there is adequate skin in the area to achieve primary closure after free tissue transfer. A technique of flap transfer which incorporates a permanent pedicle (radial flap transfer) or a preliminary pedicled groin flap may be used to provide skin cover in addition to the free tissue transfer. The advantage of the permanent pedicle is the importation of a lasting source of blood supply.

3. If the amputation is proximal to the metacarpophalangeal joint, but the intrinsic muscles are relatively undamaged, the first choice is a thumb-lengthening procedure.

4. When the intrinsic muscles or the carpometacarpal joint have been destroyed, it may be better to amputate the damaged remnants of the thumb and pollicise the index finger (Fig. 13.14) (see Ch. 15). Even a damaged index finger may be suitable (or another damaged finger may be used).

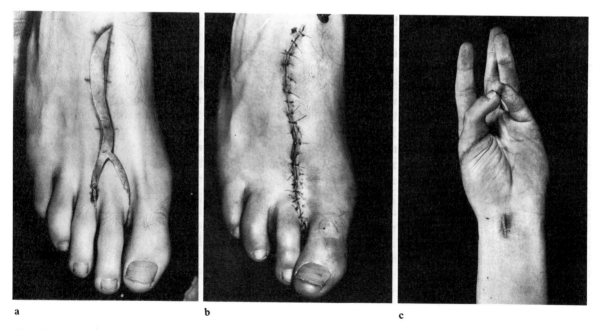

a                                    b                                    c

**Fig. 13.13** Thumb reconstruction by second toe transfer. **a** Harvesting the second toe. **b** Closure of the foot. **c** Late result

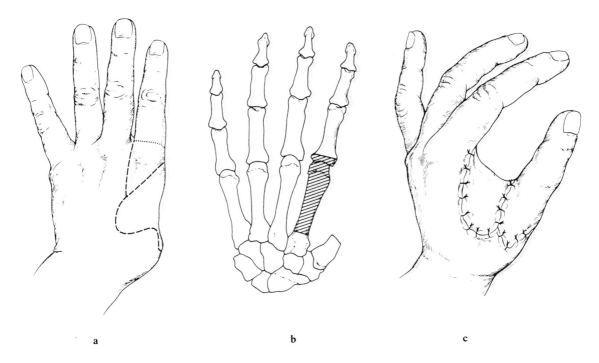

**Fig. 13.14** Thumb reconstruction by pollicisation. **a** Incisions used. **b** Bone removed. **c** The index is shortened and rotated and moved to the thumb position

Many of the techniques of thumb lengthening require the insertion of bone graft. Interpositional bone grafts are capable of being incorporated, but onlay bone grafts tend to resorb. The precise reason for this is unclear. Vascularised bone transfers may be preferable. The radius offers a local source of vascularised bone, part of which may be transferred on an inferiorly based pedicle of the radial artery and venae comitantes (Fig. 13.15).

If the thumb and index are both lost, pollicisation is contraindicated and a toe transfer is preferred. Restoration of prehension becomes less likely if there is an associated middle finger loss.

### Ulnar loss

The loss of the ulnar half of the hand is less significant than radial loss, as pinch and fine manipulation will often be preserved between the thumb, index and middle fingers. Power grip is, however, weak. There is therefore no indication for reconstruction of the missing ulnar part of the hand.

### Distal transverse loss

Distal transverse loss or amputation of the finger-tips is rarely amenable to reconstruction, although secondary procedures may be required for neuroma pain. Reconstruction of a single finger-pulp is possible (but rarely indicated) by vascularised tissue transfer using the techniques described by Foucher. Parts of the nail-bed and digital pulp may be replaced or a second toe transfer used to elongate a finger end, but it must be appreciated that the appearance of the finger may be ambiguous (Viktor Meyer has coined the term 'Tinger'). Cosmetic prostheses may improve function as well as appearance and have a wider application than has been previously recognised. Equalisation of finger lengths to correct a 'battlement hand' is occasionally required by amputation,

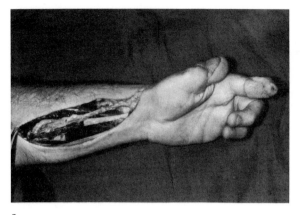

a

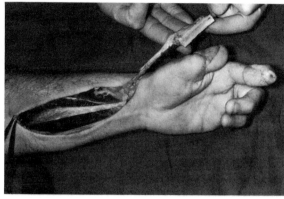

b

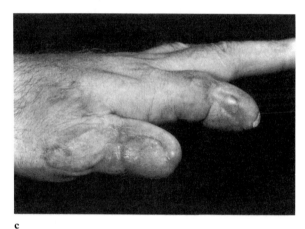

c

**Fig. 13.15** Thumb reconstruction by pedicled transfer of the radius on a vascular pedicle. **a** A 4 cm length of radius has been harvested on an inferiorly based pedicle including the radial artery and venae commitantes. The blood supply of the bone is maintained through a cuff of the flexor pollicis longus. **b** The bone peg is turned downwards and tunnelled to reach the thumb. A free toe-pulp transfer had previously been applied to the thumb reconstruction. **c** Late result

augmentation or telescoping the digit. Careful counselling and analysis of the functional demands are necessary.

**Proximal transverse loss**

Amputation through the metacarpophalangeal joints results in a functionally awkward hand. It may be preferable to widen the first web space to allow the patient to grip between the thumb and third metacarpal. It must be appreciated, however, that excision of the index metacarpal head will produce a more unsightly hand. Where cover is poor, innervated flaps may be migrated to cover the metacarpal heads. When the amputation is through the shafts of the metacarpals,

elongation of some of these by an on-top plasty may permit pinch (if the thumb is normal). This is a procedure whereby metacarpal remnants are migrated on top of others as vascularised or non-vascularised transfers. Skin cover may be difficult. Transfer of a toe or two toes allows reconstruction of a pinch or tripod (chuck) grip respectively. Both second toes may be moved separately, or a two-toe *en bloc* transfer of second and third toes from one foot is possible. Such surgery is rarely indicated if the patient has a normal contralateral upper limb.

**Total loss of the hand**

Total loss of the hand would generally be managed

by prosthetic replacement. If the loss is bilateral the patient is severely disabled. The Krukenberg operation separates the forearm bones and provides them with individual skin cover forming a rudimentary pinch. The appearance is unacceptable to most patients.

## SUMMARY

For judicious reconstruction the surgeon must be the master of the literature and all available techniques. He must keep his knowledge of the subject up to date and be aware of the expanding frontiers in the field. His knowledge and technical ability must be equalled by his judgement and timing.

# 14. Tendon transfers

*Principal author:* **F. D. Burke**

Absence of power in one muscle group may be compensated by transferring active muscles to replace the function that has been lost. Beasley has described this as a redistribution of the remaining functioning parts. The procedure may be indicated following injury to peripheral nerves, brachial plexus or spinal cord. Transfers may also be required following polio, cerebral palsy or leprosy. Tendon rupture following attrition or rheumatoid synovitis may merit tendon transfer.

## GENERAL PRINCIPLES

### Motor power

The tendon muscle unit to be transferred must be of adequate strength. In practice, this means normal muscle power. Transfer of a motor that is already weakened or reinnervated after injury is unlikely to achieve satisfactory function. Muscle power is graded on the Medical Research Council scale as:

0   No contraction.
1   A flicker of activity in the muscle.
2   A contraction of the muscle but inability to overcome gravitational forces.
3   Contraction that does overcome gravitational forces.
4   Contraction against resistance.
5   Normal function.

Useful function following transfer can only be obtained by using motors of strength 4 plus and 5. The maximal contractile force of a normal muscle is related to its cross-sectional area. It is approximately 3.5–4 kg/cm² of muscle.

### Tendon excursion

Tendon excursion varies considerably in the upper limb. The flexor profundus tendon's maximal excursion is approximately 70 mm, the digital extensors 50 mm and the wrist extensors 30 mm. The excursion of some muscles may be increased by extensive mobilisation prior to transfer but the increase achieved in this way is not great. Full wrist motion provides the digital tendons with optimal function. Power grip is strengthened by wrist extension; finger extension is augmented by wrist flexion. This 'tenodesis effect' plays a critical role in hand function — movement of the wrist adjusting the effect of the digital tendon excursion. Wrist fusion destroys this form of adjustment and is rarely of benefit if tendon transfers are to be considered.

### The direction of transfer

This is critical to the success of the procedure. The line of pull of the musculotendinous unit used for transfer should be as close as possible to that of the deficient motor. Extensive mobilisation of the muscle is often needed to achieve the necessary change in alignment. Care must be taken to preserve the neurovascular supply. Pulleys may be required to reroute the tendon but will reduce the power of the transfer.

### The tissue bed

The bed in which the transfer lies must be capable of permitting tendon excursion. Some loss of excursion must be expected even when a tendon is transferred in the most favourable of circumstances, thus reducing power. Dense fibrosis will prejudice the chances of satisfactory movement. If gross damage has occurred to the tissues, sufficient time must be allowed to elapse for the oedema and scarring to settle. Tendon transfers are often tunnelled through subcutaneous fat to minimise the chance of dense adhesions developing. If a transfer is passed through the interosseous membrane, a wide window is required to minimise the risk of tendon adhesion.

## Joint mobility

No transfer will achieve a greater range of motion at the joint than was passively available preoperatively. Therefore, several months' rehabilitation therapy may be required before the tissues are suitable for tendon transfer. There should be no, or minimal, joint contracture and a soft supple hand.

## Synergism

Synergism has been considered as an important factor in the choice of a tendon for transfer. This concept is now felt to be of more minor significance. Wrist extensors potentiate and are synergistic with the finger flexors. As the fingers flex the wrist extends. If a synergistic muscle is available for transfer, it is probably more readily incorporated into subsequent hand function. However, antagonists are frequently used with good effect, since the direction, force and amplitude of the transfer are more important factors.

## Functional consideration

Each tendon transferred should only be required for one function. Attempts to produce a variety of functions from a single tendon are unlikely to be successful. In the assessment of a possible tendon for transfer, the disadvantages of losing its original function must be outweighed by the benefit that its new action will bring to the hand.

## The timing of tendon transfers

The role of early tendon transfers following nerve injuries is controversial. Such early transfers may produce subsequent tendon imbalance if reinnervation occurs. Additionally, they will sacrifice function needlessly and revision of the transfer may be required. However, where the prospect of reinnervation is remote, transfers may be considered as soon as the limb is supple.

When assessing a patient for transfer, it is prudent to draw up a list of those functions that have been lost in the upper limb and an adjacent list of possible tendons that could be used to motor the deficit. Muscles are then chosen for the transfers based on the previously mentioned factors (Table 14.1). It is beyond the scope of this book to detail all the varieties of tendon transfers for peripheral nerve injuries. Absence of available motors or inability to use certain routes justifies several options for each transfer. Some examples of transfers are included to clarify the preceding section.

## TENDON TRANSFERS FOR RADIAL NERVE PALSY

Under favourable circumstances, the results of radial nerve repair or graft are gratifying. Where possible, function should be regained by reinnervating the existing muscles. If this is inappropriate (distal nerve avulsion, extensive muscle damage or poor reinnervation following repair), consideration may be given to tendon transfers. The tendon transfers for radial nerve palsy shown in Table 14.1 produce excellent functional results:

*1. Pronator teres* requires little rerouting to pull in the appropriate direction, but the excursion of the muscle is small and only a limited range of motion results from this transfer. Nevertheless, it

**Table 14.1**   Tendon transfers for radial nerve palsy

| Function lost to the upper limb | Transfers |
| --- | --- |
| 1. Wrist extension | Pronator teres to extensor carpi radialis brevis |
| 2. Finger extension | Flexor carpi ulnaris to extensor digitorum communis |
| 3. Thumb extension | Palmaris longus to extensor pollicis longus |

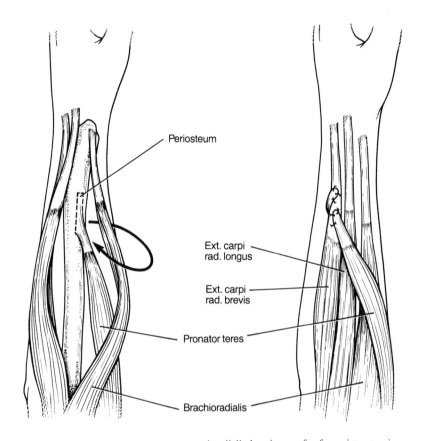

Fig. 14.1   Pronator teres to extensor carpi radialis brevis transfer for wrist extension

places the wrist in a dorsiflexed position and permits the finger flexors to grasp firmly. The pronator teres is sutured to the extensor carpi radialis brevis tendon, which inserts into the third metacarpal base, and this tends to avoid any significant radial or ulnar deviation in dorsiflexion (Fig. 14.1). Pronator function is maintained by pronator quadratus. The loss of donor function in these cases is so slight and the benefits of early active wrist extension so great, that in this particular case the early transfer of pronator teres may be considered, even though reinnervation is anticipated (thereby breaking the general rule). An element of metacarpophalangeal joint extension is achieved through the tenodesis effect of wrist flexion. If this effect is inadequate, a tendon transfer is indicated.

*2. Flexor carpi ulnaris* requires extensive mobilisation to permit realignment around the ulnar border of the forearm (Fig. 14.2). A large incision is required on the volar aspect and the muscle is dissected proximally until satisfactory mobility is achieved. The neurovascular supply is proximally based and is preserved. The tendon is then brought around the forearm and sutured to the four extensor communis tendons. In the past the distal end of the tendon was sutured to extensor pollicis longus to produce a mass action of thumb and finger extension.

*3. More recently, palmaris longus,* if available, has been used to achieve thumb extension. The extensor pollicis longus is divided proximally and mobilised distally. It is rerouted to be joined to palmaris longus in the forearm (Fig. 14.3) This

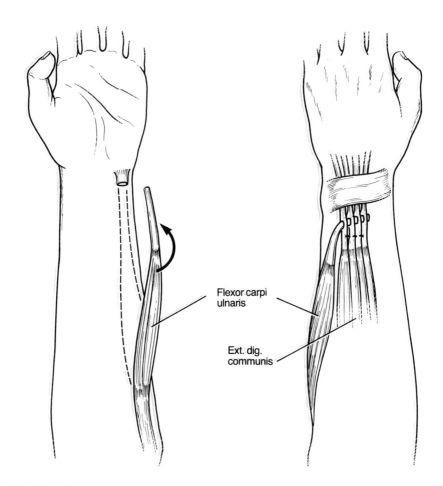

**Fig. 14.2** Flexor carpi ulnaris to extensor digitorum communis transfer for finger extension

permits the thumb to be extended and abducted from the palm, independent of finger extension.

## MEDIAN NERVE PALSY

Damage to the motor branch of the median nerve may result in loss of thumb opposition (the ability to radially abduct and pronate the thumb out of the palm). In median nerve injury the degree of opposition loss is variable. A surprising number of patients maintain active opposition due to variations in thenar muscle innervation. If opposition is lost, the thumb lies in the palm and cannot be effectively drawn over to oppose to the fingers. Pinch grip tends to be between the ulnar border of the thumb, rather than the full pulp. The disability will be compounded if the thumb is allowed to lie in an adducted position in the postinjury period, permitting a first web space contracture to develop. Opposition loss does cause significant disability and many tendon transfers have been devised to overcome the problem.

The most popular transfer is that described by Bunnell, where the superficial flexor of the ring finger is rerouted around flexor carpi ulnaris near the pisiform and passed across the palm to the thumb (Fig. 14.4). The tendon may be inserted into the abductor pollicis brevis tendon, the base of the proximal phalanx or the insertion of extensor pollicis brevis. The latter will result in

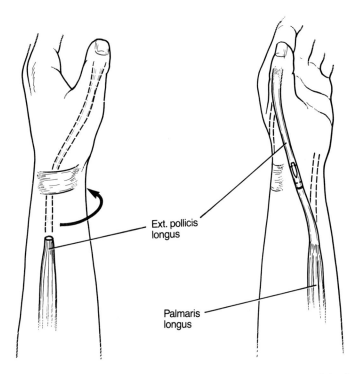

**Fig. 14.3**  Palmaris longus transfer to a distally re-routed extensor pollicis longus for thumb abduction and extension

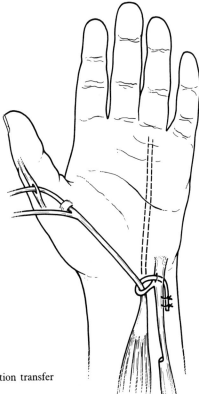

**Fig. 14.4**  Ring superficialis opposition transfer

more satisfactory rotation of the thumb. The direction of pull of superficialis around its pulley lowers its efficiency but the muscle remains sufficiently powerful to achieve opposition. The transfer is generally successful in isolated median nerve palsy, but if there is a total intrinsic paralysis (combined median and ulnar nerve injury) grip strength is significantly reduced and the superficial flexor is more valuable in its original role. In such cases, a single opposition transfer will not permit the destabilised thumb to function satisfactorily.

Extensor indicis proprius can be used as an opposition transfer. Extensor indicis is divided at the level of the metacarpophalangeal joint and freed proximally in the forearm. Very extensive mobilisation of the tendon and muscle is required

to achieve sufficient length to reach the thumb. However, the line of action of the rerouted tendon around the ulnar border is excellent and no pulley is required (Fig. 14.5).

The Camitz transfer has proved of benefit in patients presenting with longstanding carpal tunnel syndrome with marked wasting of the median innervated thenar musculature. Palmaris longus is used as the motor, but it has insufficient length to reach the thumb. At the time of carpal tunnel decompression, a strip of palmar fascia is raised in continuity with palmaris longus to achieve the necessary additional length. The tendon transfer is then sutured to the insertion of abductor pollicis brevis. Carpal tunnel decompression is achieved with return of thumb abduction (Fig. 14.6).

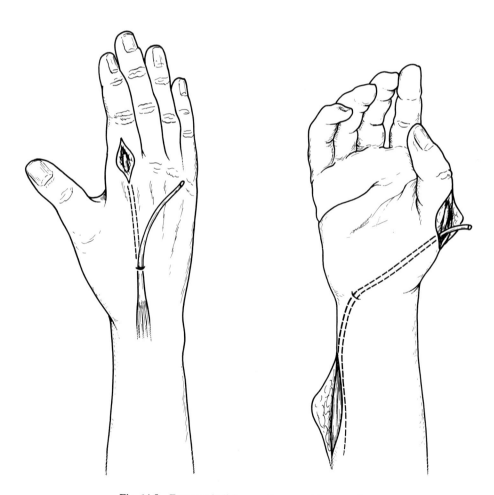

**Fig. 14.5**   Extensor indicis proprius opposition transfer

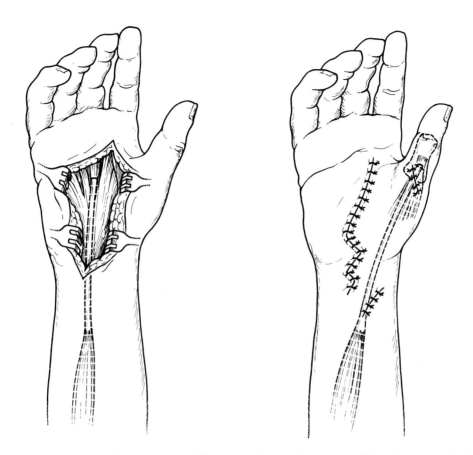

**Fig. 14.6**   The Camitz transfer: palmaris longus mobilised in continuity with a portion of the palmar fascia for thumb abduction

## LOW ULNAR PALSY

A low ulnar nerve palsy causes loss of thumb adduction, loss of index abduction and clawing of ring and little fingers.

*1. Loss of thumb adduction.* The brachioradialis may be mobilised, lengthened with a tendon graft and passed through the interspace between the third and fourth metacarpals. It is then attached to the abductor insertion (Fig. 14.7a). Alternatively the superficialis of the middle or ring finger (if the profundus is of normal power) may be passed across the palm to insert in like manner (Fig. 14.7b). The distal end of the palmar fascia forms the pulley. If the superficialis tendon is used, further weakening of grip occurs. Pinch grip is improved by both types of tendon transfer, but thumb metacarpophalangeal joint fusion is frequently required to achieve adequate first ray stability.

*2. Loss of index abduction.* First dorsal interosseous function may be regained by transferring a tendon to the interosseous insertion. Extensor indicis, a slip of abductor pollicis longus or a flexor superficialis have all been recommended for this transfer. Extensor indicis proprius needs considerable radial rerouting to produce strong abduction. The flexor superficialis is more valuable in its correct role. A slip of abductor pollicis longus can be spared and has a more suitable line of pull (Fig. 14.8).

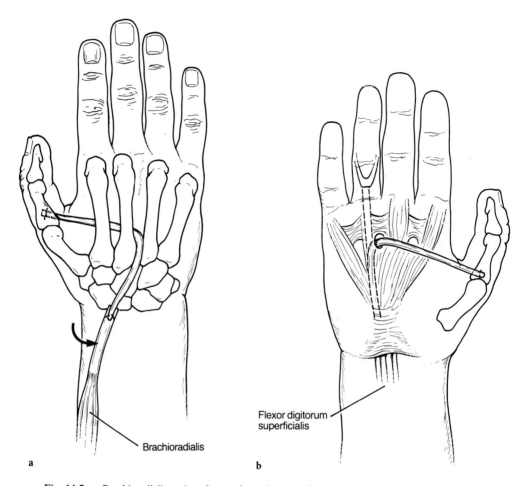

**Fig. 14.7**   **a** Brachioradialis and graft transfer and **b** superficialis transfer for thumb adduction

*3. Clawing of the ring and little fingers.* In early clawing, where the deformity is still correctable, active extension of the proximal interphalangeal joint can be achieved by blocking hyperextension at the metacarpophalangeal joint. The clinical test can be reproduced surgically by the Zancolli I procedure (Fig. 14.9). The volar plate is reefed to produce a block to further extension at a position of 30° of flexion. The foreshortened volar plate tends to slowly stretch out with use. A dynamic transfer is preferred. The Zancolli II procedure involves lassooing the flexor superficialis around the A2 pulley and suturing it to itself, thus limiting full metacarpophalangeal joint extension and allowing the central slip of the extensor

tendon to produce full proximal interphalangeal joint extension (Fig. 14.10). Clawing is corrected by this means.

*4. Inability to grasp large objects because of poor finger roll-up.* This is due to intrinsic dysfunction and a dynamic intrinsic transfer into the paralysed intrinsics is required.

## THUMB EXTENSION

Isolated rupture of extensor pollicis longus occurs following a minimally displaced Colles' fracture, or more commonly from rheumatoid synovitis under the extensor retinaculum. The ruptured tendon is frequently attenuated over a consider-

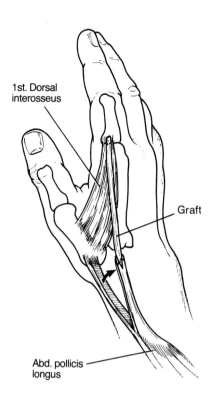

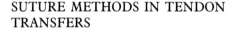

**Fig. 14.8**  A slip of abductor pollicis longus with graft for index abduction

able distance and direct repair is inappropriate. In these cases, the extensor indicis proprius is divided at the level of the index metacarpal head and drawn back to a small incision at the wrist. It is then rerouted to the base of the thumb and sutured to the distal portion of extensor pollicis longus.

## SUTURE METHODS IN TENDON TRANSFERS

Tendons may be joined in a variety of ways:

*1. The Pulvertaft weave.* This is a much stronger repair than the simple end-to-end apposition used in trauma. The adjacent tissues must be released over a sufficiently wide area to permit adequate excursion of the tendon junction. One tendon is passed at right angles through the other

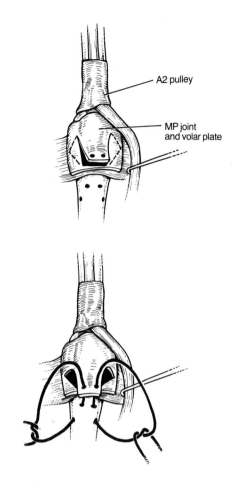

**Fig. 14.9**  The Zancolli I procedure: reefing of the metacarpophalangeal joint volar plate

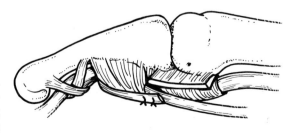

**Fig. 14.10**  The Zancolli II procedure

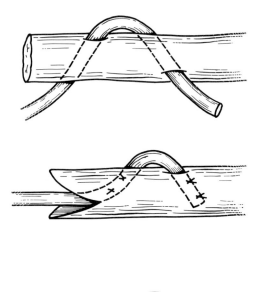

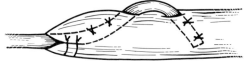

**Fig. 14.11**    The Pulvertaft weave

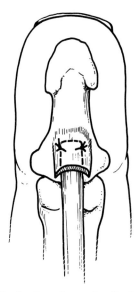

**Fig. 14.12**    Tendon insertion to the distal phalanx

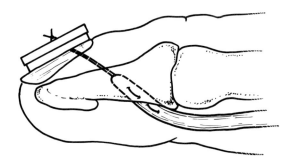

**Fig. 14.13**    Tendon insertion to bone

two or three times in different planes and sutured with non-absorbable material (Fig. 14.11).

*2. End-to-side repair.* This is particularly appropriate if reinnervation is possible, or several tendons are being motored by a single transfer (e.g. flexor carpi ulnaris to the finger and thumb extensors).

*3. Tendon insertion to bone.* A variety of techniques may be used. In the case of the profundus tendon, the stump is usually preserved. The remnant can be elevated at its proximal end and the tendon graft sutured beneath it (Fig. 14.12). A wire suture may be inserted into the tendon, passed through drill holes in the distal phalanx and tied over a button on the dorsal aspect of the finger. A variation of this technique is to drill a hole in the distal phalanx on the volar side, where the tendon is to be inserted. The distal end of the tendon graft has a stitch passed through it and then the suture and graft are drawn into the hole in the distal phalanx. The suture is brought out on the dorsal side and tied over a button (Fig. 14.13).

## POSTOPERATIVE MANAGEMENT

Tendon transfers are usually placed in sufficient tension to produce mild over-correction in the resting limb. On completion of the transfer, a tenodesis test (passive flexion and extension of the wrist) is performed to ensure that the tension is not excessive, preventing full passive range at the involved joint. The test ensures that the excursion of the transfer is unrestricted. The position of immobilisation should ensure that the tendon transfer is not under tension. The transfer is statically immobilised for a minimum of 4 weeks and thereafter protected by dynamic splintage during the continuing healing phase. Physiotherapy and rehabilitation are of prime importance in establishing the use of the transfer.

# SECTION 5

# 15. Congenital hand deformities

*Principal author: P. J. Smith*

The birth of a child is an eagerly awaited event. The presence of an obvious deformity is a traumatic experience for the parents. They are subjected to a mixture of emotions ranging from disbelief, anger and guilt, to anxiety regarding the child's future. Concern about future limitation in the child's abilities is foremost in their minds. Many parents have unrealistic aims, expecting the surgeon to produce a normal hand. It is at this stage, while still in the nursery or maternity unit, that the initial consultation with a surgeon who is familiar with the problem should occur, as this can have a reassuring influence. Detailed discussion is best left until a later outpatient appointment, when the realistic aims should be carefully explained and a programme of reconstructive surgery outlined. Such a programme may require the use of a wide variety of surgical techniques involving orthopaedic, plastic and microsurgical procedures. The surgeon providing this advice must have up-to-date information about the rapid pace of development in reconstructive surgery. Early well-informed contact encourages parental confidence — an essential aid when a child requires numerous operative procedures to achieve the maximum correction of a complex deformity. The presence of multiple anomalies requires close co-operation between the hand surgeon and his paediatric colleagues.

## DEFORMITY AND DISABILITY

Attitudes to deformity vary. In western civilisation, patients with hand deformities are no longer ostracised and are more readily accepted by society. However, the patient is made more aware of his deformity by the high expectation of normality by the community. Although informed adults now have a more tolerant attitude to obvious deformity, children do not. For a child with an uncorrected deformity, the psychological stresses are considerable, especially in early school life and adolescence. Surgeons concern themselves with the functional disability of such patients, but the patients themselves are more often concerned with their appearance.

Children with congenital hand deformities present with differing levels of disability. With minor degrees of structural deformity, inability to perform precision pinch may be the only loss of function. In the spectrum of hand function, this ability lies at the more sophisticated end. Its loss is related to digital disproportion or disarray. With greater degrees of structural deformity more basic hand functions are lost. Inability to grasp may be related to digital absence. In the most severe deformities, prehension (the ability to reach out and grasp) becomes bimanual. It is at this level that independence is impaired. Thus the grades of deformity form a ladder of functional ability. Surgery may help a child ascend this ladder. Demonstrations of amazing dexterity from severely deformed children, such as those with bilateral single digits who are capable of tying their shoe laces, mean little if they are incapable of attending to personal hygiene. Such dependence strikes at the very root of their developing personality. If it is possible to improve their functional independence by the judicious use of surgery, treatment should be undertaken, but this may be a difficult decision. While there are many surgical ladders, there are also surgical snakes.

## PRINCIPLES AND PLANNING OF SURGICAL TREATMENT

The aims in the treatment of congenital hand deformities are:

1. Restoration of the basic functions of a normal hand; grasp and precision pinch.
2. Unrestricted growth.
3. A cosmetically acceptable hand.

In assessing these children, the first question to ask is 'should anything be done?' If the aims are already achieved, then clearly the child requires no treatment. Careful annual review is required, even in these children, to allow repeated assessment of growth, functional adaptation and deformity. If no treatment is possible, a child is forced to adapt to the limitations imposed by its deformity.

In other children, orthotic, prosthetic or surgical treatment may be required. Splintage is more effective the earlier it is instituted. It is of particular value in the treatment of radial club hand, where it may achieve pre-operative passive correction of the deformity, allowing later surgical stabilisation. Splintage has a role to play in the management of many congenital deformities, correcting deformity, maintaining corrections achieved surgically, and preventing postoperative scar tissue contractures in their early dynamic phase. In certain circumstances, reconstructive procedures may improve function, but produce such a cosmetically unacceptable result that the patient will prefer a prosthetic alternative. In other deformities prosthetic augmentation is the only option (e.g. complete agenesis at the wrist level or more proximally is best treated by the provision of a powered prosthesis). Recently, there have been significant developments in this field and liaison with a prosthetic service specialising in hands is desirable.

Careful observation of the child's hand function is necessary before any conclusions can be reached about the advisability of surgery. This may involve the redistribution, augmentation or realignment of structures, in order to correct structural deficiencies and deformities. Correction of deformity may require osteotomy, tendon transfer, release of skin shortages or provision of good skin cover. Correction of deficiencies involves tissue augmentation using a range of reconstructive procedures from bone grafting and flap cover techniques to the transfer of composite tissues by microsurgical means. Unsuspected anatomical abnormalities frequently complicate congenital hand surgery. Motors for tendon transfer may be poor or absent and vascular anomalies are common. Growth may be redirected by the release of tissue shortages which tether growing bones. Epiphysial plates should be protected during surgical procedures. It should be appreciated that sensation is normal in the congenitally deformed hand, alteration in its quality is only secondary to surgery. Established abnormal prehensile patterns influence cortical representation. These prehensile contact areas of the deformed hand should remain undisturbed by surgery.

The timing of surgery is governed by many factors. Urgent surgery may be required in the neonatal period in cases of congenital ring constriction syndrome with severe distal lymphoedema. Surgery in the first year of life should be undertaken for complex syndactyly between digits of differing length. The treatment of radial club hand should be commenced early. These problems will be discussed in detail later. Pollicisation, if indicated, should follow shortly. The child only becomes aware of the abnormal appearance and function of his own hand when he first leaves his protected family environment to enter playgroup or school. Surgical treatment should, if possible, have been completed prior to the child commencing school, in the hope that the taunts of his classmates will be minimised. If further surgical treatment is necessary, it should be so timed as to limit the loss of schooling.

The ability to undertake co-ordinated purposeful movement in the hand is a milestone of development dependent upon postnatal maturation of the peripheral nervous system. A primitive grasp reflex is present from birth, but precision pinch develops later. Early surgery allows the incorporation of the reconstructed precision pinch mechanism into the emerging patterns of prehension and manipulation. Early pollicisation allows the child to develop dexterity with the reconstructed thumb. Later pollicisation necessitates a relearning process as patterns of dorsal prehension have been established.

*The hand rapidly increases in size during the first four years of life.* Microsurgical reconstruction using small recipient vessels is best left until this age unless larger vessels are to be used. The age at which these procedures are undertaken may also be modified according to the experience of the surgeon. Arteriography should be performed prior to any microvascular procedure in the congenital hand, as vascular anomalies are frequent and vessel size may be much smaller than expected. In procedures where detailed postoperative rehabilitation is required, reconstruction is delayed until the child is old enough to co-operate.

Like the face, the hand is an important cosmetic unit. It is an area of the body on constant display. Without pockets, deformed hands would have nowhere to hide. Gloves are often worn to cover scarred or grafted areas. It is essential that the results of surgery should be cosmetically acceptable.

## INCIDENCE

Congenital deformities of the upper limb are not unusual. There is approximately one anomaly for every six hundred live births. Syndactyly is the commonest of these deformities followed by polydactyly. The relative incidence of the various deformities varies from country to country, but in the UK a frequency table (Table 15.1) has been established.

## EMBRYOLOGY

The limb buds make their first appearance during the fourth week of intra-uterine life on the ventro-lateral surface of the embryo, opposite the eighth to twelfth myotomes (these correspond to the lower sixth cervical and the two upper thoracic vertebrae) (Fig. 15.1a). The upper limb buds develop marginally in advance of the lower limb buds.

The first indication of the presence of musculature in the limb is found in the seventh week, as a condensation of mesenchyme at the proximal portion of the limb bud. It is not known whether the muscle differentiates in situ, or if it migrates from the cervical myotomes (Fig. 15.1b). As the

**Table 15.1** Incidence of congenital upper-limb defects[a]

| Defect[b] | No. of infants[c] | Fraction of total (per 10 000) |
|---|---|---|
| 1. Failure of formation | | |
| 1.1 Transverse | | |
| Transcarpal | 3 (1) | 0.6 |
| Below elbow | 2 (0) | 0.4 |
| Shoulder | 1 (1) | 0.2 |
| 1.2 Longitudinal | | |
| Radius | 4 (4) | 0.8 |
| Ulna | 1 (1) | 0.2 |
| Hand | | |
| Preaxial | 8 (8) | 1.5 |
| Central | 13 (11) | 2.5 |
| Postaxial | 9 (8) | 1.7 |
| 2. Failure of separation of parts | | |
| Syndactyly | 8 (5) | 1.5 |
| Radioulnar synostosis | 1 (1) | 0.2 |
| 3. Duplication | | |
| Polydactyly | | |
| Preaxial | 18 (1) | 3.5 |
| Postaxial | 28 (13) | 5.4 |
| 4. Overgrowth | | |
| Forearm/hand | 1 (1) | 0.2 |
| 5. Undergrowth | | |
| Forearm/hand | 2 (2) | 0.4 |
| Brachydactyly | 8 (6) | 1.5 |
| 6. Constriction band syndrome | | |
| Hand | 3 (3) | 0.6 |
| 7. Others | 3 (3) | 0.6 |
| Total | 113 (69) | 21.6 |

[a]Derived from the Edinburgh Register of the Newborn (1964–1968) accepted by the International Federation of Hand Societies.
[b]Using classification by Swanson et al.
[c]The first figure in the column shows the total number of infants affected. The second figure (in parentheses) indicates those within the total in which the specified limb defect is present along with other limb abnormalities, for example, malformations of the lower limbs, or as part of a known syndrome.
Reproduced with permission from Lamb DW & Law HT, Upper-limb deficiencies in children: prosthetic, orthotic and surgical management. Little, Brown and Company, Boston, MA.

limb ventral buds elongate, the muscular tissue divides into central and dorsal components. Muscles may have origins from more than one segment. The spinal nerves penetrate the base of the limb buds early in their development. It may be necessary for the spinal nerves to come into

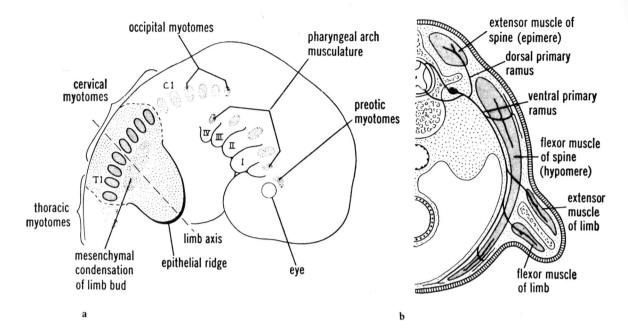

**Fig. 15.1** **a** Transverse section through the cervical myotomes showing mesenchymal condensations. **b** Transverse section through the developing limb bud showing the origin of the extensor and flexor muscles

contact with the differentiating muscle cells early, as a prerequisite for their complete development. These nerves are also responsible for the sensory distribution to the limb. As time progresses and development proceeds, fusions may occur between the various branches.

Differentiation begins and continues in a proximodistal sequence, with the arm and forearm appearing before the hand. By the fourth week, a constriction is present separating the upper arm from the forearm and towards the end of this week, the digital swellings first become evident. By the fifth week, the hand plate, with prominent digital swellings, is clearly demarcated from the forearm and arm. The skeletal framework is represented by areas of hyaline cartilage. By the end of the seventh week, the arm, forearm and hand have achieved their recognisable adult form, although internal differentiation is still proceeding. Form is established before the pregnancy is confirmed.

At the time of birth, all structures within the hand are fully differentiated, except for the nervous system. Prenatal movement may have a profound influence on the development of tissue planes.

## POSTNATAL DEVELOPMENT OF HAND FUNCTION

Shortly after birth, the hands begin to play an important role in the exploration of the environment. Early movements are unco-ordinated and are performed as mass actions or as individual muscles contracting in isolation. At this stage, the hand has two basic functions; grasp, as seen in the grip reflex, and the use of the flat hand. This is occasionally seen in breast-fed infants, who rest their hands on the maternal breast. As the child matures, patterns of co-ordinated use develop. By the first birthday, the child is able to oppose his thumb and pick up objects. He can also position the hand and grip firmly. Postnatal peripheral and central changes in the nervous system lead to an improvement in strength and dexterity. The brain is a sophisticated computer capable of self-programming. Sensory and visual stimulation lead to central software development and this ability is age related. Peripheral physical changes (myelination) represent hardware alterations which are most rapid during the first 2 years. Software programming, however, continues throughout life as the individual strives to acquire new skills.

## AETIOLOGY

'What caused the deformity?' is a frequent and early parental enquiry. It is a difficult question for a clinician to answer, but he should have some basic understanding of the principles involved. A congenital deformity can arise in two ways: inheritance of faulty genetic coding, or due to an alteration in intra-uterine environmental factors. In most cases, the cause remains unclear.

The faulty genes are located in the chromosomes of the fertilised ovum from which the individual develops. Such abnormalities may affect a single gene, multiple genes or the chromosome as a whole. The pattern of single gene inheritance, or Mendelian inheritance, may be dominant, recessive or sex-linked. Where the affected gene is dominant, the deformity will appear in heterozygous offspring. Syndactyly and polydactyly are inherited in this way. If the heterozygote marries a normal person, then there is a 50% chance of each child having the defect. Recessive abnormalities tend to be more severe than the dominant ones, e.g. acrocephalopolysyndactyly. In these abnormalities, both parents have been carrying a recessive gene. Of their children, 25% will show the defect, 25% will be normal, and half of their children may become carriers. In sex-linked inheritance, the affected gene lies within the X chromosome (orofaciodigital syndrome Type I).

Congenital hand deformities associated with chromosomal defects tend to be part of major syndromes, for example, Turner's syndrome (X0) in which there is a short fourth metacarpal. There are also autosomal chromosomal defects, the commonest being trisomy 21 (Down's syndrome).

Congenital deformities, due to changes in the internal embryological environment, account for the remaining abnormalities. The internal milieu may be influenced directly and indirectly by anoxia, irradiation, hormones, drugs and some viral infections. The physical intra-uterine environment may lead to congenital amputation or ring constriction syndrome. The aetiology of most congenital hand anomalies is, however, unknown. Questioning the mother regarding the possible intake of teratogens, viral infections, or other events occurring within the first 7 weeks of pregnancy is unlikely to yield any useful information and may exacerbate any feelings of guilt. It cannot be emphasised too strongly that this enquiry should be avoided in the immediate postnatal period and left until the parents request genetic counselling. Great sensitivity is required by the attending physicians.

## CLASSIFICATION

Classifications are arbitrary and are constrained by the limits of current knowledge. They are never perfect and boundaries will always be blurred. At present the classification proposed by the American Society for Surgery of the Hand has been adopted by the International Federation of Societies for Surgery of the Hand. This classification is based on the supposed embryological failures related to the production of any particular deformity.

1. Failure of the formation of parts (arrest of development).
2. Failure of differentiation or separation of parts.
3. Duplications.
4. Overgrowth (gigantism).
5. Undergrowth (hypoplasia).
6. Congenital constriction band syndrome.
7. Generalised skeletal abnormalities.

There still remain areas of confusion and conditions which defy precise classification.

## FAILURE OF FORMATION OF PARTS — GROUP 1

In this group, where arrest of development has occurred, the failure may be transverse or longitudinal (Fig. 15.2). Transverse arrest of development produces a so-called 'congenital amputation'. Amputation in the presence of a

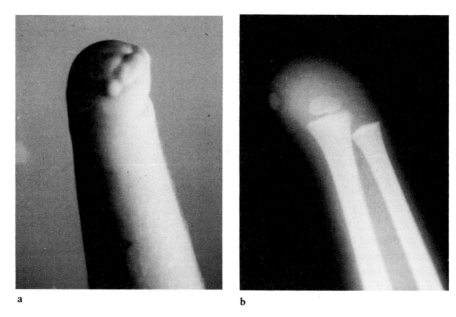

a                                    b

Fig. 15.2  a, b Congenital transverse arrest of development

constriction ring is not included in this group. Transverse arrest may occur at any level. Common sites include the transverse forearm defect occurring just below the elbow joint and transverse carpal defects. All failures of development which are not congenital amputations form the longitudinal group. Such defects may include isolated failure of the radial, central or ulnar components of the limb or total segmental failure. In recent years, total segmental failure has been associated with the intake of thalidomide used in an attempt to control nausea during the first trimester of pregnancy. The alternative term is 'phocomelia', derived from the Greek and implying similarity to a seal flipper. If complete, the hand is directly attached to the trunk. If the arm is missing and the forearm and hand are attached to the trunk, the defect is described as proximal phocomelia. In distal phocomelia the forearm is absent with the hand being attached at the elbow.

Failure of development of the pre-axial or postaxial segment of the limb may result in radial club hand, or its ulnar equivalent. Distal to the wrist, central defects produce cleft hand deformities. In the mildest cases, there may be absence of the third ray. With progressively more severe involvement, the second, third and fourth rays may be absent, producing a 'lobster claw hand'. In the most severe forms, central deficiency may be combined with radial or ulnar failure.

## Radial club hand

The term 'radial club hand' describes radial deviation of the wrist, producing an appearance similar to a golf club (Fig. 15.3). This is associated with thumb hypoplasia, or with total absence of the thumb, first metacarpal, scaphoid, trapezium and the radius. There are varying degrees of involvement. The index and middle fingers are stiff. The deformity is not confined to the pre-axial border of the limb. The ulna is always abnormal. It never achieves normal size and is often short and curved. The remnants of the pre-axial bones and muscles may be condensed into a vestigial counterpart — the so-called Anlage (German derivation). There may be neurovascular abnormalities which must be considered where pollicisation proves necessary. Associated elbow stiffness is pronounced during the first 2 years, but may diminish as time progresses, with many children achieving a 90° range of movement. Early elbow stiffness is thus

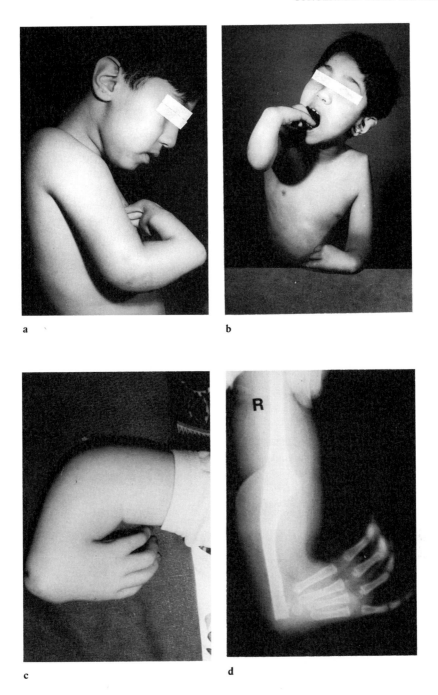

**Fig. 15.3** **a** Radial club hand. Note the shortness of the forearm, the radial deviation and hypoplasia of the thumb. **b** The child is still capable of reaching his mouth and feeding himself. **c** Another example of radial club hand with the thumb completely absent. **d** Radial club hand with an absent thumb

not an absolute contraindication to surgical realignment of the wrist. Precision pinch is always impaired. Affected children use dorsal prehension and are incapable of unilateral fine manipulative tasks. If the thumb is absent, pollicisation may be indicated to provide this mechanism. Grasp may be improved by wrist centralisation as the power of the digital flexors is thereby increased. The short forearm and radial deviation of the wrist permit hand-to-mouth function. Wrist realignment, although contributing to improved hand posture, may prevent the hand reaching the mouth, especially in the presence of a stiff elbow. Many children with this deformity achieve a surprising functional ability. Surgery on both hands in bilateral deformities must be carefully considered. There may be a conflict between the desire for cosmetic improvement and the possibility of functional impairment. Cosmesis, however, is of such significance, that many adult patients with established deformity will request wrist realignment in an attempt to improve their appearance.

### Treatment

**Splintage**. Splintage should be commenced shortly after birth. The aim is to achieve a full passive correction of the deformity and to prevent secondary shortening of the soft tissues. Serial plaster casts are used initially, extending above the flexed elbow. A ratchet-type splint is useful. Manipulative treatment, similar to that used in the management of club foot, may be undertaken at a later stage, or for less deformed cases. Two years of splintage may be necessary to achieve positioning of the carpus on the distal end of the ulna. If progress is being maintained, conservative treatment should be continued until wrist centralisation is undertaken (Fig. 15.4).

**Wrist centralisation**. If no improvement occurs with splintage, or progress ceases, this may be attributable to tethering of the radial structures due to soft tissue tightness, or the presence of an Anlage. Radiographs may reveal bowing of the ulna. Early surgical release of the soft tissues is indicated in such cases. Growth may aggravate the situation, increasing the taughtness of the soft tissues and thus the curvature of the ulna. To achieve centralisation of the wrist, osteotomy of the ulna and carpal bone excisions may be required in addition to soft tissue release. Maintaining the position of the centralised carpus on the distal end of the ulna is difficult. Tendon transfers are required to prevent recurrent deformity. There is some controversy as to whether centralisation can be maintained by such techniques. Bone fusion is advocated by some authors and is more likely to obtain permanent correction. In achieving this, the growth zone of

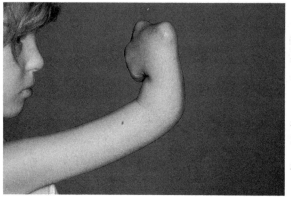 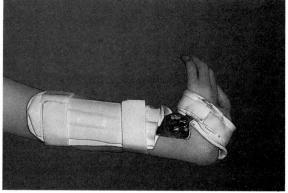

a                                                        b

**Fig. 15.4  a** Radial club hand. The deviation is so severe that one can see thinning of the skin on the ulnar side of the wrist. **b** The use of a ratchet type splint should be commenced shortly after birth in order to attempt to correct the deformity. If progress is arrested then surgical release of the structures on the radial side of the wrist may be necessary

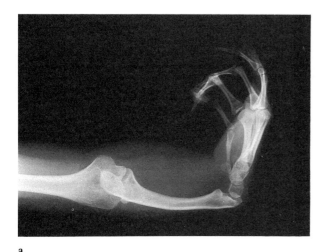 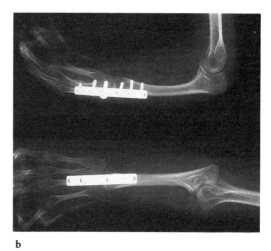

a b

Fig. 15.5 a Radial club hand with marked wrist deviation. b AO plating has been used to achieve wrist centralisation and fusion

the ulna is destroyed leaving the bone shorter. This may not be disadvantageous, as it allows the hand and corrected wrist to reach the mouth because of the short forearm. The mobility of the elbow often increases following wrist centralisation. Some surgeons now overcorrect the deformity by undertaking a radialisation of the carpus to prevent the problem of recurrent deformity. Others have replaced the absent radius using vascularised fibula transfers in an attempt to stimulate radial growth and produce a dynamic correction of the deformity (Fig. 15.5).

*Pollicisation*. Having corrected the position of the hand, attention may be directed towards the function of prehension, particularly precision pinch. In most cases no thumb is present and in others it is so hypoplastic as to be non-functional (Fig. 15.6a). Pollicisation is the creation of a new thumb from an existing digit. Despite its stiffness, the index finger is most commonly used. It is a complex operation with repositioning of the index finger as a thumb, based upon its neurovascular pedicles (Fig. 15.6b,c). The metacarpal is shortened and rotated. The metacarpophalangeal joint becomes the new carpometacarpal joint. Tendon transfers are required to produce a 'balanced thumb'. A satisfactory first web space is created by the use of local skin flaps. Because of the stiffness of the index finger, it has been suggested that the finger should not be shortened to the length appropriate to the normal thumb–index relationship. For the same reason, the ring finger should not be pollicised for this disturbs the normal function of the ulnar side of the hand. Pollicisation should only be undertaken after the vascular status of the digit to be transferred has been ascertained. The digital Allen's test can be used clinically in children old enough to co-operate, but in general, arteriography is necessary, especially in the more severe deformities. Doppler ultrasound may be useful. These techniques provide an anatomical assessment of the vessels. At operative exploration, a functional assessment using vascular clamps should be undertaken.

The timing of these procedures is of importance. Wrist centralisation may be delayed in an attempt to preserve forearm length. However, it is now felt that little is lost by early intervention. It is therefore undertaken as soon as passive correction proves possible. If pollicisation were to be performed prior to centralisation, the tendon balance would be subsequently altered by the wrist procedure. It is therefore usually performed about 6 months after operation on the wrist.

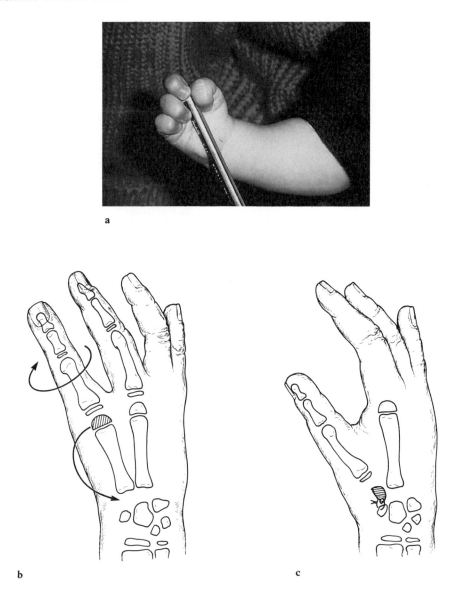

**Fig. 15.6** Pollicisation. **a** A minor degree of radial club hand, but associated with absence of the thumb. **b, c** Plan of pollicisation showing rotation of radial digit and shortening of second metacarpal with rotation of its head to make the carpometacarpal joint

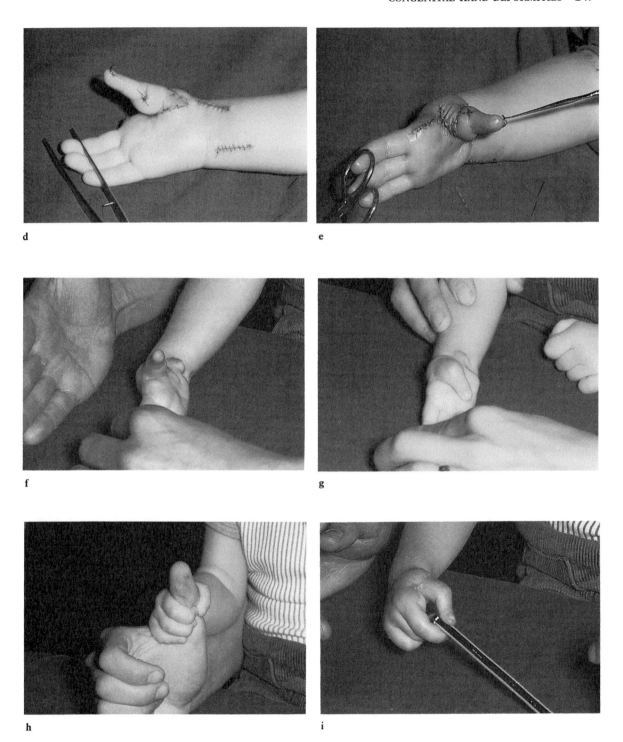

**Fig. 15.6** **d** Appearance of the thumb at the end of the pollicisation. **e** A good first web space has been obtained. **f** The web space has been maintained and active abduction of the thumb is possible. **g** Showing flexion of the pollicised thumb. **h** The child can grasp reasonably large objects and **i** pick up smaller objects

## Cleft hand and central defects

This terminology covers a wide spectrum of deformities arising as a longitudinal failure of development of the distal central portion of the upper limb. It has been suggested that the second, third and fourth rays develop embryologically at a different time from the radial and ulnar rays. 'Typical' cleft hands have the central ray alone missing, with the metacarpal absent or present in a disrupted state (Fig. 15.7a–e). Such anomalies are familial with dominant inheritance, often bilateral and with simultaneous involvement of the feet. The more severe the defect, the more likely the presence of syndactyly of the border digits. Syndactyly is more frequent between the ring and little fingers than between the thumb and index, but when the latter does occur, there may be a significant adduction contracture of the thumb requiring early release.

In 'atypical' cleft hand, there is absence of more than one central ray. If fully developed, there is a central defect with only border digits. The term 'lobster claw hand' particularly describes this group, but this term is offensive and its use should be avoided.

Hands in which a central metacarpus is present together with border digits, but with intermediate finger nubbings, should not be classified in the cleft hand group. The presence of vestigial fingernails implies a different mechanism of production and it would seem sensible to include these in an alternative group; for the purposes of the present classification, they are included in the group known as symbrachydactyly, which essentially describes short, stubby and stiff fingers.

Central defects are not common, forming less than 3% of all congenital hands. Despite considerable deformity, these hands may function well. However, the cosmetic appearance leads many patients to seek advice about surgery.

### Surgical treatment

The first priority is to correct any associated syndactyly of the border digits. This is particularly important if the thumb–index web is affected. In the cleft hand, an ingenious method of correcting the cleft and deepening the first web space has been described (Fig. 15.7f–k). The index finger ray is transposed on to the base of the third metacarpal. The deep transverse metacarpal ligament is reconstructed. The first web space is adequately released and lined by the skin from the original cleft which is transposed as a flap based on its palmar blood supply. This may be regarded as a huge Z-plasty in which one limb is a palmar flap and the other contains a digit.

In the treatment of atypical cleft hand, the presence of transverse metacarpals in the metacarpus may impair pinch between the two halves of the hand. These bones should be removed. If the thumb is hypoplastic, rotational osteotomy, tendon transfers and even pollicisation may be necessary to achieve some degree of function. Syndactyly release and pollicisation should not be undertaken simultaneously because of the high incidence of vascular abnormalities in this condition. Conversely, for the more severe central deficiencies, closure of the cleft is not recommended as it tends to diminish function (Fig. 15.7l–o). The cleft may even require deepening. Digital rotation osteotomy may be necessary to permit some form of opposition. Such procedures should be performed early.

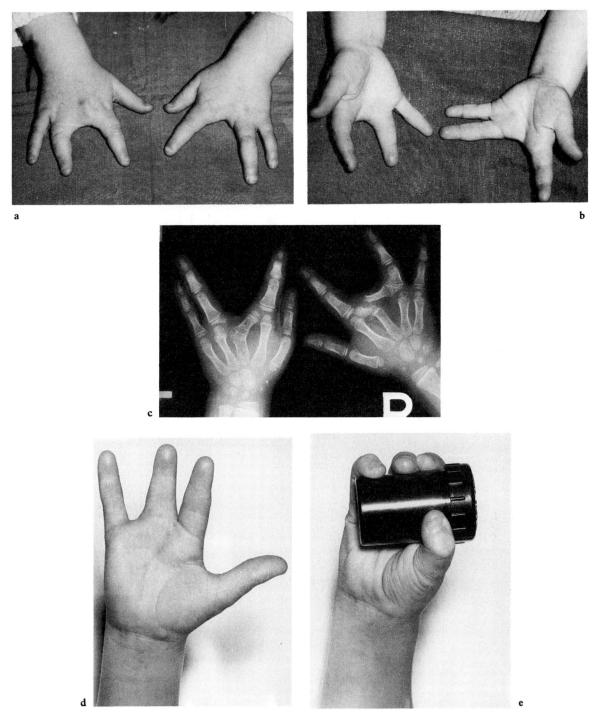

**Fig. 15.7** **a** Cleft hand (dorsal view). **b** Cleft hand (volar view). **c** The bony structure of the cleft hand shown in **a** and **b**. Note the abnormal widened metacarpals and the transverse metacarpals which link in with adjacent metaphalangeal joints and would seriously interfere with function if allowed to develop in this manner. **d** The appearance of the hand after transfer of the web space skin to create a new web. The second metacarpal has been transferred onto the base of the third metacarpal. **e** Showing the child now grasping large objects

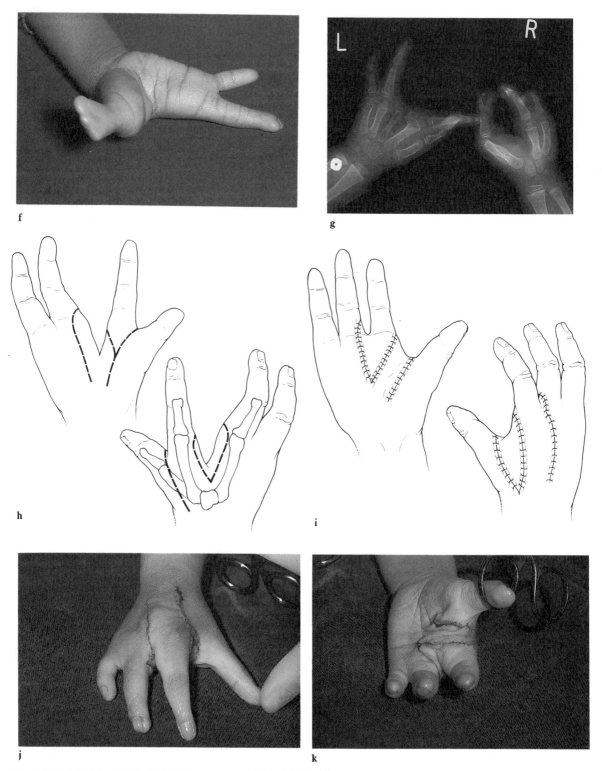

**Fig. 15.7**   **f** Cleft hand. **g** Radiological appearance of the cleft hand in **f**. Volar (**h**) and dorsal fusion of the cleft hand prior to and after operative treatment. **j, k** Completion of the operative procedure outlined in **h** and **i**. **k** The index finger has been transferred and the second web space now lines and creates a good first web space.

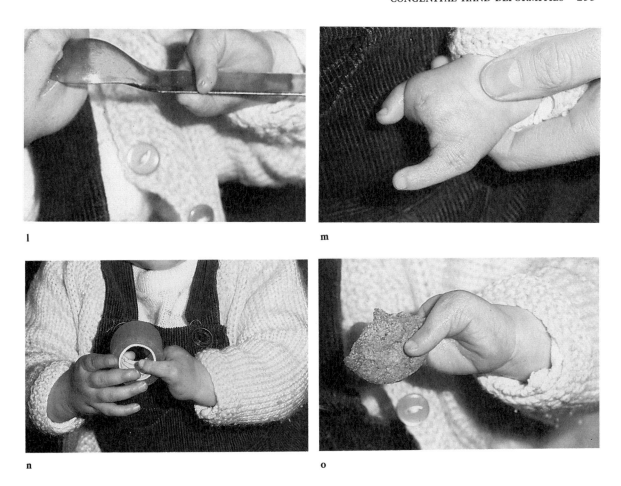

l                                                              m

n                                                              o

**Fig. 15.7  l** A severe cleft hand, in which the cleft should not be closed as function is good. The child is able to pick up small spoons (**l**) and manipulate larger objects (**n**). **o** She can feed herself and such good function should not be impaired.

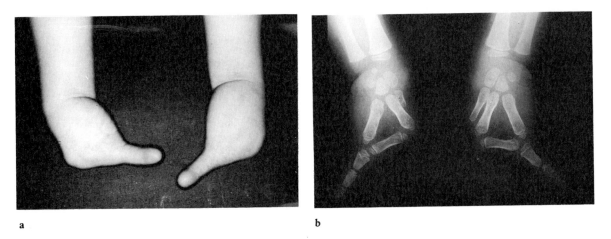

a                                                              b

**Fig. 15.8  a** Severe supression syndrome with complete aplasia of the radial side of the hand. **b** Note again the abnormal transverse metacarpals.

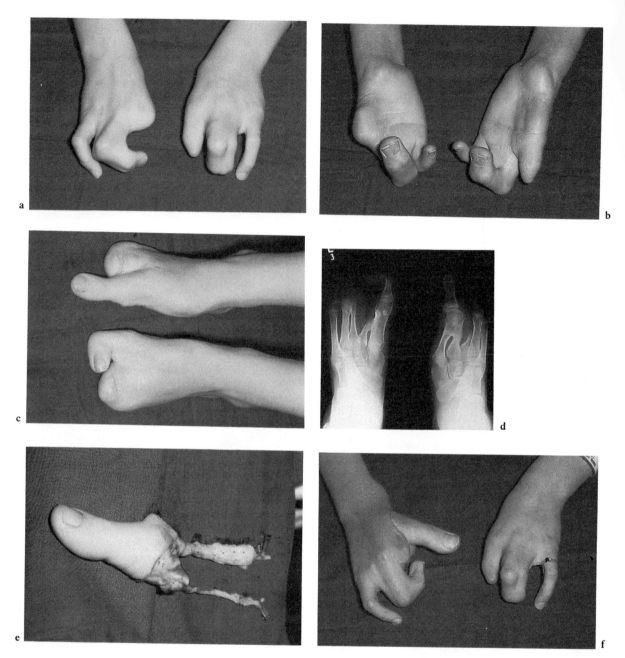

**Fig. 15.9** **a, b** Microsurgical reconstruction of the missing thumb in a case of a complex deformity involving syndactyly and hypoplasia of the radial side of both hands. This had been left untreated for many years, but was referred for consideration of surgery by the orthopaedic surgeon who was about to treat the child's feet (**c**) and who suggested that some of the troublesome toes which were about to be removed in order to allow the child to wear satisfactory foot wear, could be utilised in the hand reconstruction. **d** Radiological appearance of the feet. Note the bifid first metacarpal. This is always a danger sign, as the vessels penetrate between the junction of the first and the second metacarpals and therefore run through the crux of the 'Y' shaped bone. **e** The great toe of the right foot detached. **f** The great toe has been reattached. Optimum function takes at least 6 months after this procedure, and secondary procedures to increase the range of movement in the tendons are often necessary.

### Severe suppression deformities

These deformities have been interpreted as representing a distal central defect with an associated partial or complete radial or ulnar deficiency (suppression). Often these defects are symmetrical. Patients with bilateral severe suppression syndromes lack the ability to perform tasks independently with either hand (Fig. 15.8). Consideration should be given to the construction of an opposition post against which the remaining digit is able to pinch. Such posts may be constructed using skin flaps and bone grafts. Neurovascular free flaps may provide sensation at key points on an established opposition post. Microsurgical procedures, such as toe-to-hand transfer, may achieve in one stage what in the past would have required several stages (Fig. 15.9). They rarely function as actively as expected because they are being transferred to a site where there may be tendon hypoplasia with inadequate

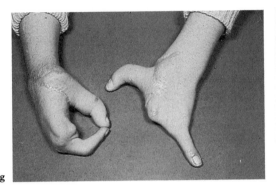
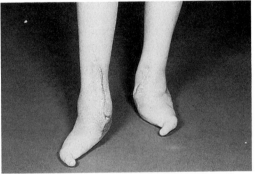
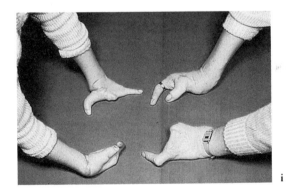

**Fig. 15.9 g** Bilateral toe-to-hand transfers used to reconstruct the hands of a child who was born with severe suppression syndrome affecting the radial half of both hands. The donor sites are seen in **h. i** The patient in **g** is shown on the left. One hand is able to grasp large objects, the other hand is able to participate in fine pinch. The patient's mother is on the right. She had a similar deformity, and on the right hand had toe-to-hand transfer undertaken some 40 years ago, using the Nicoladoni procedure

residual motors. Reinnervation of these transfers requires the sacrifice of a cutaneous nerve at the recipient site in the hand. Such nerves are difficult to find. Many such transfers are therefore poorly innervated. There is limited proprioceptive and sensory feed-back. Motion is imperative for good sensory interpretation, but is often impaired in these cases. The real advantage of such composite tissue transfers is that they achieve, in one stage, an opposition post which is more finger-like in appearance than that achieved by any other method. The active digit on the hand may require repositioning to achieve contact with the opposition post. Osteotomy to rotate the digit, tendon grafting to mobilise it and fusion to stabilise it, may all be required. In markedly hypoplastic digits, with a poor passive range of movement, tendon hypoplasia may be associated with absent pulleys; tendon grafting would be unlikely to achieve a satisfactory result in such cases.

## FAILURE OF SEPARATION OR DIFFERENTIATION OF PARTS — GROUP 2

Failure of differentiation of the soft tissues may lead to isolated absence of a muscle, or to more complex deformities such as arthrogryposis. In the latter there is no differentiation between muscle, ligaments and skin, each merging gradually into the other, producing soft tissue contractures. The involved structures may fuse together as in syndactyly or synostoses. Skeletal synostoses may affect the elbow, radius and ulna, carpal bones and metacarpals. They rarely require surgical treatment, but occasionally, if there is severe limitation of pronation and supination at the elbow, surgical release may be considered.

### Syndactyly

This is the commonest of all congenital hand deformities and involves the failure of separation or differentiation of two or more adjacent digits (Fig. 15.10a–d). The incidence is between 1:1000 and 1:3000 live births. If familial, it is inherited as a dominant gene of varying penetrance and the deformity is usually symmetrical. Males are affected twice as frequently as females.

The third, fourth, second and first interdigital webs are affected in decreasing order of frequency. Syndacatyly may be complete or incomplete. If complete, the involved digits are united throughout their length. Within this group, the degree of nail-bed fusion will influence the quality of the final result. In incomplete syndactyly, the common web extends to a variable extent along the length of the adjacent digit, but not as far as the distal interphalangeal joint. The deformity may be simple or complex. In simple syndactyly soft tissue webbing is present, but the bones of affected digits remain separate. In complex syndactyly there is bony fusion between adjacent digits. This may affect all the adjacent phalanges, or occur only at the fingertips (acrosyndactyly). The difference is not academic, but practical — growth in complex syndactyly tends to aggravate the deformity and so early release should be undertaken to permit unimpeded growth of the affected digits. Syndactyly is commonly associated with other hand deformities such as severe cleft hand and symbrachydactyly as well as with other generalised congenital deformities (Fig. 15.10).

Incomplete syndactyly affects only the proximal web space and surgery is optional, depending upon the parents' attitude to the cosmetic deformity. This also applies to simple syndactyly affecting the whole web. However, the majority of patients will seek correction of the deformity in later life, if correction is not effected in childhood.

### Treatment

Provided growth is unimpeded, there is no urgency about division of a syndactyly. The earlier surgery is undertaken, the greater the potential for disaster. Great skill is therefore required to achieve satisfactory results in a young child.

Early treatment in syndactyly is indicated in certain situations, in complex syndactyly and acrosyndactyly where the deformity would become progressively worse if left alone; in simple syndactyly between affected rays of unequal length, particularly the thumb–index web. Scar contractures may be due to poorly placed incisions or inadequate skin provision. However, even in the

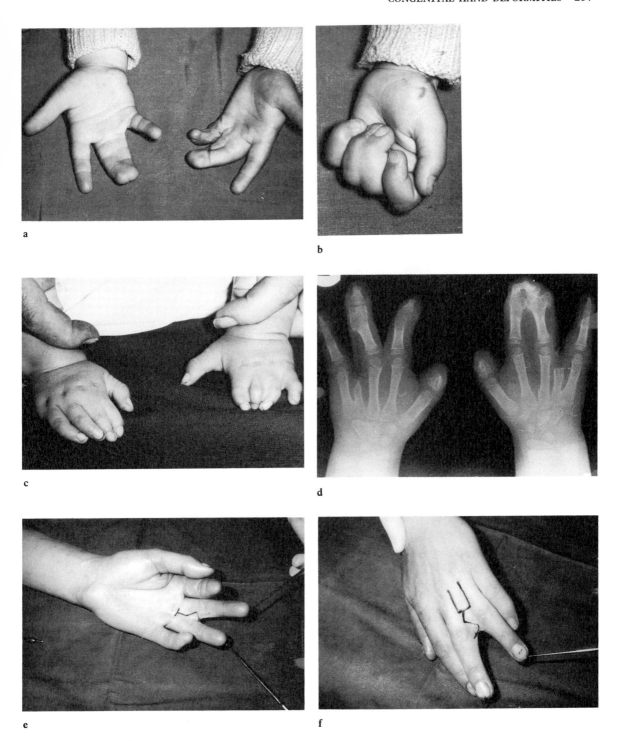

**Fig. 15.10  a, b** Simple syndactyly. **c** Simple syndactyly associated with brachydactyly. **d** Complex syndactyly with bony fusions in a patient who has already had treatment (continued overleaf).

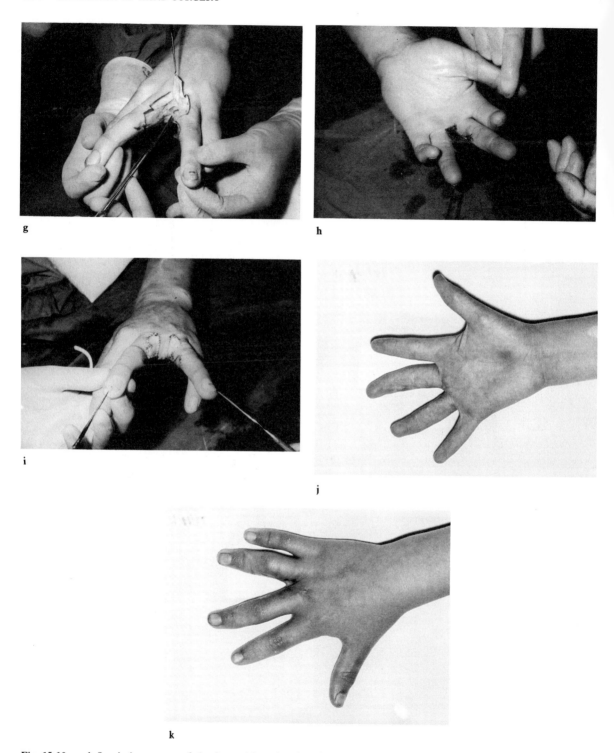

g

h

i

j

k

**Fig. 15.10   e–k** Surgical treatment of simple partial syndactyly using zig-zag dorsal and volar flaps and a dorsal rectangular flap. Wolfe grafts are applied to the secondary defects and the result of a similarly treated case is shown 2 years after treatment (**j, k**). Even with the most careful technique using conventional methods, it is difficult to avoid repeated operations in these children

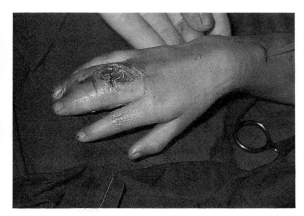

**Fig. 15.11** An example of simple syndactyly treated by a purpose-built tissue expander designed by the author. Note: tissue expansion is associated with a high rate of complications.

presence of adequate skin cover, the rapid growth of the hand, prior to 4 years of age, may lead to numerous surgical revisions. Some surgeons, therefore, feel that it is wiser to wait until just prior to the child starting school to correct simple syndactyly using current techniques. Tissue expansion techniques may have a role in the future (Fig. 15.11).

The aims in surgical correction of syndactyly are:

1. The creation of a commissure using a flap.
2. The separation of the involved digits using a volar and dorsal zig-zag approach.
3. The provision of adequate skin cover using full thickness grafts.

The new commissure should have a natural appearance. There should be no transverse web scars which would limit abduction and restrict the child's span. After separation of the digits, the marginal scars surrounding the raw surfaces should be oblique. Volar and dorsal zig-zag scars are essential to prevent linear scar contractures. Such contractures may produce lateral deviation of the digits and advance the new commissure distally. There is always a shortage of skin, even in the simplest of syndactylies. Adequate skin cover means the use of full thickness grafts. The principle is 'do not stretch the flaps, but graft the defect'. If adequate grafting is undertaken there is no need to distribute the skin flaps preferen-

tially to one digit. Partial thickness grafts contract more and should not be used.

When attempting to provide a commissure of normal depth, it is occasionally necessary to divide the digital artery to one side of the cleft distal to the common digital bifurcation. For this reason, adjacent involved web spaces should not be released simultaneously. The common digital nerve is split in a proximal direction and the deep transverse ligament may require division. Careful haemostasis is essential prior to suturing of the flaps and full thickness grafts. A well-padded dressing is applied beneath a volar slab keeping the fingers in abduction and extension. The first dressing is performed 1 week later under adequate anaesthesia in an operating theatre. If further grafting is required it can be undertaken immediately.

## Symphalangism

Symphalangism is the failure of interphalangeal joint differentiation. The proximal joints are commonly affected. Flexion creases are absent opposite the missing joint. Radiographs may show some semblance of the joint space due to the presence of a solid cartilage block (Fig. 15.12). Multiple digits are affected. The pure form of this disease is extremely rare. There is distal joint function and limited tendon activity. Usually, the digits are short. There may be an associated syndactyly (symbrachydactyly).

Attempted surgical correction of this condition has proved unsuccessful. The lack of normal stabilisation and motor tendons renders such attempts non-functional at best, and destabilising at worst. Most patients adapt well to this deformity, and surgery to restore motion or to place the digits in a more 'functional position' should not be undertaken in adults. In the cases where there is an associated syndactyly, early release of the conjoined digits is undertaken if it is believed that there will be a restricting influence on their growth potential.

## Contractures resulting from failure of differentiation

These include the relatively common congenital

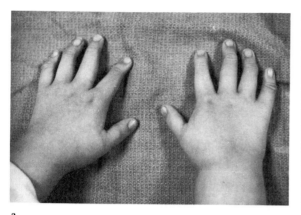

a

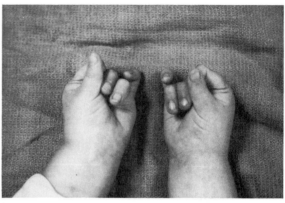

b

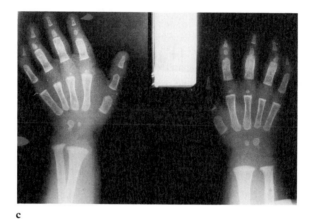

c

**Fig. 15.12   a, b** Symphalangism. Note the absence of the flexion and extension creases opposite the proximal interphalangeal joints. Note also the excellent flexion that occurs at the distal interphalangeal joints of the affected digits. **c** Radiographic appearance of symphalangism. Some semblance of the joint space occasionally occurs, but it is non-functional

clasped thumb, camptodactyly and arthrogryposis multiplex congenitum. If the skeleton has been involved in the failure of differentiation, lateral deviation of the digits may occur (clinodactyly).

### Congenital trigger thumb

The interphalangeal joint is held in marked flexion and attempted passive extension produces pain in these infants (Fig. 15.13). The parents notice that the child does not extend the thumb. There is a thickening of the tendon sheath at the level of the metacarpophalangeal joint with underlying nodu-

larity of the flexor pollicis longus. The condition is initially intermittent and in one-third of cases, will resolve spontaneously. In the remainder it remains troublesome and may become fixed. Occasionally splinting is successful, but if there is no response within 6 months, surgical release should be undertaken. Release or excision of a small area of thickened sheath should be performed leaving the nodule in the tendon to resolve spontaneously. Surgical interference with the tendon will lead to adhesions. Its excursion should be seen to be full, prior to closure.

Congenital trigger finger is a similar condition, but is much more rare.

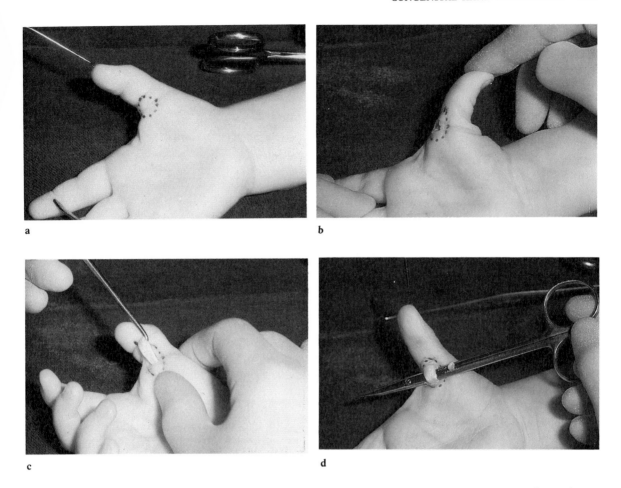

**Fig. 15.13** **a, b** Congenital trigger thumb. **c, d** Showing release of the flexor pollicis longus and full flexion and extension

## Congenital clasped thumb

These children present with an adducted thumb which is in full flexion at the metacarpophalangeal joint. It is a postural deformity, not an isolated condition, and there may be many underlying causes, ranging from hypoplasia to absence of extensor pollicis brevis. Sometimes it is associated with abnormalities of extensor pollicis longus. On rare occasions, flexion contractures may also be responsible for thumb hypoplasia and muscle deficiencies. Treatment is directed towards the cause. It is unusual for there to be complete absence of the tendons. More often they are atten-

uated. In such cases, prolonged splintage may protect the hypoplastic tendons from the powerful flexor forces. Splintage will only work in the least affected cases where full passive extension is possible. Flexion contractures will require release and grafting. Associated extensor tendon hypoplasia, or absence, requires tendon transfer. Local tendons, such as extensor indicis proprius, may also be affected and therefore are unavailable for transfer. Some flexion deformities prove resistant to all forms of surgical treatment except fusion in a position of function. Some patients may have a mild form of arthrogryphosis.

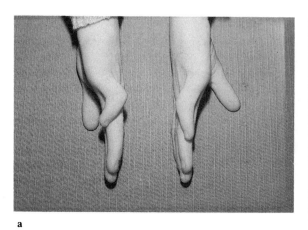

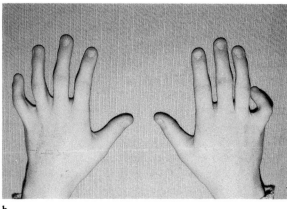

a                                           b

**Fig. 15.14   a, b** Camptodactyly

*Camptodactyly*

This is a congenital flexion deformity of the
proximal interphalangeal joint, involving the little
finger most commonly and the other digits with
decreasing frequency towards the radial side of the
hand (Fig. 15.14). In early life, the deformity is
minimal or not apparent and does not interfere
with function. There are two groups of patients,
those with a static deformity and those in whom
the deformity may progress rapidly during
adolescence, but become static again in adult life.
The aetiology is uncertain and may be multifact-
orial. Abnormalities of the flexors, extensors or
lumbricals as well as fascial shortening have been
implicated. The surgical treatment of this condition is as yet unsatisfactory and should be
embarked upon only when rapid progression leads
to functional impairment. In such cases, soft
tissue release and correction is of no benefit if
secondary joint changes have occurred. X-ray of
the proximal interphalangeal joint is of crucial
importance in assessing the subsequent treatment.
Osteotomy, or arthrodesis may be required.
Where the joint is normal the central slip test (see
Ch. 20) should be performed to ascertain whether
or not the patient has an active extensor mechanism capable of producing full extension at the
proximal interphalangeal joint. In such cases,
exploration of the volar surface of the finger may
reveal tendon abnormalities which, if released,

will allow the patient to actively correct the
deformity. If there is no functioning extensor
mechanism, a tendon transfer is required into the
lateral bands in addition to release of volar structures. An adjacent uninvolved sublimis may be
used for the transfer.

Although our understanding of this condition
has improved, functional results remain disappointing and surgery in these patients should be
approached with caution.

*Clinodactyly*

Clinodactyly is a congenital lateral deviation of the
digit from its normal longitudinal alignment (Fig.
15.15). There is malalignment of the interphalangeal joint surfaces from their normal orientation
at 90° to the long axis of the finger. Abnormal
development of the middle phalanx is commonly
responsible. It rarely requires treatment unless so
severe as to interfere with function. In normal
length fingers, a closing wedge osteotomy is indicated. In short fingers, attempts at an opening wedge
osteotomy may be undertaken. These may fail due
to the presence of soft tissue contracture on the
shorter side of the digit. Often the deformity is
due to the presence of an abnormally shaped delta
phalanx, in which the proximal epiphysis is C-
shaped, extending along the length of the bone
and continuous with the distal epiphysis. The

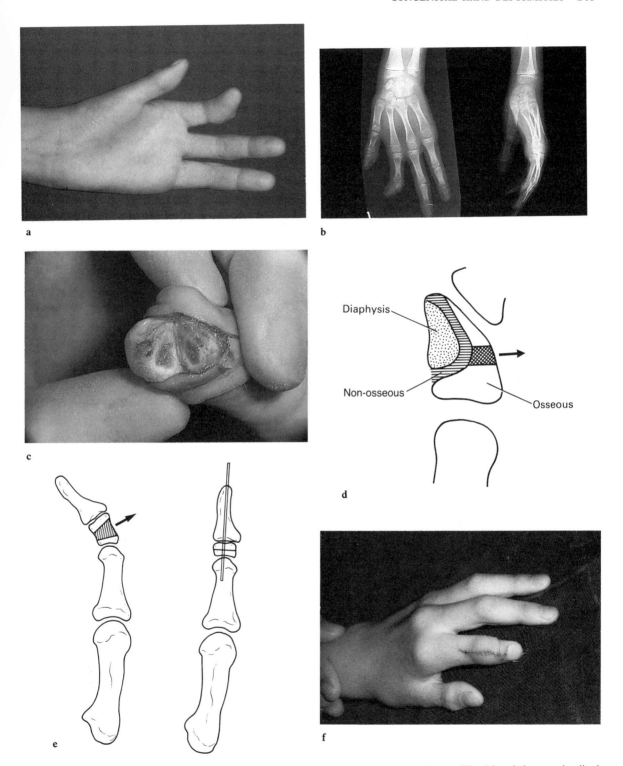

**Fig. 15.15   a** Clinodactyly. **b** The underlying cause can be seen to be a small delta phalanx. **c** The delta phalanx as visualised at operation showing its bevelled surface. **d** Diagram of delta phalanx. **e, f** After osteotomy and realignment, a straighter digit is obtained. It should be noted, however, that some loss of range of movement may occur following such procedures

deformity increases until skeletal maturity. Ossification proceeds in a proximodistal sequence. Epiphysiodesis under magnification is the most logical surgical procedure, but remains to be evaluated. Until its role is established, osteotomy remains the mainstay of treatment. Osteotomy should not be undertaken until ossification has established the definitive shape of the so-called longitudinally bracketed diaphysis. Opening wedge osteotomy and insertion of bone grafts may lead to recurrent deformity with shortness of the soft tissues. Closing wedge osteotomy shortens the digit. A wedge with an angulation of half the

required correction may be taken from one side, and inserted into the other. Such a reversed wedge is technically difficult, but more likely to yield longer term success. All surgery for this condition is difficult and the results unpredictable. Shortness of the finger, non-union and tendon adhesions may occur. Surgery should, therefore, be avoided in minor cases of clinodactyly. Major cases are usually due to delta phalanges. If the delta phalanx is supernumerary it should be removed in toto and a reconstruction of the collateral ligament undertaken. This is the situation in the triphalangeal thumb. Where

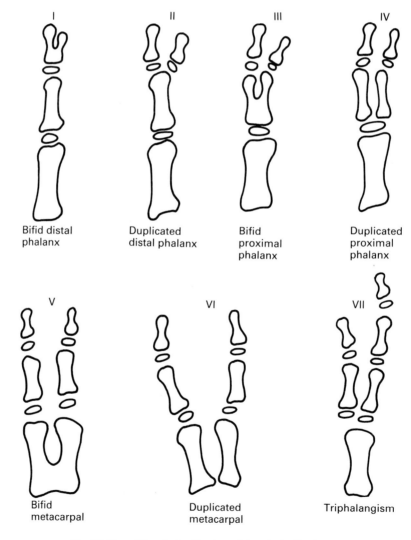

a

Fig. 15.16   a Wassell classification of thumb duplications.

pronounced deformity is present in the little finger, the phalangeal complement is usually normal and late osteotomy is the treatment of choice.

## DUPLICATIONS — GROUP 3

Duplication is one of the commonest malformations in the hand. In the American negro population the incidence is as high as 1:300 with frequent involvement of the little finger. It is less common in the European population with the thumb being the most frequent site. Index duplication is exceedingly rare. In the past, it has been described in error when a triphalangeal thumb was present. Duplication of the whole hand is even more rare. Central polydactyly is seen in association with complex syndactyly.

The feet may also be involved, and an associated syndactyly is frequent. Patients with polydactyly require careful pre-operative assessment, as the condition is associated with numerous systemic congenital malformations. Modes of inheritance are therefore various and genetic counselling is required to predict the involvement of future offspring.

There are three degrees of polydactyly:

Type 1 — an extra soft tissue mass not attached to the skeleton.
Type 2 — an extra digit, or part thereof containing normal components articulating with a metacarpal or phalanx.
Type 3 — an extra digit with normal components articulating with an extra metacarpal.

Treatment is governed by the type of duplication. Simple amputation of the extra digit is inadequate except in type 1. In other cases, surgery may

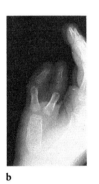
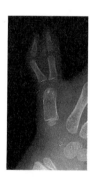

b

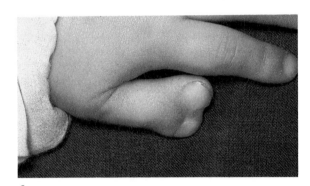

c

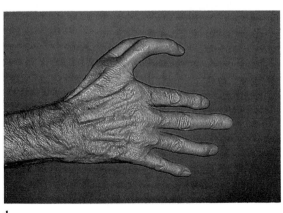

d

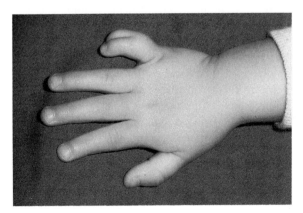

e

**Fig. 5.16  b** A Wassell type IV duplication of the thumb, showing a shared metacarpophalangeal joint. **c** A more distal duplication of the thumb. **d** A more proximal duplication of the thumb. **e** Ulnar polydactyly

involve osteotomy to thin a thickened metacarpal or phalanx, or to re-orientate its joint surface. In addition, Y-shaped abnormal tendons or neuro-vascular bundles may be split off. Collateral ligament reconstruction may be required with thenar muscle reattachment. Where there is dupli-cation, there is inevitably hypoplasia of both component parts. The parents should appreciate that the remaining digits will be smaller than normal.

## Radial (thumb) polydactyly

Duplication of the thumb most commonly occurs at the level of the metacarpophalangeal joint. However, it may occur at virtually any level within the thumb, arising either from a common joint, or from an abnormal but bifid bone at phal-angeal or metacarpal level. The Wassell classification is useful in that treatment is essentially governed by both the level of duplication and the relative size of the two duplicated thumbs:

Type 1 — bifid distal phalanx 2%.
Type 2 — two distal phalanges arising from the interphalangeal joint 15%.
Type 3 — bifid proximal phalanx 6%.
Type 4 — bifid thumb arising at the metacarpophalangeal joint 43%.
Type 5 — bifid metacarpal 10%.
Type 6 — bifid thumbs arising at the carpometacarpal joint 4%.
Type 7 — any thumb with triphalangia 20%.

In the distal duplications of types 1 and 2, where there is a common interphalangeal joint and the two components are equal in size, the Bilhaut–Cloquet technique is used. This involves the resection of a central wedge, but the basal epiphysis may be damaged by this procedure. Nail deformities are invariable and can be reduced by taking one complete nail from one thumb, although this will be slightly smaller than normal. If one of the thumb components is significantly smaller, its removal is justified. For more proximal duplications the presence of dual interphalangeal joints prevents the satisfactory application of the above technique. In type 4 duplication the radial digit is sacrificed if the two are of equal size and function. This preserves normal sensation on the important contact ulnar

side of the thumb and maintains stability in pinch as the ulnar collateral ligament of the metacarpo-phalangeal joint remains undisturbed. Reinsertion of the thenar muscles is required along with radial collateral ligament reconstruction. The metacarpal head is wedge shaped, like the roof of a house, and osteotomy to realign its articular surface is necessary. The head is also wider than usual and should be contoured. The long flexors and exten-sors may contribute to malalignment at the interphalangeal joint level through abnormal inser-tions on the distal phalanx.

In cases where there is a pronounced difference in size and function, careful observation will indicate which thumb should be removed. In triphalangeal thumb, a delta phalanx, if present, is best excised. If one of the triphalangeal thumbs is similar to an extra index finger, formal pollicis-ation may be necessary and the creation of a first web space may require the use of a skin flap from the extra thumb to be sacrificed.

## Central and ulnar polydactyly

Central involvement is more difficult to treat than ulnar duplications. It is often associated with a syndactyly and a hypoplastic extra digit may thus be hidden. The early removal of this digit is required to achieve maximum function in the hand. However, the anatomical complexity of the polydactyly may be such that the remaining digit functions poorly, despite a relatively normal appearance. There may be abnormal transverse metacarpals in this condition. Ulnar polydactyly is usually quite simple to treat, based on the previously described principles.

## OVERGROWTH OR GIGANTISM — GROUP 4

### Macrodactyly

This is a congenital, localised, pathological enlargement of skeletal and soft tissues (Fig. 15.17). It is rare and does not occur in association with other deformities. It is usually unilateral, affecting the index finger most frequently, but if multiple, the involved digits are adjacent. Involve-ment may be limited to the digits, or extend to the hand and forearm. Occasionally, the feet are

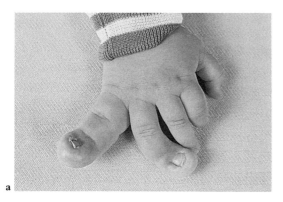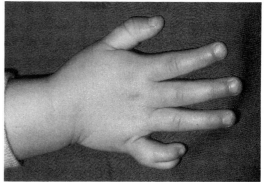

a                                                       b

**Fig. 15.17  a, b** Macrodactyly affecting the little and ring fingers

affected. No genetic relationship has been established. When there is digital involvement, the fingers are curved in a palmar direction. Growth may produce an increase in curvature. There seems to be progressive loss of movement with advancing age.

There are two clinical types of macrodactyly:

1. Static — the digital involvement remains in the proportions established at birth.
2. Progressive — there is an aggressive enlargement of the involved digits changing the proportions established at birth.

There is an associated involvement of the nervous system with an adjacent abnormal digital nerve in the area of hypertrophy in the majority of cases. There may be a link between macrodactyly and neurofibromatosis. In both conditions, there is fatty and fibrous proliferation. Some patients with macrodactyly display *café au lait* spots, neurofibromas or lipomas. The digital nerves are usually enlarged. The term 'nerve territory-orientated macrodactyly' reflects this relationship.

Treatment of this condition is extremely difficult. Medical treatment has nothing to offer and radiotherapy is contraindicated. Surgery may be ablative or corrective. Corrective procedures may involve epiphysiodesis to arrest growth. This produces bone shortening, but circumferential thickening of the shaft continues. Longitudinal osteotomy will thin the bones. Neurectomy, in an attempt to prevent growth, has been attempted.

Fat reduction may be required on several occasions, but care is necessary in performing these procedures as the blood supply to the skin flaps is poor. Whatever surgical procedures are undertaken, the range of joint motion is invariably compromised, and although a significant cosmetic improvement may be obtained, the final result is likely to be a relatively stiff, abnormal looking finger. In isolated digital involvement, amputation may therefore be preferable.

## UNDERGROWTH OR HYPOPLASIA — GROUP 5

The most common type of hypoplasia seen in the hand is that affecting the thumb. If the fingers alone are involved, surgical treatment is rarely required. The presence of a short digit which is functional is not an indication for ablative surgery. Short metacarpals are often seen and these are associated on occasion with systemic syndromes such as Turner's (X0). Short phalanges (brachydactyly) most commonly affect border digits. Short digits are often seen in association with syndactyly.

### Thumb hypoplasia

This deformity has a spectrum ranging from the minimally short to the functionally inadequate or absent thumb. Short thumbs occur in many different syndromes. The shape and size of the phalanges and metacarpals will suggest the appropriate diagnosis. Surgery to the skeleton is rarely required. Web space deepening is usually adequate to achieve a relative increase in length. The Blauth classification of these defects is useful as surgical treatment is governed by the degree of hypoplasia.

Grade 1 — The thumb is slightly small, but has normal components. Surgery is not required for this group as function is not impaired.

Grade 2 — The thumb is as above, but in addition there is hypoplasia of the thenar muscles. This leads to an adducted first web. There may be associated insertional abnormalities of the extrinsic tendons. Release of the first web space, opponensplasty and reinsertion of the extrinsic tendons may be required. The metacarpophalangeal joint is lax, requiring ligamentous reconstruction.

Grade 3 — The thenar muscles are absent. The extrinsic tendons are abnormal or absent. There is associated skeletal hypoplasia and poor function of the carpometacarpal joint limiting possible abduction and opposition. In such circumstances, reconstruction of the existing thumb is unlikely to produce useful function. Pollicisation of the index finger should be considered.

Grade 4 — 'Pouce flotant': a floating thumb attached only by the skin and having no function. Pollicisation undertaken within the first year of life is appropriate for grade 4. The principles of this procedure have been described already.

Grade 5 — Total aplasia of the thumb. Pollicisation is also indicated.

## CONGENITAL CONSTRICTION BAND SYNDROME — GROUP 6

Ring constrictions occur in about 1 : 15 000 live births. They consist of grooves running around the fingers at 90° to the long axis of the digit, or more proximally (Fig. 15.18). The depth of these grooves varies, but the deepest part of the ring may consist of granulation tissue constricting the phalanx. The portion of the digit distal to the groove may appear to be hypoplastic, or swollen due to lymphoedema. Autoamputation may occur at the same level as a ring constriction affecting

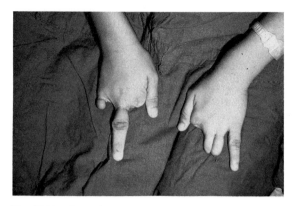

**Fig. 15.18** Congenital ring constriction syndrome, showing congenital amputations and ring constrictions

adjacent digits. Ring constriction syndrome is often associated with webbed, short and fused digits. Other more generalised abnormalities such as club feet, cleft lip and palate are associated with some 40–50% of cases.

The aetiology of this condition is a matter of some debate. Since the time of Hippocrates, it has been assumed to be due to the constricting effect of bands of amnion in intra-uterine life. However, in the early part of this century it was postulated that these abnormalities were the results of focal dysplasia of the germinal tissue, i.e. the mesoderm. It is interesting to note that the short border digits are the least commonly affected with the longer digits more frequently involved. Patterson has classified ring constriction syndrome into four types:

1. Simple ring constriction.
2. Ring constriction associated with distal deformity.
3. Ring constriction associated with fusion of the distal parts (acrosyndactyly).
4. Autoamputations.

The treatment is surgical. For type 1 (simple ring constrictions) surgery is not urgent. Progressive damage does not occur and operative treatment can be undertaken at any time, but preferably prior to attendance at school. In type 2, the ring constriction is associated with distal deformity. This implies that the constriction ring compresses the bony component of the finger and that there is functional impairment of venous and lymphatic drainage. Surgery should be undertaken early to prevent distal progressive lymphoedema producing severe damage, occasionally leading to autoamputation. In some cases, surgery is urgently required in the neonatal period. In this group, staged Z-plasties are the treatment of choice. Where the ring is more superficial (as in type 1), one-stage circumferential multiple Z-plasties can be safely performed. Care must be exercised to avoid injury to the digital nerve branches and vessels. In type 3, where there is associated acrosyndactyly, release of the tips of the involved digits should be performed by the time the child is 1 year of age. In the case of the thumb, the procedures normally used for the reconstruction of the traumatically injured thumb should be considered. There may be an associated need to release the web space.

## SUMMARY

The surgery of the congenital hand is complex. During the early years, the developing hand is in a state of dynamic, anatomical and physiological equilibrium. Care must be taken not to destroy this balance by injudicious intervention. The structures affected are small but their rate of change is rapid. Growth must not be impaired by surgery. Early redistribution or augmentation of tissues will allow their incorporation into the developing patterns of behaviour. Repeated surgery may be necessary and patient and parental confidence in the surgeon must be maintained.

# 16. Arthritis

*Principal author: F. D. Burke*

## INTRODUCTION

Rheumatoid arthritis is a generalised inflammatory process of unknown aetiology. It is a systemic disease that may affect hand function in a variety of ways. Joint synovitis is the most obvious feature of the process but assessment of the rheumatoid hand must include many other tissues which may also be involved. Detailed evaluation is required in order to elucidate the precise mechanism by which the rheumatoid process is producing dysfunction in the upper limb.

There are three broad subgroups within adult rheumatoid arthritis. The *monocyclic* group runs the most benign course, presenting with a single episode of synovitis which fully resolves without subsequent exacerbations. In the more characteristic *polycyclic* group, exacerbations follow remissions with a gradual deterioration of function. A minority of cases present with rapid and *relentlessly progressive* deterioration in function, associated with marked deformity. If rheumatoid arthritis develops in children, the epiphyses are involved in the disease process (Still's disease or juvenile rheumatoid arthritis). Premature epiphyseal arrest results in marked shortening of the digits (Fig. 16.1). A majority of patients with rheumatoid arthritis have IgM rheumatoid factor in their serum, and this seropositive group tends to develop severe varieties of rheumatoid arthritis with generalised systemic involvement.

## PATHOLOGICAL FEATURES OF RHEUMATOID ARTHRITIS

### Joint synovitis

Massive hyperplasia of the synovial layer occurs.

Initially the peripheral cartilage adjacent to the thickened synovium is eroded, exposing subchondral bone which may itself be further eroded, causing large bony defects and in some cases total joint destruction. In addition, painful distension of the capsule by bulky synovial tissue and fluid reduces motion at the joint. Adjacent ligaments may be stretched, or themselves eroded by synovial tissue, rendering the joint unstable. The unopposed action of the surrounding tendons may result in further joint subluxation or dislocation. Even if the inflammatory process halts at an early stage, the cartilage or bone damage may lead to the development of late deformity. Secondary osteophytic lipping of a joint may erode adjacent flexor or extensor tendons. This is most commonly seen at the head of the ulna where the extensors to ring or little finger are ruptured, producing loss of metacarpophalangeal joint extension (Fig. 16.2). In the flexor compartment the commonest tendon to rupture is flexor pollicis longus, frayed at the trapezioscaphoid joint.

### Tendon synovitis

The synovial lining of tendon sheaths may also hypertrophy, causing local pain and swelling that restrict motion. Extensor tendon synovitis is the more obvious variety, presenting as a soft tissue mass under the extensor retinaculum. Infiltration of the tendons frequently follows with attenuation or rupture. If one of the extensor tendons ruptures, it is likely that further tendons will follow suit in the succeeding days or weeks. Flexor tendon synovitis is equally common but less obvious and careful clinical examination is required. There is fullness over the flexor tendon

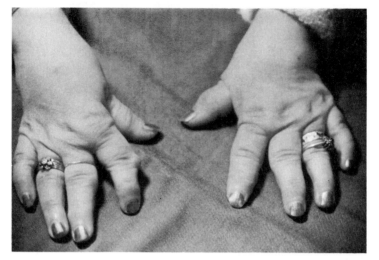

a

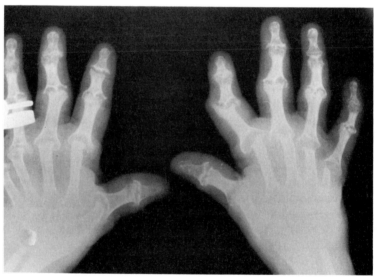

b

**Fig. 16.1**   Stills Disease—the appearance at skeletal maturity. **a** Clinical.
**b** Radiological

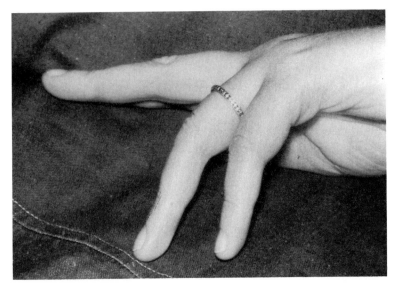

a

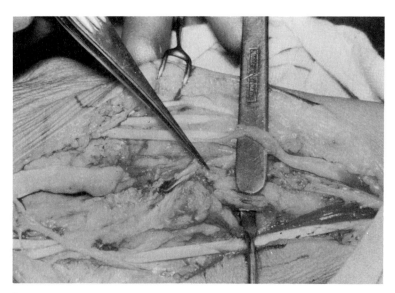

b

**Fig. 16.2** Extensor tendon rupture. **a** Loss of extension to ring and little fingers. **b** Synovial proliferation with tendon rupture

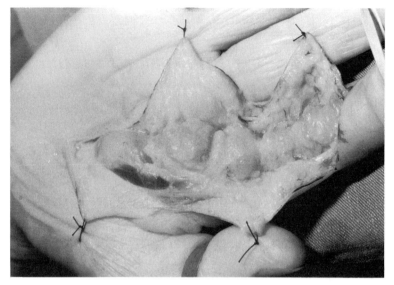

a

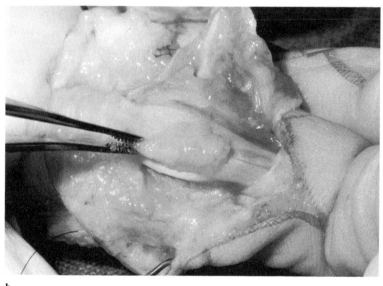

b

**Fig. 16.3** Flexor synovitis in the finger. **a** Attenuation of the flexor tendon sheath. **b** Synovium infiltrating the flexor tendon

sheath and motion of the fingers is frequently accompanied by crepitus. The synovial bulk commonly reduces the patient's ability to flex the fingers into the palm. The tendons are infiltrated by the synovium, particularly within the flexor tendon sheath (Fig. 16.3). Flexor tendon rupture is uncommon but may be found in the more severe cases.

## Muscle lesions

Wasting of the associated muscle groups occurs when joints are painful and stiff. There is also an inflammatory process which directly damages muscle fibres, reducing power. Muscle biopsy may reveal areas of perivascular lymphocytic infiltration. Focal fibrinoid necrosis may be present, associated with small vessel thrombosis and surrounding muscle degeneration. The power of the muscle is reduced by this process. The resulting clinical picture may be of quite marked wasting of the hand musculature.

## Nerve lesions

Abundant rheumatoid synovium may produce local nerve compression. The median nerve in the carpal tunnel is most frequently involved (Fig. 16.4), but ulnar nerve compression at the elbow or wrist may occur. A diffuse distal neuropathy is found less frequently. There is lymphocytic infiltration of the nerve, particularly around the intraneural blood vessels. Glove and stocking anaesthesia is present, rather than sensory loss limited to one specific nerve territory. Nerve conduction studies fail to reveal an area of localised slowing at wrist or elbow and indicate a more diffuse disease within the nerve itself. In some older seropositive patients, there may be numbness of the fingertips or hypoaesthesia along one side of the digit. Cervical root compression from spondylosis may also affect power and sensibility in the hand.

## Vasculitis

The accumulation of perivascular inflammatory cells and subsequent thrombosis is not restricted to muscle and nerve, the cutaneous vessels are

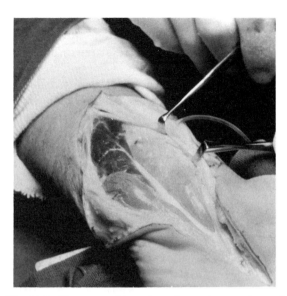

**Fig. 16.4** Flexor synovitis at the wrist causing carpal tunnel syndrome

involved also. Splinter haemorrhages may be apparent around the nail and the skin is commonly thin. It is particularly important that the quality of the skin is adequately assessed if surgical intervention is under consideration. Any procedure, particularly joint replacement, would be jeopardised by delayed wound healing.

## Nodules

Nodules are subcutaneous aggregations of collagenous material which occur over bony prominences (e.g. the subcutaneous border of the ulna and dorsal aspect of the fingers). Histologically they can be recognised as having features pathognomonic of rheumatoid arthritis. They may be tender and cosmetically unsightly.

## PATTERNS OF DEFORMITY IN RHEUMATOID ARTHRITIS

### Zig-zag deformities

As the capsule and ligaments of a joint are weakened, characteristic deformities occur. These result in part from the action of the adjacent muscles and tendons loading a joint that is deprived of the stability which the capsule and ligaments normally provide. The stresses arising from the normal activities of daily living are the most significant cause of deformity (e.g. hammering or opening jars).

In a skeletal system of intercalated joints, loaded under axial compression, deformity may be initiated at one joint, but under the laws of physics there will be an inevitable zig-zag collapse. This is analogous to a child's model train which, on crashing, will collapse in this pattern. Once established it is difficult to ascertain which is the initial joint responsible for precipitating the deformity. Zig-zag collapse in the sagittal plane produces boutonnière and swan-neck deformities. In the coronal plane the deformity produced at the metacarpophalangeal joint is ulnar drift with radial deviation of the carpus. The external forces applied to the hand in everyday use ensure that the reverse of these deformities does not occur.

## The wrist

The carpal rows buckle. This is particularly evident on the lateral radiograph (Fig. 16.5). The lunate moves volarly with the capitate approaching the radius. The scaphoid takes up an axis perpendicular to that of the radius (see Ch. 7).

## The metacarpophalangeal joints of the fingers

The forces produced by the digital flexors have a tendency to displace the proximal phalanx in a volar direction relative to the metacarpal head (Fig. 16.6). In normal circumstances this force is partly resisted by tension in the collateral ligaments. In the rheumatoid hand, ligamentous laxity frequently leads to volar subluxation at the joint. Patients with metacarpophalangeal joint subluxation often have associated swan-neck

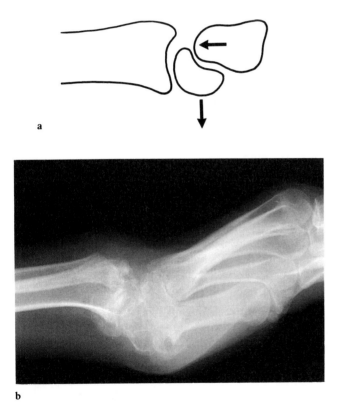

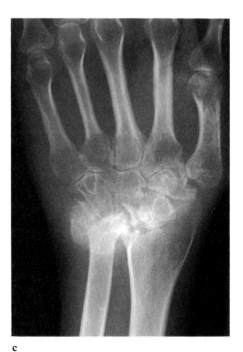

**Fig. 16.5** Rheumatoid carpal collapse with volar subluxation of the lunate (**a**) and proximal migration of the metacarpal bases (**b, c**)

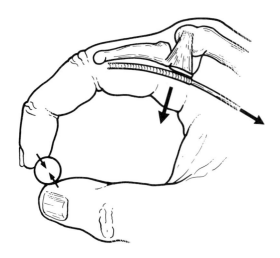

**Fig. 16.6** Volar subluxation of the proximal phalanx base

deformities and have poor grasp. If ulnar drift is prominent, surprisingly good grasp remains, although pinch and key grip are diminished.

## Ulnar drift

There are several causes of ulnar drift. Many activities of daily living involve the application of powerful ulnar deviating forces to the fingers. The carpus frequently drifts into radial deviation, increasing the tendency for the fingers to move in an ulnar direction. The lateral fibres restraining the extensor tendons on the dorsum of the metacarpophalangeal joints may be eroded and permit the extensor tendons to slip off the metacarpal heads into the gulleys on the ulnar side (Fig. 16.7). Laxity of the radial collateral ligament may also contribute to the deformity. All these factors may be responsible for the development and persistence of ulnar drift.

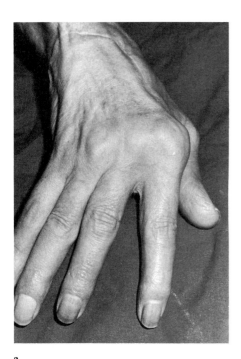

a

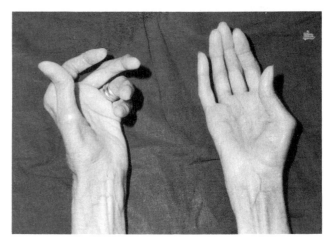

b

**Fig. 16.7** **a** Ulnar drift with dislocation of the extensor tendons. **b** The extension loss that frequently occurs in such cases

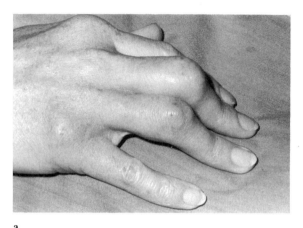

a

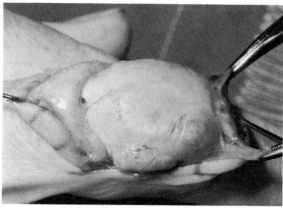

b

c

**Fig. 16.8** Rheumatoid boutonnière deformity. **a** Proximal interphalangeal joint flexion with distal interphalangeal joint hyperextension. **b** Abundant synovium with attenuation of the central slip. **c** Volar subluxation of the lateral bands

## The proximal interphalangeal joints of the fingers

*Boutonnière deformity* (Fig. 16.8)

Exuberant synovium erodes the central slip at its insertion at the base of the middle phalanx. The transverse fibres maintaining the dorsal position of the lateral bands are also eroded. The lateral bands migrate volarly, beyond the centre of rotation of the joint, thus forcing the proximal interphalangeal joint into flexion, with hyperextension at the distal interphalangeal joint.

*Swan-neck deformity* (Fig. 16.9)

Swan-neck deformity is incompletely understood but seems to arise from an imbalance of the normal forces acting upon the proximal interphalangeal joint. 'Tightness' of the intrinsics has been considered important but is probably secondary. The powerful external forces from the activities of daily living are the major deforming agent. Weakness, attenuation or rupture of the flexor digitorum superficialis may be a cause, or there may be erosion of the volar plate insertion by the bulky joint synovium. Metacarpophalangeal joint subluxation is often found in association to complete the zig-zag pattern and may be a cause of swan-neck deformity. The finger assumes the position of hyperextension at the proximal interphalangeal joint and flexion at the distal interphalangeal joint. Initially the deformity is reversible, and passive flexion from beyond the normal position of full extension permits further active flexion into the palm. If the position of

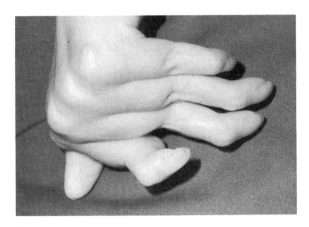

a

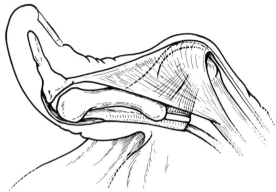

Fig. 16.10 The Nalebuff Type I deformity: metacarpophalangeal joint flexion and interphalangeal joint hyperextension

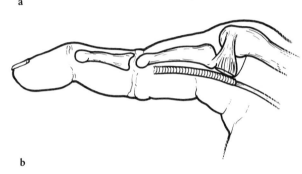

b

Fig. 16.9 Swan-neck deformity. **a** Proximal interphalangeal joint hyperextension with distal interphalangeal joint flexion. **b** Volar subluxation of the proximal phalanx base

hyperextension is allowed to persist, the dorsal capsule rapidly contracts and passive and active flexion are lost.

## Thumb

The deformities of the thumb form a reproducible series of patterns, the commonest of which have been described by Nalebuff.

### The Nalebuff Type I deformity (Fig. 16.10)

This is analagous to the boutonnière deformity in the finger but, in the case of the thumb, the flexion deformity occurs at the metacarpophalangeal joint. Attenuation of the extensor mechanism, particularly the extensor pollicis brevis insertion, results in metacarpophalangeal joint flexion, with hyperextension at the interphalangeal joint.

Extensor pollicis longus may displace ulnarwards and becomes a less effective extensor. The action of the long and short flexors produces volar subluxation of the proximal phalanx base.

### The Nalebuff Type II deformity

The distal deformity (metacarpophalangeal joint flexion and interphalangeal hyperextension) is the same as Type I, but the metacarpal is adducted against the palm. This is the least common variety of zig-zag collapse of the thumb.

### The Nalebuff Type III deformity (Fig. 16.11)

Instability of the carpometacarpal joint produces progressive adduction of the first metacarpal. Compensatory hyperextension occurs at the metacarpophalangeal joint, with a flexion deformity at the interphalangeal joint. This is analagous to the swan-neck deformity in the finger, although in this case it is the metacarpophalangeal joint that hyperextends.

### The Nalebuff Type IV (Fig. 16.12)

This may be regarded as a variety of gamekeeper's thumb. Carpometacarpal subluxation causes metacarpal adduction. This deformity throws added stresses on the metacarpophalangeal joint ulnar

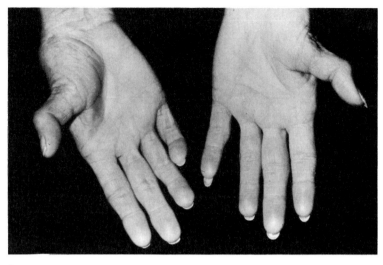

a

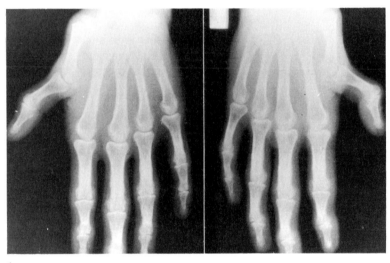

b

**Fig. 16.11** The Nalebuff Type III deformity. Metacarpal adduction. Metacarpophalangeal joint hyperextension and interphalangeal joint flexion. **a** Clinical. **b** Radiological

collateral ligament, which becomes attenuated, rendering the joint unstable.

The collapse patterns described by Nalebuff are but part of a broader spectrum of deformities as shown in Table 16.1. The individual joints of the thumb may deform as follows: the interphalangeal joint may flex or extend, radially deviate or become totally unstable. The metacarpophalangeal joint may undergo similar deformities, but ulnar

deviation is not seen at either joint because of the pattern of external forces.

The thumb is capable of a wide range of motion pivoting around the carpometacarpal joint. An internationally agreed terminology has been established to describe these positions (Fig. 16.13). When the thumb moves from a position of adduction to that of palmar abduction, automatic pronation of the thumb metacarpal occurs,

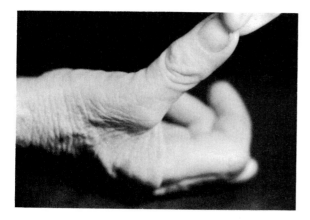

**Fig. 16.12** The Nalebuff Type IV deformity

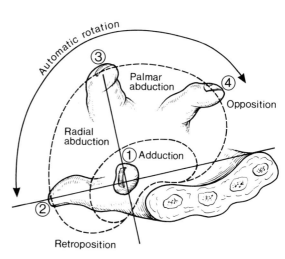

**Fig. 16.13** The clinical term 'adduction' indicates that the thumb metacarpal lies in close proximity to the index metacarpal (1). From this position, the thumb may move away from the index finger either parallel to the plane of the palm (radial abduction 2) or at right angles to the palm (palmar abduction 3). Additionally, at any point in space the thumb may flex or extend at interphalangeal or metacarpophalangeal joints. As the thumb moves around an arc of maximal abduction it undergoes automatic rotation (pronation) with the result that the thumb pulp is apposed to the digital pulps (opposition 4)

rotating the thumb to permit pulp to pulp contact. The automatic rotation stems in part from the saddle-shaped carpometacarpal joint.

## ASSESSMENT OF FUNCTION IN THE RHEUMATOID UPPER LIMB

A broad approach is required when evaluating hand function. The hand can only function properly if it is freely mobile in space. Pain or stiffness

**Table 16.1** Pattern of thumb deformity

|  | One-joint deformity | Zig-zag deformity |
|---|---|---|
| Interphalangeal | Flexion — — — — — — — — — — — | Swan-neck (Nalebuff III) |
|  | Extension | Boutonnière (Nalebuff I) |
|  | Radial deviation |  |
|  | Total instability |  |
| Metacarpophalangeal | Flexion |  |
|  | Extension — — — — — — — — — — — — | (Nalebuff II) |
|  | Radial deviation - - - - - - - - - - - - - - | Gamekeeper (Nalebuff IV) |
|  | Total instability |  |
| Carpometacarpal | Adduction (supination) - - - - - - - - - - - - - - |  |
|  | Abduction (pronation) |  |
|  | Total instability |  |

at shoulder, elbow or wrist may greatly reduce the ability of the hand to perform the activities of daily living. The crucial significance of pronation/supination motion is frequently overlooked. Comprehensive assessment of upper limb function involves evaluation of the interrelationship between both limbs. Function in one upper limb may complement deficiencies in the other. This is most commonly seen in the hands, where one may be suitable for grasp and lack extension, whereas the other is held in extension and unable to flex. The patient will perform grasp activities with one hand and functions requiring finger extension (e.g. washing) with the other. Hand dominance is less significant than the functional ability of each hand. Care should be exercised, if surgery is contemplated, to ensure that such a balance of function is not disturbed.

## Assessment of hand function

Deformity in the rheumatoid hand is common, but what role does the deformity play in everyday use of the hand? Marked deformity may cause little functional difficulty, while minor deformity may greatly incapacitate the patient. The patient's functional difficulties must be accurately analysed, and if surgery is contemplated it must be planned with a clear idea of the likely benefit to hand function. Several upper limb assessment forms have been designed in an attempt to evaluate disability and monitor progress. It is inevitable that ranges of motion, grip strength and dexterity tests predominate. The critical section of any such chart, however, is the portion that relates to the activities of daily living. In clinical practice, questions such as 'What difficulties are you experiencing?' remain crucial to full evaluation.

Grip and pinch function in the hand comprises an infinite variety of digital configurations. In addition, such functions are dynamic and the hand is under constant motion. In clinical usage the complexity of function has been arbitrarily classified into a series of standard positions of precision pinch, key pinch and power grip.

*Precision pinch* (Fig. 16.14)

Precision pinch is required for picking up small

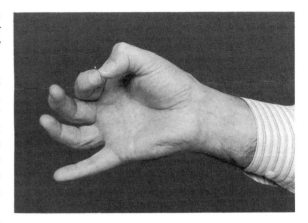

**Fig. 16.14**  Precision pinch

objects and fine manipulative skills. It requires moderate flexion of the interphalangeal joints of thumb and index finger. Joint deformity of the thumb or index may result in difficulty approximating thumb and index pulps. Power may be reduced by synovitis, pain or tendon rupture. Adequate sensibility is an essential part of precision handling and it is always prudent to ensure that carpal tunnel syndrome (due to flexor synovitis) is not limiting fine manipulative skills in the rheumatoid patient. Broad pulp pinch is a variant of the above (Fig. 16.15). This grip is used for handwriting and other precision skills. The interphalangeal joints of the thumb and index must be straight for this form of grip to take place. There is a broad area of contact between the pulp of both finger and thumb. The metacarpophalangeal joint of the

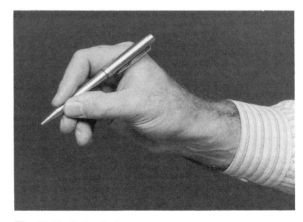

**Fig. 16.15**  Pulp pinch

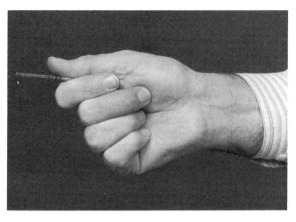

**Fig. 16.16** Key pinch

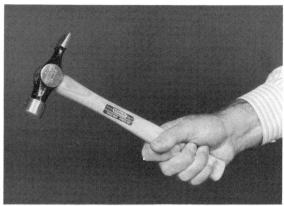

**Fig. 16.17** Power grip

thumb is slightly flexed and the carpometacarpal joint is held in abduction. The middle finger may work with the index and thumb to produce a three-point chuck grip.

*Key pinch* (Fig. 16.16)

This is one of the most important forms of grip available to the rheumatoid arthritic, as finger joint disease (particularly swan-neck deformity and ulnar drift), combined with loss of thumb abduction, may restrict contact between thumb and finger pulps. In this variety of pinch, the thumb flexes against the radial side of the index finger, which is stabilised by the first dorsal interosseous.

*Power grip* (Fig. 16.17)

Grip is weak in all rheumatoid patients and this may be due to a variety of factors. Pain alone will reduce power but there are also many contributory mechanical causes. The muscles are frequently weakened either by the disease process directly, or by atrophy arising from persistent pain and disuse. Wrist synovitis or extensor tendon rupture may result in a flexion deformity of the carpus. The relative lengthening of the flexor tendons so produced reduces their power. Flexor synovitis, triggering, or tendon rupture may all present as weakened power grasp. Joint synovitis, subluxation or intrinsic muscle tightness may also reduce

finger flexion. Combinations of such causes are frequently present in individual cases, making management more difficult. For these reasons it is not possible to fully restore power grasp to the rheumatoid hand.

## THE RADIOLOGICAL ASSESSMENT OF THE RHEUMATOID HAND

Routine radiographs will in most cases reveal the extent of damage to the joint. Standard views of the metacarpophalangeal joints, however, are by themselves inadequate, and an additional view described by Brewerton will also demonstrate early rheumatoid involvement. The fingers are laid on a cassette, palm upwards, with the interphalangeal joints extended and the metacarpophalangeal joints flexed to 65°. The beam is angled 15° from the ulnar side. The view skylines the metacarpal head and neck revealing the degree of erosion under the collateral ligaments. Cervical spine X-rays are indicated when general anaesthesia is contemplated to exclude atlanto-axial instability.

## MANAGEMENT OF RHEUMATOID ARTHRITIS OF THE UPPER LIMB

### Conservative management

Conservative management forms the mainstay of treatment in the rheumatoid upper limb. The rheumatologist co-ordinates a rehabilitation team that includes occupational therapists, physiotherapists, orthotists and surgeons. In an acute exacerbation of the disease the involved joint should be supported in a functional position with a light orthoplast splint. Analgesics and non-steroidal anti-inflammatory drugs are usually required. Specific disease-modifying antirheumatic drugs, such as gold, penicillamine or cytotoxic agents, may be prescribed for progressive active disease. Systemic steroid therapy is only considered in severe cases that fail to respond to other treatment, or if the patient's independence is threatened. Intra-articular steroid injections are frequently used when the exacerbation is limited to a single joint. Steroid infiltrations may be of benefit for flexor or extensor synovitis. No treatment is without its hazards and occasionally depigmentation, fat atrophy or tendon rupture may occur after local injection. A precise knowledge of the local anatomy is essential when performing such injections.

Night splintage of involved joints helps to preserve them in a functional position. Physiotherapy will often help to maintain muscle power and joint range. Home assessment by occupational therapists and social workers may be indicated. The occupational therapists will also instruct the patient in the techniques of joint preservation and protection. Shock loading, such as the use of hammers, should be avoided. Opening jars and similar activities produce marked ulnar deviation forces at the metacarpophalangeal joints and should be minimised by the use of aids.

## The surgical management of the rheumatoid upper limb

### Introduction

The surgeon should not make his evaluation and decision in isolation but in co-ordination with the rheumatologist who has supervised the patient's conservative management. Both should be guided by the assessments of hand therapists. The combined clinic forms the ideal environment in which to plan rheumatoid surgery. Consideration must also be given to lower limb dysfunction and the additional strains that this may place on the upper limbs, due to the use of sticks or crutches.

The combined clinic may also be used for postoperative review so that the benefits and limitations of surgery are appreciated by all involved in patient care.

The patient's confidence must be gained before surgery is offered. While this is true for all forms of elective surgery, it is perhaps most important when dealing with patients who have rheumatoid arthritis, as they often require multiple procedures performed over several years. The initial interview will provide a general assessment of disability. It is important that a balanced view of the benefits and limitations of surgery is presented. It is prudent to conclude the first interview at this stage, advising the patient to consider the options available and to return for further discussion. A decision about surgery may then be made, or even deferred to further meetings if necessary.

The broad principles of surgical treatment are:

1. Think function — not anatomy.
2. Procedures must be well timed.
3. Operative treatment should not be performed in an acute exacerbation of the rheumatoid process.
4. Soft tissue procedures to correct joint deformity provide no lasting benefit.
5. There should be rapid postoperative mobilisation.

Our current philosophy of the management of rheumatoid joint disease is that once deformity has commenced, it must inevitably progress. The ideal management would be early soft tissue correction but the collagenous structures are inadequate. Surgical intervention is delayed until there is significant functional loss. Skeletal realignment is undertaken by arthrodesis or arthroplasty, re-establishing musculotendinous balance.

Patients frequently present with multiple joint disease to a single upper limb and several joints may merit surgical intervention. The order in which these procedures are performed depends on individual preference and particularly on the likely functional benefit. Gain the patient's confidence by ensuring that the first procedure is a winning operation. Multiple simultaneous procedures require considerable surgical experience with appropriate rehabilitation skills. Once the decision has been made, surgery should follow without undue delay. The rheumatoid process frequently follows the path of gradual deterioration and prolonged periods on surgical waiting lists will undermine any benefits that might have accrued from surgery.

In conclusion it must be stated that the function of the rheumatoid hand cannot always be improved by surgery and intervention in such cases is inappropriate.

## The shoulder joint

The glenohumeral joint is commonly involved in the rheumatoid process. Moderate stiffness is tolerated quite well by the patient without enormous loss of function in the upper limbs. There is a useful range of scapulothoracic motion which the rheumatoid patient retains. However, a minority of patients complain of persistent severe pain and are considerably incapacitated. If the symptoms cannot be controlled by conservative means, joint replacement or interposition arthroplasty may be considered. Both techniques have limitations; implant loosening in the case of the former and fragmentation of the silicone rubber in the latter. A near normal range of motion is rarely achieved, the objective being to obtain good pain relief and a moderate range of motion. Arthrodesis is rarely performed.

## The elbow joint

Degenerative changes between the head of the radius and the humerus result in a reduced pronation/supination range. This may be far more disabling for the patient than any reduction in extension or flexion. If significant degenerative changes are confined to the radiohumeral joint, a simple excision of the radial head may dramatically improve the range of rotatory movements, with good pain relief. Many rheumatoid patients gradually lose flexion/extension range at the elbow. It is not uncommon for the patient to be left with a 40° arc of motion with the midpoint at about 90° of elbow flexion. Despite the limited range of motion, it is usually possible to feed, wash and perform personal toilet. If the flexion/extension arc at the elbow is such that the hand cannot be used effectively, or use is limited by persistent severe pain, elbow arthroplasty may be considered. The constrained replacements with metal stems, cemented into humerus and ulna, have tended to loosen. A new generation of smaller implants requires minimal bone resection and cement. They rely on the existing elbow ligaments for their stability. Loosening appears uncommon and there is good pain relief, with an average range of motion around 60°. Radial head excision is performed as part of the procedure with improved pronation/supination. The procedure is well tolerated by the patient, and may produce long-lasting benefit. It should be considered for those patients with persistent severe elbow pain, or an inappropriate arc of motion.

## The wrist

Discomfort over the ulnar styloid may greatly disable the rheumatoid patient. Pronation and supination are restricted. Excision of the ulnar styloid, with or without a silicone elastomer cap, relieves pain and may improve movement. Synovitis of the wrist joint may produce rapid loss of motion with progressive joint subluxation or bony ankylosis. The end position that the wrist assumes is commonly around the neutral point. Persistent pain, or volar flexion of the wrist, will reduce function. In the past, stabilisation of the wrist has been the preferred surgical treatment. The Mannerfelt technique, using a metal pin from third metacarpal to radius, is currently popular (Fig. 16.18). The technique is simple to perform, well tolerated by the patient and allows early mobilisation without the prolonged use of plaster casts. The alternative surgical treatment is wrist arthroplasty. The most common variety is the Swanson silicone rubber replacement (Fig. 16.19). This is simply a stemmed silicone elastomer spacer. No cement is used and bone resection is minimal. The replacement can be converted to an arthrodesis if complications arise. The intention is to produce limited pain-free motion at the wrist with an arc of approximately 60° around the neutral point. Some wrist extension permits firmer grasp and this feature is much appreciated by the patient. Wrist fusion and replacement have an underestimated role in surgery of the rheumatoid upper limb, as the gain in hand function is often considerable.

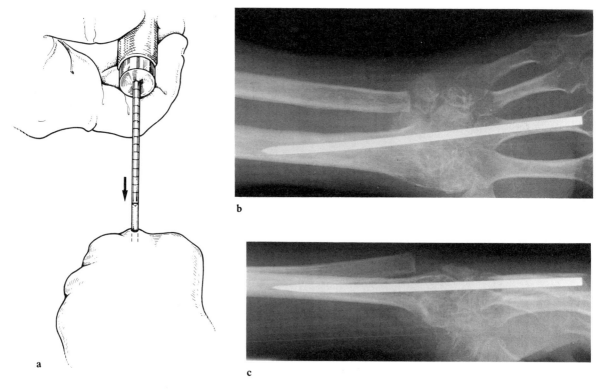

**Fig. 16.18**  Wrist arthrodesis with the use of an intramedullary metacarpal pin. **a** Introduction of the pin into the third metacarpal. **b, c** Anteroposterior and lateral radiographs

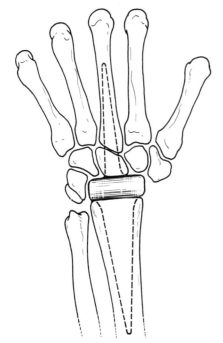

**Fig. 16.19**  Swanson arthroplasty of wrist

## Surgical procedures in the rheumatoid hand

### Extensor tenosynovectomy

Synovitis around the extensor tendons at the level of the retinaculum may provoke tendon rupture. A dorsal rim of radius or ulna may protrude into the extensor tendon compartments and cause an attrition rupture of the tendons. Exploration, synovectomy and rerouting of the retinaculum deep to the extensor tendons will protect them from further synovial infiltration or attrition. Early operation is necessary to avoid further tendon rupture. It is rarely possible to perform a direct repair of the ruptured tendons and the distal portion is normally sutured to an intact adjacent extensor tendon. Extensor tenosynovectomy is well tolerated by the patient, provides long-lasting benefit and is one of the more effective soft tissue procedures available for the rheumatoid arthritic.

*Flexor tenosynovectomy*

At wrist level, synovitis may cause carpal tunnel syndrome. Decompression is performed in conjunction with a synovectomy of the involved tendons. The results of surgery at this level are gratifying, with good relief of symptoms and retention of a satisfactory range of motion. Distal flexor tenosynovectomy is less rewarding. It is difficult to achieve effective clearance of synovium from the digital flexor sheath, and the patients experience greater difficulty mobilising the fingers in the postoperative period. An intensive rehabilitation programme is required if satisfactory results are to be achieved.

*Joint synovectomy*

**Metacarpophalangeal joints.** Early synovitis with minimal damage to the articular surface and without joint subluxation may be benefited by synovectomy. However, soft tissue reconstruction confers no lasting benefit in rheumatoid arthritis and the majority of patients present with established joint changes which merit replacement rather than synovectomy.

**Proximal interphalangeal joint.** Synovectomy may relieve pain and arrest articular degeneration if performed at an early stage, but some loss of motion of the joint frequently occurs. Synovectomy is most beneficial if there is no stretching of the central slip. However, a mild boutonnière deformity may be apparent, in which case the procedure may be coupled with a reefing of the central slip and the patient mobilised in a Capener, or similar splint. Late-established boutonnière deformity may require fusion of the proximal interphalangeal joint in an appropriate degree of flexion (from 20° at the index finger to 40° at the little finger).

Swan-neck deformity may arise from attenuation of the volar plate following synovial hyperplasia. If synovectomy is performed in the early cases, it should be supplemented with a tenodesis of one slip of the flexor superficialis to maintain the proximal interphalangeal joint in mild flexion. The excision of a transverse ellipse of volar skin (dermadesis) at the level of the proximal interphalangeal joint is an alternative procedure which limits hyperextension. Late-established cases may benefit from manipulation or dorsal capsular release, supplemented with temporary Kirschner wire stabilisation. The joint is held in mild flexion. An arthrodesis is indicated in severe cases.

**Distal interphalangeal joint.** Distal interphalangeal joint synovectomy is rarely required.

*Ulnar drift*

A variety of soft tissue procedures has been used in an attempt to control ulnar deviation of the fingers. The cross intrinsic transfer reroutes ulnar intrinsics to act as radial deviators of the adjacent fingers. Digital extensors which have dislocated ulnarwards off the metacarpal heads may be relocated with reefing of the lateral fibres. If radial deviation at the carpus is felt responsible for ulnar drift, extensor carpi radialis longus can be transferred to extensor carpi ulnaris. Although on occasion a satisfactory correction of deformity may be obtained in the short term with these procedures, recurrence of ulnar drift is inevitable if the disease is progressive. Further deterioration of the metacarpophalangeal joint often necessitates joint replacement.

*Arthroplasty*

True digital joint replacements have been plagued by loosening at the cement–bone interface, and the implant which is currently most widely used is the type devised by Swanson — a stabilising interpositional arthroplasty which promotes capsule formation. The spacer makes no attempt to achieve fixation to bone. The stems of the implant simply lie in the medullary canal of metacarpal and phalanges (Fig. 16.20). A fibrous capsule develops around the implant which gives satisfactory stability and a moderate range of motion.

The main indication for metacarpophalangeal joint replacement is deformity, associated with significant loss of function. Examples of deformity associated with functional loss are:

1. Volar subluxation caused by ligamentous laxity. Joint incongruity may progress to dislocation (Fig. 16.6).

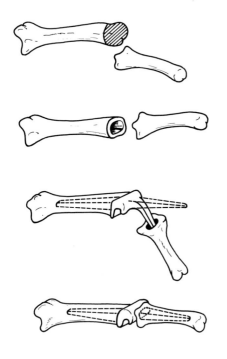

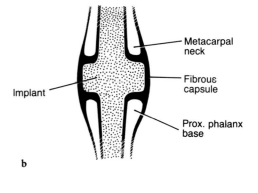

Fig. 16.20 Swanson arthroplasty of the metacarpophalangeal joint. **a** Metacarpal head resection, reaming and implant insertion. **b** Stability regained by the fibrous capsule which develops around the implant

2. Ulnar deviation in association with poor grip strength (Fig. 16.7).

The restoration of skeletal alignment reduces functional loss. Pain, alone, is an early symptom and not an indication for joint replacement. Satisfactory results will only be obtained by a precise and intensive programme of postoperative rehabilitation. However, the limited arc of motion at the metacarpophalangeal joint following replacement means that patients with poor mobility of the more distal joints may achieve a less satisfactory functional result. The procedure will have the best results in those with good mobility at the interphalangeal joints, and unimpeded tendon excursion. The improved appearance of the hand is greatly appreciated by the patient.

Proximal interphalangeal joint replacements with silicone rubber spacers are less frequently indicated. Stability of the implant may be difficult to achieve in border digits, especially the index. An arthrodesis of the joint may be preferred in such cases.

### Arthrodesis

Joint arthrodesis may be required at proximal interphalangeal or distal interphalangeal joint level in the fingers and most frequently at metacarpophalangeal and interphalangeal joint level in the thumb.

***The thumb.*** Arthrodesis of the thumb metacarpophalangeal or interphalangeal joint may be required if zig-zag deformities are present. Joint replacement at these levels rarely provides sufficient stability for effective thumb function. Arthrodesis produces excellent long-term improvement, both functionally and cosmetically, and is greatly appreciated by the patient.

There are several ways of achieving an interphalangeal joint fusion. Kirschner wires may be used but they require good bone stock. They are easy to insert, offer moderate stability but do tend to restrict the use of the digit in the weeks following surgery. The Herbert scaphoid screw may be used to achieve a stable fusion. The procedure is more complicated than some techniques but permits the early mobilisation of the thumb postoperatively without the restriction of external splintage or Kirschner wires. The screw is completely buried in the bone and does not require to be removed. For similar reasons, the mini-fragment AO plate may be used for thumb metacarpophalangeal joint fusions. Excellent stability is achieved immediately and the patient is allowed to mobilise the thumb at an early post-operative stage. The Harrison peg is another popular form of fixation, especially for soft bone. The bone ends are trimmed to the appropriate angle and the peg introduced through both cut surfaces to splint the fusion in the desired position.

Arthrodesis of the carpometacarpal joint at the base of the thumb is rarely indicated. Although excision arthroplasty is a satisfactory procedure in the osteoarthritic, it may produce instability in the rheumatoid. Silicone elastomer replacement arthroplasty may be of benefit but difficulty is sometimes experienced in obtaining satisfactory capsular stability.

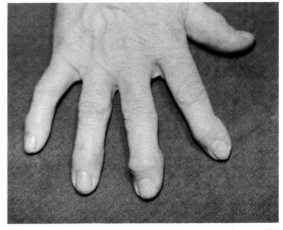

**Fig. 16.21** Heberden's nodes at the distal interphalangeal joints

# OSTEOARTHRITIS

## PRIMARY OSTEOARTHRITIS

Women are more commonly affected, often with a previous family history. Although the precise mechanism is unclear, there are biochemical changes in the cartilage which fissures and fragments. The principal upper limb joints involved are the distal interphalangeal joints and the first carpometacarpal joints.

### The distal interphalangeal joints

The patient complains of swollen and stiff distal joints. The proximal interphalangeal joints are less commonly involved and flexion of the fingers into the palm is only slightly reduced. Swellings develop on the dorsal aspects of the joints (Heberden's nodes) (Fig. 16.21). They are, in part, bony exostoses, in association with synovial hyperplasia. Radiographs reveal joint space narrowing, subchondral sclerosis and cyst formation. Surgical intervention is rarely required. Persistent pain is uncommon but the nodules and joint stiffness persist. Painful instability of the index distal interphalangeal joint may limit pinch grip and justify arthrodesis.

### The first carpometacarpal joint

Primary osteoarthritis, although common, is not always symptomatic. The patient experiences pain on stressing the first ray when performing pinch grip. Hand function is significantly impaired. The grinding test is positive (rotatory motion of the first metacarpal in compression, producing crepitus and discomfort), and radiographs reveal degenerative changes within the joint. Stress radiographs may indicate laxity of the joint (Fig. 16.22). Conservative management (splints or the use of a scaphoid plaster) may relieve discomfort, but relapse is frequent. Intra-articular steroid injections are particularly effective in gaining a remission. A subtle alteration of the patient's lifestyle, avoiding activities which provoke discomfort, will maintain the majority of patients in remission. Surgery is reserved for that group of patients who remain significantly incapacitated. Arthrodesis of the first carpometacarpal joint is difficult to achieve and may not adequately control the discomfort if the arthritis extends to all bones adjacent to the trapezium. In such cases arthroplasty of the first carpometacarpal joint is more frequently required. Trapezial excision arthroplasty provides excellent pain relief but pinch grip may be reduced compared with replacement arthroplasty.

A proportion of cases with first carpometacarpal arthritis develop progressive adduction of the first

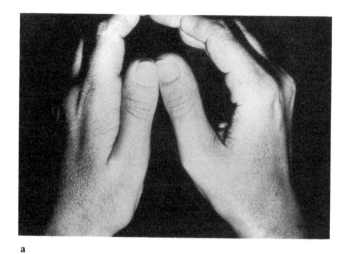

a

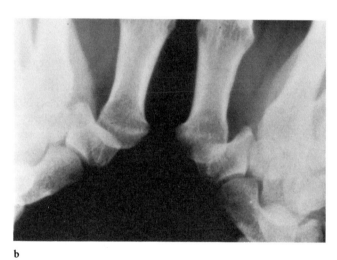

b

**Fig. 16.22**   Stress radiograph of the first carpometacarpal joints revealing moderate laxity. **a** Clinical. **b** Radiological

metacarpal across the palm reducing thumb function. This tendency can be countered by careful capsular reefing and advancement or plication of the abductor pollicis longus. However, once established, the deformity is extremely difficult to reverse.

Trapezial replacement arthroplasty is most commonly performed using a silicone elastomer spacer. This may take the form of a partial replacement where the bulk of the trapezium is left in situ. A hemi-arthroplasty (a Silastic disc with a stem in the first metacarpal) is placed in the joint and the trapezium contoured to accommo-

date the implant. More extensive degeneration requires total removal of the trapezium and the use of a larger implant (Fig. 16.23). Satisfactory containment of the spacer within the capsule is essential and removal of a portion of the trapezoid is usually required. The capsule may be buttressed with a strip of flexor carpi radialis and plication of the abductor pollicis longus is of benefit. Replacement arthroplasty is a more complex procedure but probably produces a more stable thumb with greater pinch grip, if containment of the implant can be achieved.

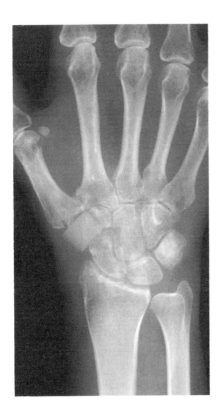

Fig. 16.23 Swanson trapezial replacement

# GOUT

Hyperuricaemia results from a disorder in purine metabolism. The majority of patients overproduce uric acid primarily, but secondary overproduction may occur (e.g. in reticulosis or leukaemia). Inadequate renal function may result in low clearance of uric acid. Gout affects males predominantly, commonly with a strong family history. Urate crystals are laid down in the joints and soft tissues, provoking synovitis. Erosions of articular cartilage are followed by secondary osteoarthritis. An acute attack without previous history may readily be confused with a septic arthritis. The patient is toxic, often with a mild leucocytosis. There may be exquisite tenderness over the involved joint, an effusion and absence of voluntary movement. Radiographs reveal osteoporosis adjacent to the joint. Aspiration of synovial fluid fails to reveal organisms but will show urate crystals in polarised light. Non-steroidal anti-inflammatory agents are used to gain control in an acute attack. The involved joint is rested and splinted, if appropriate. Surgery is not indicated. Maintenance therapy with hypo-uricaemic drugs is required if

## SECONDARY OSTEOARTHRITIS

Secondary osteoarthritis in the upper limb is most frequently due to trauma. Degenerative arthritis may follow any intra-articular fracture but should not be regarded as the inevitable sequela. Isolated fractures of finger joints often develop degenerative changes. The joint may be stiff but persistent severe pain is uncommon. Arthrodesis or arthroplasty is infrequently indicated. Intra-articular fractures of the lower end of the radius are common and a minority of these will, in the longer term, require either wrist arthrodesis or arthroplasty for persistent pain. Healed, displaced scaphoid fractures or non-unions may produce degenerative changes limited to the radius and scaphoid. If symptoms justify intervention, a silicone elastomer scaphoid replacement may be indicated. More extensive carpal arthritis would require either a wrist replacement or arthrodesis.

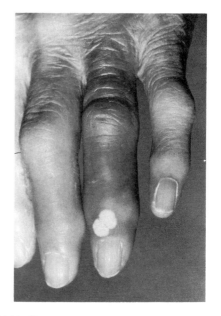

Fig. 16.24 Urate deposits in acute gouty arthritis

multiple attacks occur and the uric acid level remains raised. Repeated episodes of synovitis lead to the development of secondary arthritis with joint space narrowing and sclerosis. Punched-out lytic areas close to the articular surface are characteristic of gouty arthritis. Urate deposits in the soft tissues (tophi) (Fig. 16.24) may become calcified and visible on radiographs. Large tophi in the pulp of the fingers may cause gross deformity in the most severe cases.

# PSORIASIS

Psoriatic arthropathy is an uncommon cause of dysfunction in the upper limb. Less than 10% of patients with psoriasis involving the skin develop psoriatic arthropathy. The condition is characterised by joint stiffness and a tendency to spontaneous fusion of the wrist, proximal interphalangeal and distal interphalangeal joints. Severe flexion contracture at the proximal interphalangeal joint is common. Metacarpophalangeal joint involvement is less frequent and joint synovitis less evident in comparison with rheumatoid arthritis. The results of joint replacement are less satisfactory when compared with rheumatoid arthritis. There is less postoperative joint mobility and an increased incidence of infection. Disappearing bone disease is occasionally seen in which there is gross instability and shortening of the digits with pronounced loss of bone stock. Such digits may telescope giving the appearance described as opera-glass hand. Treatment is difficult, but comprises attempts at fusion to maintain bone length.

# 17. Dupuytren's disease

*Principal author: D. A. McGrouther*

In 1831, Baron Gauillaume Dupuytren, Surgeon at the Hotel Dieu in Paris, described to his students the results of surgical treatment of two cases of 'Permanent Retraction of the Fingers'. In both cases, he attributed the contracture to tightness of the palmar fascia. *La maladie de Dupuytren* came to be known in English literature as 'Dupuytren's contracture'. More recently it has been recognised that certain features of the condition (e.g. palmar nodules) may exist in the absence of finger contracture and the term 'Dupuytren's disease' has been adopted. There is no definite evidence, however, of a distinct disease process. Many of the phenomena can be explained on the basis of biological processes akin to wound healing. There is no specific test or unequivocal histological appearance and the diagnosis is therefore based on clinical features. Contractures of the palmar fascial ligamentous bands may represent the final common pathway of many different conditions.

Dupuytren's attribution of the cause of the contracture to the palmar fascia has, regrettably, focused the major therapeutic attention on this layer. The lesions, however, involve not only the connective tissues of the hand, but also the skin and even the joints. The surgeon must choose a co-ordinated plan of management for each of these structures.

## NATURE OF THE DISEASE PROCESS

Dupuytren's disease may be defined as a condition of the hand characterised by the contraction of bands of palmar or digital fascia (Fig. 17.1). There is bunching of the skin with distortion of the palmar creases and skin pits. Flexion contractures may occur at the metacarpophalangeal or proximal interphalangeal joints and are most common in the ulnar digits. The thumb may adduct. Clinical signs which may be found in association with palmar disease are knuckle pads, plantar fascial nodules and occasionally Peyronie's disease (see below). The palmar nodule has been suggested to be the earliest clinical sign, but this is not invariable, and it is essentially a secondary phenomenon following contraction of the underlying fascia.

A concept of the pathogenesis is necessary in order to establish principles of treatment. The pathological process in Dupuytren's contracture is incompletely understood, but has cellular and biochemical features indistinguishable from those seen in the healing of wounds. It is considered likely that Dupuytren's disease develops as a biological reactive process in certain genetically susceptible individuals in response to systemic, vascular and/or mechanical factors which are incompletely understood. It does not appear to be a neoplastic cellular process. An alternative suggestion is that it is an autonomous cellular process (fibromatosis) with a curious biological behaviour in between a reactive process and a benign neoplasm.

The nodule may represent a variety of pathological processes including, bunching of the skin, or the deposition of masses of new fibrous tissue.

The rate of progression is variable, but may be measured in months or years. It is more rapid in the younger patient. Once the disease has begun, however, the delicate ligamentous structures of the palmar fascia become tethered by masses of new tissue composed of immature collagen and fibroblasts. The normal movement between the fascial ligamentous bands, which should accompany

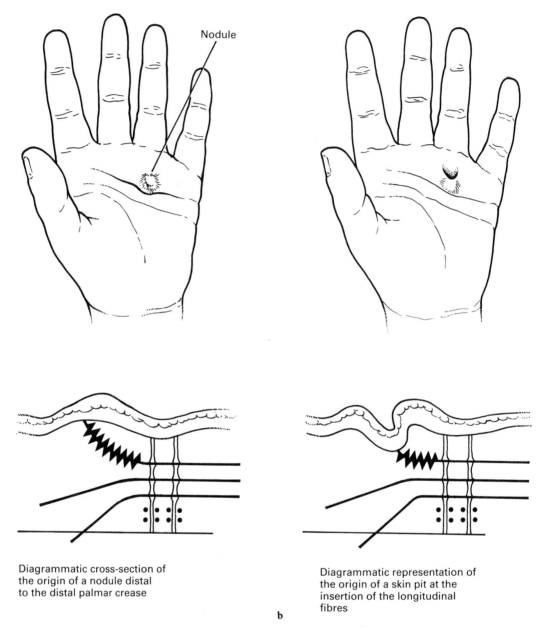

Nodule

Diagrammatic cross-section of
the origin of a nodule distal
to the distal palmar crease

Diagrammatic representation of
the origin of a skin pit at the
insertion of the longitudinal
fibres

a

b

**Fig. 17.1** Features of the disease. **a, b** In the early stage a nodule forms distal to the distal palmar crease. A longitudinal section through the palmar fascia at this point shows tethering of the skin with the formation of a nodule.

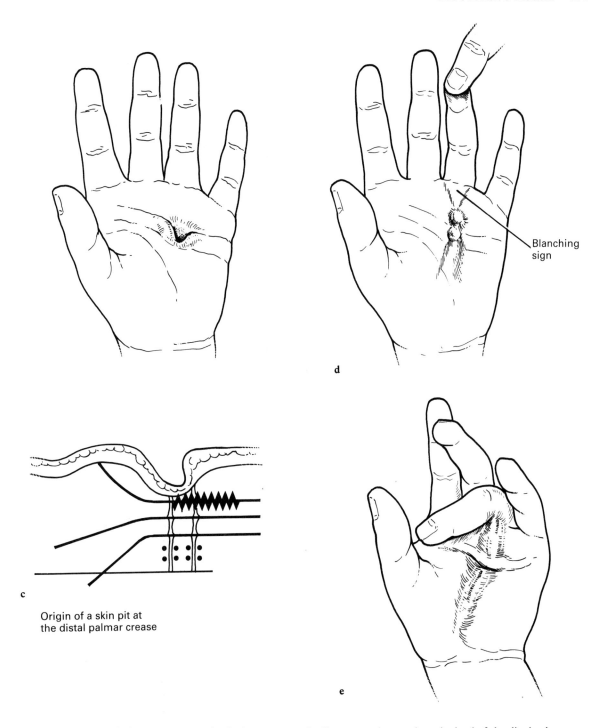

Blanching
sign

d

c

Origin of a skin pit at
the distal palmar crease

e

**Fig. 17.1  c** Alternatively, a contracture developing more proximally may produce a pit at the level of the distal palmar crease. **d** Once the longitudinal bands of the palmar fascia are tethered, forced extension of the digit will blanch the skin distal to the area of tethering producing a characteristic sign. **e** As the disease progresses the finger will become flexed at the metacarpophalangeal or interphalangeal joints

the folding of the palmar skin on flexion, is prevented. Tension develops in these ligamentous bands as the hand extends and this pulls on the distal ligamentous continuations (Fig. 17.1d); this may be the stimulus which propagates the contracting process of 'the disease'. It is known that immature fibroblastic tissue does respond to mechanical stimulation. Intermittent tension, in particular, is known to stimulate the deposition of collagen and influence its orientation.

There is a convention whereby the normal anatomical ligamentous structures are designated 'bands', whereas contracted Dupuytren's tissues are described as 'cords'. Dupuytren's tissue is not randomly distributed. *The cords follow anatomical pathways*, i.e. they follow normal ligamentous bands and pass from band to band at normal points of crossing or from band to dermis at points where the bands insert into skin.

Tension has a role in maintaining the tissue response, and this is shown by the biological behaviour of the condition after cord division (fasciotomy). Considerable resolution of the pathological process may occur with disappearance of subcutaneous nodules and softening of the tissues if tension is successfully released. The technique is only effective, however, when the fascial ends are prevented from re-uniting.

Dupuytren cells behave like normal palmar fascial fibroblasts in tissue culture, but produce abnormal quantities (and ratios) of glycosaminoglycans (connective tissue ground substances) when in the palm. This suggests that the cellular behaviour in the palm is in response to the local mechanical environment.

The above evidence suggests that the aim of surgery should be to produce a stable biological solution by the permanent release of tension rather than by a radical excisional approach, such as would be used in tumour surgery. The treatment philosophy can be compared with that in postburn scar contractures, where release and prevention of re-union by prolonged splintage may be effective. Total excision of all burns scar tissue is not required. Dupuytren's 'tissue' behaves in a similar way to postburn contracture tissue, but being situated in different anatomical planes, it gives rise to different clinical manifestations.

The surgical aim must be to reconstruct the palmar tissues in such a way that tension cannot subsequently be transmitted through fascial bands or the fibrosis resulting from operation. This may be achieved either by interposition of normal subcutaneous fat or by excision of involved subcutaneous tissues and application of a skin graft. However, the wound healing processes after surgery tend to promote adhesion between tissue layers producing so-called 'recurrence', and this process must be modified during the rehabilitation phase.

Surgery excises Dupuytren's 'disease' myofibroblasts and replaces these by wound healing myofibroblasts. The aim of treatment must be to minimise cellular proliferation by avoiding dead space. The wound bed is 'contractile' and should be held out to length after operation until collagen maturity is established.

## INCIDENCE

The incidence of the disease varies considerably from one part of the world to another and this seems to be based on racial rather than environmental factors, although the incidence seems higher in colder climates. The disease is common in the UK, Europe, Scandinavia and Russia. It is rare in African negroes, in China and South East Asia, and very uncommon in India and Japan. There is a high incidence in Canada, the USA and in Australia and this is thought to be due to the migration of peoples of Northern European extraction. The precise geographical roots of the disease remain obscure however, as there was almost no documentation prior to the report by Dupuytren. The incidence certainly rises with age and in the UK has been reported to be as high as 20–25% in men over the age of 70 years. The disease is twice as common in men as in women. However, there is considerable variation in incidence between recorded series and this is probably due to patient selection and the difficulty in making an unequivocal diagnosis of the condition.

Apart from this 'natural' incidence, a number of clinical conditions seem to be associated with Dupuytren's disease. There is a definite relationship to epilepsy, but a question remains as to whether the association is with the disease or with anticonvulsant drugs; phenytoin, epanutin or phenobarbitone. The incidence is increased in diabetic patients and it has been suggested that all Dupuytren's patients should be screened for diabetes. Patients in long-term institutional care for tuberculosis and suffering chronic respiratory disease have an increased incidence. A relationship has been reported with alcoholism and cirrhosis, but ethnic population selection may account for this apparent finding. No increase has been shown in cigarette smokers and the disease has been reported to be reduced in frequency in patients with rheumatoid arthritis. Dupuytren's disease may occur together with carpal tunnel or trigger finger, but it is uncertain whether this is a chance occurrence or a true relationship.

Ulnar nerve pathology and gout have been suggested as contributory factors, but this seems unlikely except in a few individual patients. Experimental measurements have shown a reduction in digital blood flow in Dupuytren's contracture; however, this may be a result of the disease rather than a causative factor. Various experimental workers have considered the role of vascular factors in the aetiology of this condition; the source of the myofibroblasts appears to be the perivascular cells. Low blood flow, oedema, reflex sympathetic dystrophy and vascular occlusions have all been suggested as contributory processes. Oedema from post-traumatic sympathetic dystrophy, such as is seen after mobilisation for treatment of Colles' fracture, does provoke a Dupuytren's-like thickening of the palm and tethering of the fascial ligaments, although this does not necessarily progress to a full contracture. Oedema and the leakage of fibrin could be a common denominator in all of these processes. Immobilisation has also been suggested to have a contributory role.

The strongest factor appears to be heredity and a strong family history is often noted, but this is not invariable. The term 'Dupuytren's diathesis' has been used to indicate a strong individual tendency. Many patients will try to associate the onset of their contracture with injury or occupational stresses such as the use of a screwdriver pressing on the palm. Dupuytren's contracture may follow a single sharp injury to the hand. Indeed there has been considerable debate about the relevance of blunt trauma or chronic repeated occupational usage as causative factors in Dupuytren's disease. In support of this hypothesis localised lesions are seen in unusual sites which the patient may attribute to particular repeated usage. The dominant hand is more often involved and when bilateral the disease is rarely symmetrical. In manual labourers the pick and shovel or the hammer and chisel do not spare the non-dominant hand, but subject the palms to different usage. The balance of evidence at present suggests that an inherited tendency is revealed, rather than that the disease is caused by mechanical factors. It seems, therefore, that there is a susceptible population and that triggering factors may interact in a complex way.

In summary, epidemiological evidence suggests that inheritance determines *if* the patient will develop the condition. *When* it commences is determined by associated diseases, drugs, injury or, perhaps occupation. *Where* the disease develops in the hand is determined by hand fascial anatomy and biomechanics (the resting posture may make the ulnar digits more vulnerable to fixation in a flexed position). The distribution of the disease in the digits may also reflect injury and, perhaps, occupational usage. The rate of progression depends mainly on age at first presentation, but personality has some influence and there is individual variation.

## PATHOLOGY

The earliest visible changes are thickening of the longitudinal fibres. Biochemical changes predate this stage and are detectable before there is any histological abnormality. The normal longitudinal bands visibly thicken to become opaque, white or gelatinous cords. From the surrounding vessels the perivascular cells proliferate and these seem to be the source of the new masses of immature fibrous tissue. Aggregations form around the cords enveloping and anchoring them. The surrounding fat and connective tissues are displaced or replaced. The skin may be heaped up by underlying cellular tissues or bunched up by tethering of the longitudinal ligamentous cords with the formation of clinical nodules.

In the early active or contractile phase, the predominant cell is the myofibroblast, a cell similar to a smooth muscle cell. These cells are recognised histologically by a crenated concertina-like nucleus having a system within the cytoplasm which is thought to permit contraction. In the later stages, the Dupuytren's tissue resembles tendon, being relatively acellular with orientated mature collagen bundles.

The mechanism of contracture is unknown. The myofibroblast may play an active contractile role rather like that seen in a healing wound. Alternatively, the fibroblastic tissue may simply act to stiffen the delicate palmar fascial bands. Thereafter extension from the neutral position is prevented. Progressive contracture may be due to incremental loss of extension range (a ratchet effect). Dupuytren's disease, like scar tissue, produces contractures on the flexion surface of the hand, as this is the concave surface in the resting position.

## ANATOMY

The clinical features of Dupuytren's disease are best understood by relating them to the anatomy of the palmar fascia. Longitudinal bundles from the palmaris longus at the wrist pass distally to the five digital rays. In the mid palm, at a deeper level, there are the transverse fibres of Skoog. Interwoven with these are vertical fibres passing downwards from the skin of the palm. The whole system forms a three-dimensional network of fibres with fat loculi in the intervening spaces. Dupuytren's disease involves the longitudinal fibre system, the distal insertions of which are in three layers (Figs 17.2, 17.3). The most superficial pass to the skin of the distal palm. The intermediate layer passes to the digits by spiralling behind the neurovascular bundle (spiral band of Gosset). The deepest fibres pass around the tendon sheath at the level of the metacarpophalangeal joints.

Early stages of the disease may present with a palpable subcutaneous thickening or a distinct nodule in the distal part of the palm. On full extension of the finger, the 'blanching sign' (pallor in the skin distal to the nodules) may be seen, indicating tension in the skin distally. Skin pits or distortion of the palmar creases may also appear. Horizontal distortion is due to tethering of the skin by contracted cords. Vertical distortion is a persistence of the palmar creases on full extension and is due to shortening of the vertical fibres.

In the digits there is also a three-dimensional system of ligamentous structures as demonstrated by McFarlane (Fig. 17.4). There is no anterior longitudinal ligamentous system in the normal digits, although longitudinal fibres do appear in Dupuytren's disease and are thought to arise from the dermis. The normal longitudinal fibres lie laterally in the digits as the lateral digital sheet (a longitudinally orientated network of fibres in the normal hand). Palmar contractures may pass to the fingers along several pathways. The *central cord* seems to form from the dermis in the digital midline and run longitudinally. There is always skin involvement over this cord and displacement of the neurovascular bundles is unlikely. A *lateral digital cord* may develop along the line of the lateral digital sheet; neurovascular bundle displacement is unusual. The cord with the highest incidence of neurovascular bundle displacement is *the spiral cord* which passes from the palmar longitudinal fibres through the spiral band of Gosset (which runs around the neurovas-

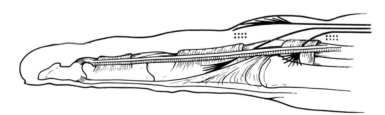

Fig. 17.2   A cross-section of the digit shows the three layers of longitudinal fibres of palmar fascia beneath the distal palmar crease. The most superficial inserts into the skin of the distal palm. The middle layer spirals around the neurovascular bundles to reach the fascia on the side of the finger (lateral digital sheet). The deepest layer passes around the sides of the flexor sheath lateral to the metacarpophalangeal joint

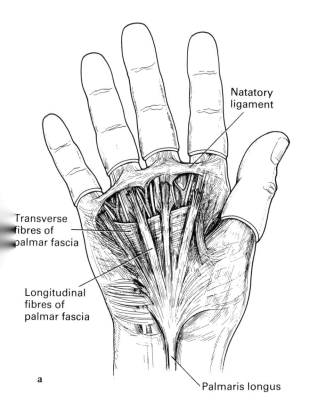

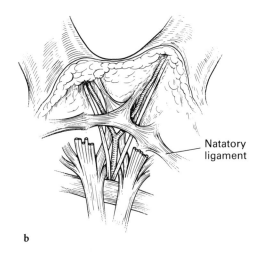

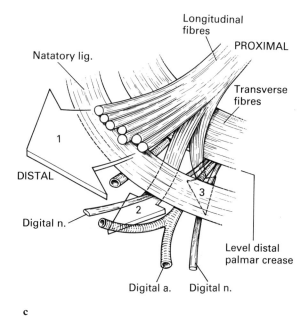

**Fig. 17.3** **a** The anatomy of the palmar fascia. The longitudinal fibres to each individual digital ray are noted. There are two transverse systems of fibres, the natatory ligaments at the base of the digital webs. A deeper transverse system (the fibres of Skoog) or transverse fibres of the palmar aponeurosis. **b** The detail of an individual web space is shown. The longitudinal fibres pass superficial to the transverse fibres of Skoog. The most superficial insert into the skin. The middle fibres spiral around the neurovascular bundles to reach the sides of the digits. The deepest fibres pass deeply into the hand around the side of the flexor tendon sheath. **c** Expanded detail of the fascia in the web. The orientation is different from **a** or **b**. Longitudinal fibres are seen passing superficial to the transverse fibres of Skoog and deep to the transverse natatory fibres. Layer 1 inserts into skin, 2 spirals around neurovascular bundles and 3 passes deeply, lateral to the metacarpophalangeal joint (Fig. 17.2).

cular bundle, see above) to reach the lateral digital sheet. A contracture following this pathway therefore spirals around the neurovascular bundle and as the cord contracts and straightens, the bundle is seen to spiral around the cord. The nerve and vessel are therefore at risk during operation. Displacement of the bundle is most likely in the proximal segment of the digit. For this reason Hueston has warned 'Beware the eccentric cord'.

On the ulnar side of the hand, cords arise from the abductor digit minimi muscle or its overlying fascia. These are commonly associated with neurovascular bundle displacement. When the thumb is involved, the Dupuytren's process may develop in the web along its free border (distal commissural ligament) or there may be a tight cord proximal and parallel to this (the proximal commissural ligament). Alternatively, the longi-

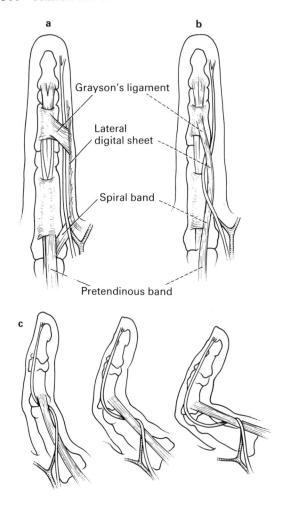

Grayson's ligament

Lateral
digital sheet

Spiral band

Pretendinous band

**Fig. 17.4** Anatomy of the digital ligaments. **a** The main fascial structure in the digit is the lateral digital sheet. **b** The formation of a spiral cord is shown when the Dupuytren's disease follows the pretendinous band through the spiral band to the lateral digital sheet and thereafter to the middle phalanx via the Grayson's ligament and flexor sheath. When contracture occurs along these structures a spiral cord is formed which displaces the neurovascular bundle. **c** As the digit becomes more flexed the displaced neurovascular bundle comes to lie more and more proximally on top of the contracting spiral band

tudinal bundle of palmar fascia leading to the radial border of the thumb may be involved. Uncommonly the interphalangeal joint flexes. The thumb rarely merits intervention on its own account. Surgery may be undertaken at the same time as procedures on other digital rays. Release of the web may require a Z-plasty. Release of

interphalangeal contracture frequently requires a graft because of skin involvement.

## 'ECTOPIC DEPOSITS'

Knuckle pads are localised thickenings over the dorsum of the proximal interphalangeal joints. Histologically the tissue has a similar fibromatous appearance to palmar Dupuytren's tissue. These knuckle pads are generally taken to indicate a strong Dupuytren's diathesis, but they can be found in the absence of palmar disease. Other associated conditions are plantar nodules (synonym Ledderhose's disease) which occur characteristically in the insole at the medial border of the plantar aponeurosis. An increased incidence of Dupuytren's disease is found in patients with Peyronie's disease. This is a localised thickening on the dorsum of the penis associated with a curvature, concave upwards.

## PRESENTING FEATURES

Nodules and progressive flexion deformity are the usual presenting factors. The condition may be noted by a general practitioner and the patient sent to a surgeon for advice on whether or not operative intervention is indicated. Symptoms are few, but tenderness over the nodules, or discomfort on heavy use, may occur. The fingers most frequently involved are the ring and little followed by the middle finger and the thumb. Flexion deformity of the index is infrequent. Contracted cords may be obvious and palpable or may lie deeply within the digits leading to confusion in diagnosis.

## FACTORS TO BE CONSIDERED IN DECIDING ON TREATMENT

Conservative treatment, for example, injection of the nodules with steroids or enzyme injection to the cords, has been tried without appreciable success. Radiotherapy, still used in some countries, is positively contraindicated as it will result in postirradiation skin changes. Splintage may retard the progression of contracture, but will not reverse the condition. Treatment is therefore by surgery. However, not all patients with Dupuytren's contracture will benefit from operation.

A balanced judgement must be reached contrasting the potential improvement in. hand function which surgery may achieve and the probable deterioration if the hand is untreated.

## TIMING OF OPERATION

Once finger contracture has commenced, it usually has a progressive course, although the rate of deterioration has considerable individual variation. *It is the rate of progression of contracture which is the single most important factor in determining when operation is indicated.* The course is generally more rapid in the younger patient and therefore the potential for deterioration in the absence of surgery is considerable. An older patient after several recurrences has a limited potential for improvement with surgery and the rate of progression of the condition will also be slower. Good clinical judgement would suggest a conservative approach.

The ideal plan of management is that all patients should be referred to a hand surgeon early and kept under regular review to judge the rate of deterioration. Postponing surgery until the digit touches the palm is disastrous. The table-top test is a useful guide to progression: the patient can usually accurately time the onset of their inability to place the palm of the hand flat on a table; it is also an indication when to intervene. *When Dupuytren's contracture reaches the stage that joint deformities are beginning to become fixed and no longer passively correctable, operation is indicated.*

Although the major indication for treatment is rapid progression of the finger contracture, the presence of a significant contraction (which cannot be passively corrected) at the proximal interphalangeal joint is an indication for surgery irrespective of the rate of progression. Metacarpophalangeal joint flexion deformity can almost always be released and there is therefore less urgency in this situation than in the case of the proximal interphalangeal joint, which once contracted can be very difficult to release. Operation is rarely indicated for palmar nodules in the absence of contracture.

## PRINCIPLES OF ALL OPERATIONS FOR DUPUYTREN'S CONTRACTURE

A co-ordinated surgical and rehabilitation programme is applied to achieve maximal improvement in hand function. There is no single operative procedure which is suitable for all patients and the appropriate procedure must be matched to the individual problem. All patients must be advised of the likelihood of recurrence. Failure to do so is a potent cause of dissatisfaction and may lead to unnecessary litigation. The factors which should be considered in making a judgement on the choice of operation are:

1. The patient: age, motivation and general health.
2. The type of hand.
3. The contracture.

### 1. The patient

*Age*: although there is general agreement that a limited operation is satisfactory in the elderly patient, a more radical operation in the younger patient will not necessarily give protection from recurrence. Younger patients often have a more aggressive and diffuse contracture. Surgery should be undertaken early and skin replacement considered. *Motivation* is an important factor and should be judged by the history and attention to such factors as hand hygiene and response to previous injuries. The patient's *general health* should be noted, particularly in relation to systemic disease or medication.

### 2. The type of hand

The *anatomy* of the patient's hand is significant. The workman's thickened hand is said to be at greater risk from postoperative stiffness, whereas long thin digits respond more favourably. The *physiology* of the hand is difficult to quantify other than by subjective impressions. The elderly atrophic hand, which is pale and cold, has a poor prognosis as has the hand which is moved little during examination. The sweating hand is at risk of postoperative oedema and the hand which shows evidence of post-traumatic sympathetic dystrophy may become stiff.

## 3. The contracture

The choice of operation is influenced by the speedy progression of the contracture and its severity. The slowly progressive contracture is likely to contain more mature cellular and fibrous tissue and respond favourably to a more limited surgical procedure.

A lasting release of the contracted fascial tissues may sometimes be possible by performing a fasciotomy. Proximal interphalangeal joint manipulation should always be gentle if performed during Dupuytren surgery. Excessive force may provoke spasm of digital vessels or cause joint subluxation rather than true extension. If the cut fascial ends retract into fat, a lasting separation may be achieved. If this is not possible because of diffuse disease or absence of fat, then a fasciectomy is required. Fasciectomy is principally aimed at excision of the nodules and involved cords, although some surgeons advocate prophylactic excision of apparently uninvolved tissue.

A broad contracture consisting of a wide cord, or group of nodules, is more difficult to release. The presence of skin involvement may indicate the need for skin replacement. The distribution of the contracture in the palm will dictate whether one or more rays require dissection. The distribution in the digit will indicate the approach required for management of the skin, the contracted fascia and the proximal interphalangeal joint.

The common principle of all operations is that healthy tissue must be interposed between the two ends of the excised or divided Dupuytren's cord to prevent the rejoining of contracted fascial structures. The aim should be to preserve a layer of fat between normal skin and deep structures. However, if the fat is lost and the dermis involved, excision of the involved skin and graft replacement is preferred.

## GENERAL POINTS IN TECHNIQUE

All surgery must be performed under tourniquet and adequate anaesthesia to allow a lengthy procedure if necessary. Loupe magnification will facilitate the identification of neurovascular bundles and the assessment of skin vascularity.

**Table 17.1** Operations for Dupuytren's contracture

*Management of the skin*
Incisions
  Zig-zag for exposure
  Linear followed by Z-plasty (for exposure and lengthening)
Skin replacement
  To replace deficiency resulting from contracture
  Prophylactically required to interrupt contracture continuity
  If excision of involved skin is necessary
Open palm

*Management of the contracted fascia*
Fasciotomy
  Open
  Closed
  Fasciotomy and Z-plasty
  Fasciotomy and graft
Limited fasciectomy
  Regional
  Selective
Radical or extensive fasciectomy
(Dermofasciectomy)

*Management of the contracted proximal interphalangeal joint*
  Release
  I    Release of tendon sheath
  II   Check-rein ligament release
  III  Volar capsulectomy
  Arthrodesis
  Arthroplasty
  Osteotomy
  Accept deformity
  Amputation

Knowledge of the anatomy of the contracted tissue is essential, particularly in relation to the possible displacement of neurovascular bundles. The surgeon must have in mind not only the excision of involved fascial tissue, but also a plan for the replacement of deficient or infiltrated skin by graft or flap cover and correction of joint contractures (Table 17.1).

## Management of the skin and subcutaneous tissues

### Incision

Incisions with a predominantly longitudinal orientation are frequently employed for these allow the neurovascular bundles to be progressively displayed without injury (Fig. 17.5). (This conforms to extensile exposure as described by A. K. Henry.) The presence of a straight longitudinal incision, however, would leave a scar which would itself

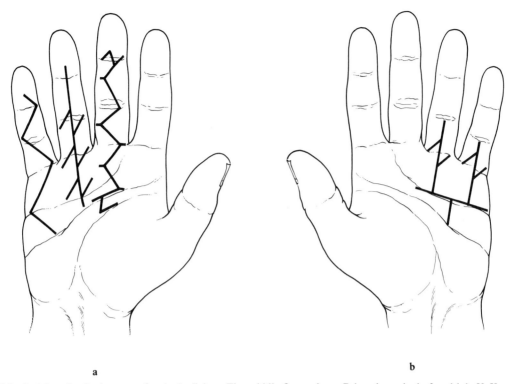

a                                                                                          b

**Fig. 17.5** Incisions for fasciectomy of a single digit. **a** The middle finger shows Palmen's method of multiple V–Y advancements. The ring finger shows a linear incision with Z-plasties. The little finger shows the technique of Bruner. **b** Skoog incision for access to two adjacent digital rays

cause contracture. The scar alignment must be interrupted by use of an initial zig-zag approach, such as that used by Bruner. Where there is skin involvement (i.e. the Dupuytren's cellular process extends into the dermis) a zig-zag incision will carry the risk of flap (tip) necrosis. All zig-zag incisions tend to straighten during wound healing.

A Z-plasty can achieve lengthening in addition to producing a zig-zag configuration (Fig. 17.5). When designing a Z-plasty, it is probably better to make a linear incision and perform Z-plasties at a later stage. In this way the distally based flap can be placed on the better vascularised side. Neutral line incisions in the digit have been used, but carry a risk of skin necrosis where there is skin involvement and, in addition, access is poor. The use of a transverse incision makes the anatomy much more difficult to visualise, but it leaves unscarred skin segments between each incision which are less likely to be a source of recurrent skin contracture. Their use is limited for

fasciectomy by the poor view that they provide. The guiding rule in the planning of incisions is to interrupt the line of future potential skin contracture.

Many patterns of skin incision are possible. In planning and raising the flaps, it is essential that the palmar skin must not be devitalised. The incision should proceed as far as the distal end of the Dupuytren's tissue. If this attachment of the cord appears to be over the middle phalanx, it may be necessary to continue the incision beyond the distal interphalangeal joint crease or even to the pulp of the digit, in order to achieve sufficient exposure to excise the tissue without damaging neurovascular bundles. Once the width and length of the exposure have been planned, the necessary skin incisions are marked out with ink. For single ray involvement, a longitudinal (zig-zag) incision is adequate. Where more than one ray is involved a transverse incision at the distal palmar crease is the usual starting

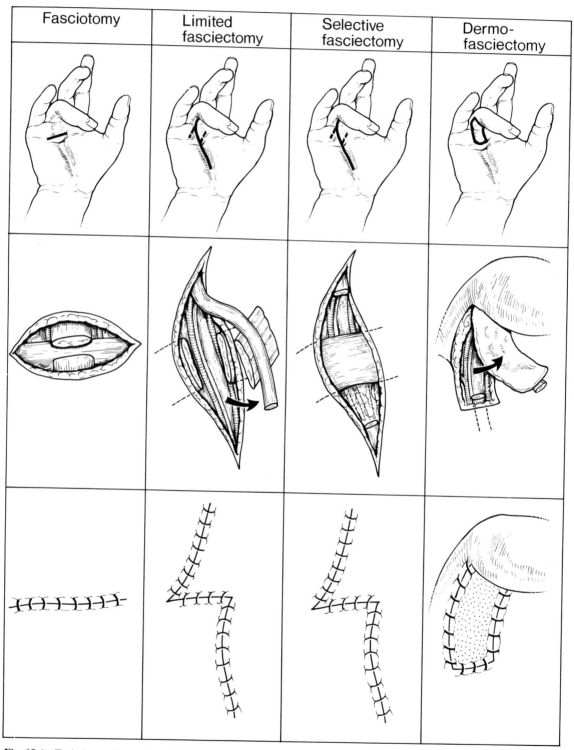

**Fig. 17.6**  Techniques of operation. A fasciotomy divides only the longitudinal fibres. A limited fasciectomy removes the longitudinal fibres together with the underlying transverse fibres. A selective fasciectomy removes only the involved longitudinal fibres. A dermofasciectomy electively excises the skin and fascia as far lateral as the neutral line of the digit. The area is reconstructed by a full thickness skin graft

point. From this a perpendicular may be extended proximally in the midline of the Dupuytren's tissue, thereby allowing retraction of equal flaps in radial and ulnar directions. Extending distally from the distal palmar crease, longitudinal extensions should be made to each of the involved digits. Preservation of the subcutaneous fat pads between these longitudinal incisions will ensure that the skin of the distal palm retains a satisfactory blood supply. It is recommended that the reader follow these rules of planning the width and length of the required operative field, rather than adhering to a preconceived geometric plan. If the palm alone is involved, a transverse incision may be adequate without extension.

*Skin replacement*

There are three indications for replacing skin in Dupuytren's disease. The *skin may be deficient* due to general contracture of the palmar tissues and this is more likely after recurrence. Release may therefore result in the creation of a deficit. A skin graft may be used to achieve wound closure, although smaller defects may heal spontaneously by the open palm method. Secondly, skin replacement may be used *to separate the ends of contracted fascia*. This is particularly indicated where the contracted fascia is left in situ. This plan was originally devised by Gonzales, who used full thickness grafts to break up the line of digital contractures. Alternative means of skin replacement are by using split skin grafts or, occasionally, a local flap. The dorsal digital skin of an amputated digit may be used in this way, spreading the skin across the palm to interrupt the line of a future potential contracture. The third indication for skin replacement arises when the dermis is 'involved' by Dupuytren's tissue or recurrent contracture and needs to be *electively excised*. This has been advocated by Hueston.

Skin involvement is apparent clinically by the strong fixation of the skin to the underlying contracted tissue. At operation, a plane can only be created artificially between involved dermis and Dupuytren's tissue by sharp dissection with a knife. The deep surface of the dermis will appear grey, there being no subcutaneous fat. The dermis is thickened and packed with myofibroblasts. This skin is liable to contract like a deep dermal burn. If such areas of skin involvement are small, it may be possible, by the design of Z-plasties, to intersperse areas of involved skin with areas of normal skin. Alternatively, the skin should be excised and replaced by skin grafts.

In the operation of dermofasciectomy (Figs 17.6, 17.7), a wide excision of involved skin is performed, usually over the proximal segment of the finger and distal palm. The excision should extend as far laterally as the midaxial line of the digit, so that subsequent contracture along the edge of the graft will not create a flexion contracture. Skin replacement is generally by full thickness skin grafts, which may be harvested from the groin crease, where the cosmetic appearance of the donor site is most satisfactory. Alternatively, the graft may be obtained from the forearm or upper arm, the donor site being closed directly or by split skin graft. Full thickness grafts should be cut to the exact size and shape using a template. Full thickness grafts on the flexor aspect of the finger necessitate splintage of the finger in extension for between 2 and 3 weeks to allow the graft to stabilise. Thereafter they must be protected from shearing for a further 2–3 weeks. A prolonged absence from work is often necessary. However, current evidence suggests that there is continuing protection from recurrence after this procedure (but not for local extension). Thinner split skin grafts are generally less satisfactory on the flexor aspect of the fingers, as they tend to contract and the resultant skin cover is less supple. Split skin grafts

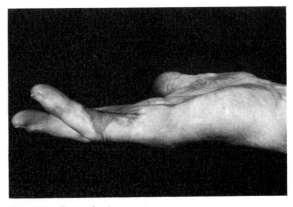

**Fig. 17.7**  Dermofasciectomy

lack sweat glands and may develop hyperkeratosis with cracking and fissuring in this site.

### The open palm technique

The 'open palm', which is a variation of post-operative management rather than an operative technique, was introduced by McCash in an attempt to overcome problems related to haematoma formation. Haemostasis is now more meticulous due to improved methods of vessel coagulation, and, thus, this is no longer the sole reason for this technique. An additional benefit lies in the release of extra skin which can be used to obtain digital cover at the expense of the palm which is left open. Gains can be achieved in this way without the need for importation of flap or graft cover. The transverse wound, at the distal palmar crease, is left unsutured and a non-adherent dressing applied which is changed daily. Antibiotic cream in the wound facilitates this. The open wound often heals by secondary intention in 8–10 days, although it may take longer. Healing is by the normal processes of wound contracture leaving a transverse linear scar.

One of the surprising advantages of the technique is almost complete absence of postoperative pain. This allows immediate mobilisation, and recovery of a full range of active motion is common within the first 48 hours of surgery. The rapid postoperative mobilisation enhances collagen orientation in the healing wound, leading to a soft and supple palmar scar, and is an essential part of the management.

The great merit of the technique is its safety. It is a reliable method of providing extra skin, minimising postoperative discomfort, and draining possible palmar haematoma — especially after extensive dissection. It is unnecessary where a limited dissection has been performed with good haemostasis.

The immediate disadvantage of the open palm technique is that it is unpopular with patients who are apprehensive about the appearance of the open wound. Careful counselling is always necessary. Advocates claim that the patient can return to full use of the hand immediately, despite the open wound and frequent dressings. This technique is not a substitute for good haemostasis.

*Haemostasis.* The underlying principle is that haematoma must not be allowed to collect in a closed dead space in the hand after fasciectomy. The exact means by which individual surgeons choose to achieve this may vary.

Possibilities are:

1. Keeping the tourniquet up until a *firm* dressing is applied. Release of the bandage is always required after several hours and the circulation must always be checked postoperatively. The authors do not recommend this technique.

2. Letting down the tourniquet and securing bipolar haemostasis prior to wound closure. The cuff should be removed from the arm. The authors advocate this technique for routine use. The bipolar coagulator should also be used throughout the operation to coagulate all small vessels which are encountered as the dissection proceeds.

3. Drains.

4. Elevation prior to wound closure.

5. Complete or partial open palm.

Most surgeons use a combination of approaches, but the measures must be effective. *Postoperative pain indicates haematoma and requires re-exploration.*

## Management of the contracted fascia

Contracted fascia may be managed either by release or by resection as follows:

### Fasciotomy

This was the operation performed by Baron Dupuytren. Fasciotomy may be either *open* (where the skin wound is made sufficiently large to identify the tendons and neurovascular bundles) or *closed*, when a more limited skin incision is made. The aim of fasciotomy is to divide tight well-defined cords producing contracture and it is only permissible under certain closely defined conditions. Longstanding palmar cords in elderly patients are most suitable. The operation is particularly indicated for the elderly, unfit patient and is (totally) contraindicated in the young active Dupuytren's patient with widespread skin involvement, as recurrence is almost certain. The cord must be divided in the palm and should be readily palpable, yet discreet from the overlying skin. The technique is reserved for release of a cord producing contracture at the metacarpophalangeal joint. The advantage of the closed operation is rapid wound healing, but there is a definite risk of injury to the digital nerve or artery, or retained haematoma. Open fasciotomy permits a better view of the cord and the adjacent neurovascular bundles, but even this procedure carries some risk, and it should be reserved for the experienced hand surgeon. *Preliminary* fasciotomy may also have a role in the severe contracture with macerated palmar skin; fasciectomy can then be performed at a later date. A short longitudinal incision will close easily, but a transverse wound will tend to gape. A small Z-plasty allows a better view of the anatomy by creating flaps which improve the exposure. A large Z-plasty is indicated for the specific technique of *fasciotomy and Z-plasty* which allows elevation of the longitudinal cords of fascia with the skin flaps. When the flaps are transposed, the fascia is also transposed, preventing re-establishment of the fascial cords' longitudinal continuity.

*Fasciotomy and grafting* is a technique reserved for a different group of patients (Fig. 17.8). It may be used primarily, but is particularly useful as a salvage procedure in the recurrent case with severe skin scarring, where elevation of skin flaps may be hazardous. The longitudinal *cords* are transected, preferably from one neutral line of the hand to the other and, after thorough release of all contracted tissues, a split skin graft is applied

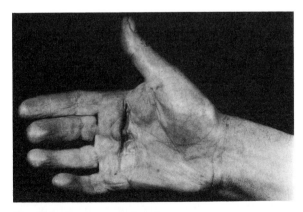

**Fig. 17.8** Fasciotomy and graft

to the defect to maintain separation of diseased fascia, rather than to make good a skin deficiency.

### Limited fasciectomy (also described as 'partial' or 'regional' fasciectomy)

There are three elements to limited fasciectomy. As soon as the transection of the involved fascia is performed at palmar level, a release rather like a fasciotomy takes place, which may produce a considerable, if not complete, correction of the contracture. The second part of the operation is the excision of the involved fascia and, thirdly, there is a limited prophylactic excision of adjacent uninvolved fascia. However, the principle aim of the operation is to excise the involved fascia in the affected ray or rays and to leave adjacent rays untouched.

Careful dissection with a No. 15 scalpel blade is 'safe' in the primary case. Great care must always be taken to identify structures before dividing them. On the rare occasions when digital nerves are accidentally cut, it is often because the surgeon believes he has safely preserved the nerve, whereas he is in reality guarding a fascial band. In densely involved areas, or recurrences, spreading the tissues with tenotomy scissors (the delicate round-pointed tips are specifically designed for spreading) is an invaluable additional technique. Beyond the distal palmar crease, there is the possibility that nerves will spiral around and pass superficial to the bands. It is therefore necessary to identify the neurovascular structures proximally and preserve them as the more distal fasciectomy proceeds.

**Selective fasciectomy (Skoog).** It is possible to retain the transverse fibres of the palmar aponeurosis as advised by Skoog. The preservation of these fibres is a useful discipline, for the nerves and vessels will always be beneath them and need not be disturbed in the proximal palm. With experience therefore, it is not necessary to identify the neurovascular bundles proximal to the distal palmar crease.

It is not always necessary to lay the bundles bare in the finger and, if possible, they should be left undisturbed if they are lying in uninvolved tissues. A recurrence around exposed bundles increases the risk of neurovascular injury on subsequent exploration.

### Radical fasciectomy

The operation of radical (or extensive) palmar fasciectomy aims to remove all of the palmar fascial structures, whether involved or not, but only involved fingers are dissected. Most of the palmar dissection is therefore prophylactic. A high incidence of fibrous contracture and joint stiffness was found in the past with this method and this was attributed to the extensive dissection of palmar fascia, with associated production of dead space and collection of haematoma. Good bipolar haemostasis, drainage, pressure dressings and elevation can prevent haematoma formation and can result in a favourable outcome to the patient. Radical fasciectomy is still widely performed in Europe and good results are achieved when attention is paid to the preservation of the skin blood supply and the avoidance of haematoma.

However, extensive dissection has not been shown to produce a lower recurrence rate. The widespread use of this method would therefore be likely to lead to an increase in complications without necessarily reducing recurrences. The development of digital recurrences or extensions is the major difficulty and a radical approach to the palm will not alter this. For these reasons radical palmar fasciectomy is not a popular operation in the UK, USA or Australia.

### Dermofasciectomy

Skin involvement is detectable clinically where the skin cannot be moved over the fascia. There is no clear plane of separation between fascia and dermis. Sharp dissection allows a layer of dermis to be elevated from underlying scar tissue, but in areas of true skin involvement, this plane can only be made by the knife. To redrape this thickened and scarred dermis over the hand seems likely to lead to further trouble. The operation of dermofasciectomy has been described by Hueston as particularly appropriate in recurrent cases, but it should also be considered in primary cases with such skin involvement.

## Management of the contracted proximal interphalangeal joint

Digital fasciectomy should permit full proximal interphalangeal joint extension if pre-operative assessment indicates that the flexion deformity is passively correctable (metacarpophalangeal flexion permitting proximal interphalangeal joint extension). If the proximal interphalangeal joint is not passively correctable pre-operatively, the release which may be obtained at digital fasciectomy is unpredictable.

Persistent contracture at the joint after fasciectomy requires evaluation of deeper structures. Further release may be achieved by division of Cleland's ligaments or the flexor tendon sheath. Good skin cover is needed to protect the exposed flexor tendons and this may require the use of a cross-finger flap.

Frequently there is residual contracture, especially in the little finger. If this is slight it may be accepted, the surgeon choosing instead to encourage maximal hyperextension of the metacarpophalangeal joint. This permits extension of the little finger pulp in line with the ring finger, but does not jeopardise flexion. A more radical release of the joint may be attempted in selected patients. A high degree of motivation will be necessary to retain the extension achieved and regain full flexion. The volar plate may be tethered proximally by two abnormal structures known as 'check-rein ligaments' which run along the volar ridges of the proximal phalanx. Check-rein ligament release may increase joint range. A more radical excision of the joint capsule of the proximal interphalangeal joint, together with partial release of the accessory collateral ligament, may be necessary to achieve full extension. If such a radical release is necessary, the joint should be held in extension by a Kirschner wire, provided that the tension in the neurovascular bundles is not so great as to obstruct the circulation. Not all patients will achieve a satisfactory result from radical soft tissue surgery.

There may be attenuation of the middle slip of the extensor apparatus secondary to the flexion deformity. Surgical shortening will increase its mechanical advantage.

Alternative salvage procedures are arthrodesis of the proximal interphalangeal joint, replacement of the proximal interphalangeal joint by a Silastic interpositional arthroplasty, or rarely, osteotomy of the proximal phalanx. Additional skin cover may be provided by grafts, cross-finger flaps or a dorsal transposition flap.

Amputation has a role in the eldery or infirm or in the patient unable to pursue his profession. If amputation of a little finger is performed through the metacarpal neck, there is the danger of scar tissue tethering the intrinsic muscles of the ring finger. This risk is less with disarticulation through the metacarpophalangeal joint. A dorsal skin flap from the little finger can be spread across the palm and this may allow interruption of residual contracted fascia. It is possible to amputate a digit through the proximal interphalangeal joint, preserving the pulp as a neurovascular island transfer. This can be migrated proximally to provide good quality skin cover over the residual proximal phalanx. By this·means, one segment of a digit can be preserved. The ring finger should never be amputated in isolation, as this produces a clumsy hand which may be avoided by reconstructive alternatives.

## FURTHER PROGRESS OF THE DISEASE

Hueston has classified further problems as recurrences (further Dupuytren's tissue in the area) or extensions (disease in different areas). A distinction between these two categories can be difficult. Additionally it must be admitted that not all unsatisfactory results fall clearly into the category of recurrence or extension. The correction of joint contracture may be incomplete at the first operation or there may be a failure of early splintage. A degree of residual joint contracture may therefore be present and may progress during the weeks or months following surgery.

Since there is no pathognomonic histology for Dupuytren's disease, it cannot be truly said that the 'disease' recurs. A deterioration or relapse in function may occur from any one of a number of causes.

Factors which conspire to produce further contractures are related to the 'trail of devastation' left by the fasciectomy operation (Figs 17.9, 17.10). If the operation should encroach on adjacent longitudinal bands, these may be tethered

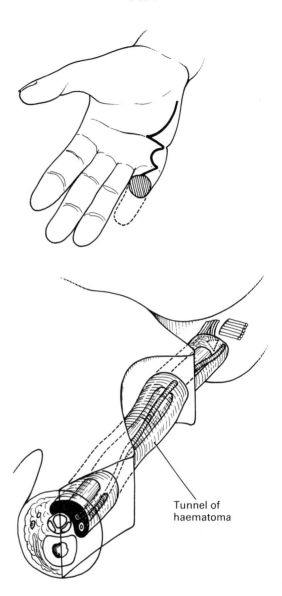

**Fig. 17.9** Schematic view through incision to show the tunnel of haematoma which is left behind by a limited fasciectomy

by the healing wound giving rise to stresses in uninvolved rays and predisposing to extension of the disease. Recurrence of deformity has traditionally been ascribed to incomplete fasciectomy. Clearance of all diseased tissue structures is probably not possible, but the concept of residual 'disease' is probably overrated. Of greater significance is the wound bed, which is a potential

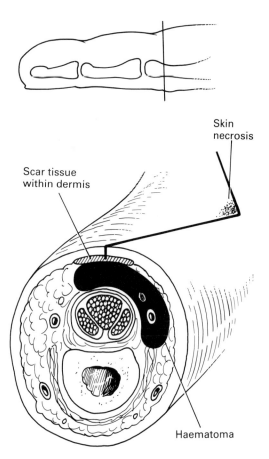

**Fig. 17.10** The causes of recurrence of contracture. Scar tissue may develop within contained haematoma or in the involved skin which is replaced on the digit. Skin necrosis will augment scarring. The haematoma is seen to encircle neurovascular bundles, such that recurrent contracture tissue is also likely to encircle the neurovascular bundles

dead space lined by traumatised cells and containing haematoma. The wound bed represents a tubular haematoma extending through the hand in the line of the excised fascia. This tubular wound will envelop neurovascular bundles and a sheet of scar will extend upwards to the skin surface. Ideally the skin wound should be a zig-zag longitudinal wound with minimal adjacent trauma. Scarring at the surface will be increased by skin necrosis or may be transmitted through involved Dupuytren's skin. The whole scar bed,

with its superficial and deep planes, produces a continuous wound with the potential to re-unite separated fascial ends proximally and distally via an active fibroblastic matrix. The tubular wound is inevitable. Its effect must be minimised by limiting its volume with drainage and gentle tissue handling techniques. In particular, dead space must be limited around joints when releases are considered. *The inevitable tubular scar must be held out to length by postoperative rehabilitation.* Finally, it must be appreciated that many of the specialised and delicate flexion mechanisms of the plamar fascia may be destroyed by either the disease or surgery. The flexor tendon sheath concertina effect may be lost, or the volar plate, the collateral and accessory collateral ligaments may become adherent. The normal relative motion between skin and skeleton is lost due to tethering by scar.

### Postoperative care

The internal scar must be held out to length. Surgeons vary greatly in their postoperative management with varying splintage periods and physiotherapy programmes. In the straightforward case, where a limited dissection produces release of contracture with adequate skin cover, the exact regimen of postoperative care is probably not critical to a successful result, provided mobilisation is rapid. Particular care is necessary where a skin graft has been undertaken. Prolonged splintage is required. A complicated dissection in which proximal interphalangeal joints have been straightened incompletely, or only with difficulty, is inevitably followed by some palmar and digital oedema. In this situation there is a possibility of early recurrence of flexion contracture or, alternatively, of general stiffness of the hand, leading to a flexion or extension loss. This is the type of hand where particular postoperative attention is necessary to achieve an adequate result, both in terms of night splintage and physiotherapy.

For palmar Dupuytren's, the dressing may be changed on the day following surgery and mobilisation commenced. No particular splintage is necessary. For digital contracture, the dressing is kept in place for a few days longer, incorporating a plaster of Paris support. After removal of the

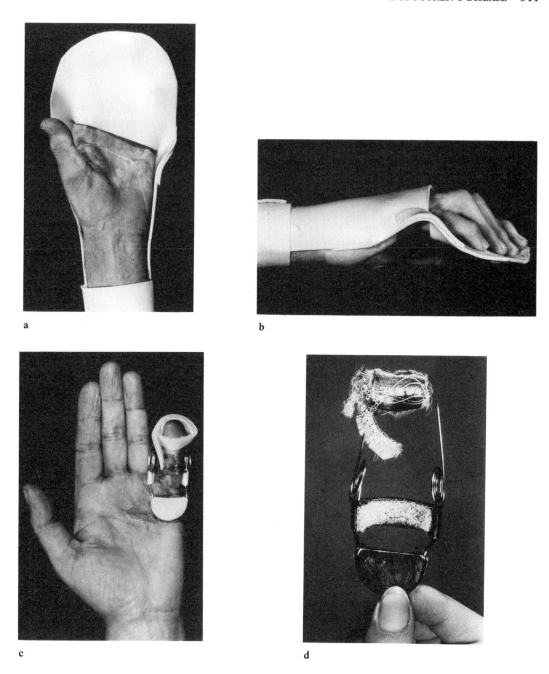

a

b

c

d

Fig. 17.11   **a, b** A night resting splint. **c, d** A dynamic Capener splint which has been worked diligently

initial dressing, a thermoplastic slot-through type of splint may be worn for most of the day (Fig. 17.11). It may then be worn only at night for a period of up to 6 months (as the scarring process is active during this time). If operative correction of the contracture has been incomplete, or there is rapid recurrence, a dynamic splint may be of benefit.

There may be further involvement of the skin, the subcutaneous tissues, or the joints at new sites. Disease 'extension' is used to describe contractures developing in other parts of the hand. The word extension has an unfortunate patho-logical connotation. It is better to consider such features as new contractures.

It seems unlikely that any particular surgical (and rehabilitational) approach can prevent the onward march of what seems to be the local mani-festation of a systemic disease process. Recurrence rates must depend on age and selection criteria as much as the operation itself.

Contracture will recur in at least 50% of cases, if followed long enough, but in the shorter term the guiding principle should be to avoid merely replacing the Dupuytren's cords with scar contracture.

# 18. Nerve 'compression'

*Principal author: P. J. Smith*

The term nerve 'compression' does not wholly convey the underlying pathophysiology, for other mechanisms produce interference in nerve function. Traction, tethering, excessive excursion, constriction by scar tissue and ischaemia may all contribute to symptoms associated with nerve 'compression' syndromes.

Nerve compression may produce a spectrum of change ranging from transient ionic block to internal architectural disruption of fibre continuity. The former may spontaneously resolve but the latter requires resection and repair. The more rapidly conducting large myelinated fibres are the first to be affected by 'compression'. The position of fibres within the nerve also influences the degree to which they are affected; peripheral fibres fail to function early with more central fibres being spared until later (Fig. 18.1).

Transient lesions (neuropraxia) may be due to ionic, vascular or mechanical abnormalities. Electrolytic imbalance of the sodium pump in the region of the node of Ranvier will inhibit nerve depolarisation. Obstruction to the venous outflow in the epineurium may raise the pressure within vessels inside the nerve, rendering the fasciculi ischaemic. Ultrastructural alterations are apparent on electron microscopy. In acute nerve compression, myelin intussusception is seen at the nodes of Ranvier. With more prolonged compression, the myelin becomes bulbous in appearance like beads on a chain (Fig. 18.2). *If compression is severe enough, segmental demyelination will occur.* However, as the internal architecture of the nerve fibres is undisturbed, with the endoneurial tubules and their axons remaining intact, remyelination occurs after decompression and there is no distal Wallerian degeneration. The return of function is

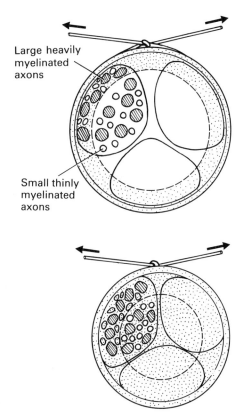

Large heavily myelinated axons

Small thinly myelinated axons

**Fig. 18.1** Location of the fibres within a nerve showing how the more central fibres are spared until late in compression

dependent on the degree of nerve damage. In ionic *neuropraxia*, rapid recovery occurs occasionally within hours of surgical release, but where there are ultrastructural mechanical alterations recovery is slower. If a segment of nerve is undergoing remyelination it usually recovers within 60 days;

313

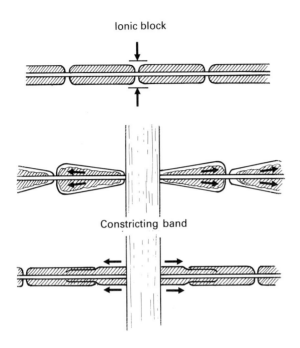

Ionic block

Constricting band

Fig. 18.2 The structural alterations associated with neuropraxia. **a** Ionic neuropraxia. **b** Myelin back-flow. **c** Myelin intussusception

this rate of recovery proceeds irrespective of the level of the lesion in the limb.

If compression is severe enough to produce *axonotmesis*, there is distal Wallerian degeneration and axonal sprouting is required for recovery (see Ch. 8). The prognosis is relatively good because the endoneurial tubules remain intact and the recovery period is related to the distance between the site of injury and the sensory and motor end-organs. Axonal regeneration occurs at approximately 1 mm per day. If Wallerian degeneration has occurred, recovery is slow compared to the more rapid recovery seen following segmental demyelination.

In the most severe forms of compression, the internal architecture of the nerve is disrupted producing intraneural fibrosis. This can be regarded as a neuroma-in-continuity in which there is complete internal disorganisation of neural tissues despite the external appearance of continuity. There is local attenuation of the nerve, usually associated with a proximal fusiform swelling. *Neurotmetic* lesions of this nature are not found in the common nerve compression 'syndromes' but may be found where compression follows major trauma such as fractures. In such circumstances, simple release of external compression is inadequate and resection of the involved area is indicated, followed by direct repair or nerve grafting. The prognosis in such lesions is dependent upon the duration of complete motor paralysis; if it is in excess of 15 months recovery is unlikely.

## DIAGNOSIS

Compression 'syndromes' in the upper limb commonly present with mild and transient symptoms. The history will often indicate the nerve involved, but sensory symptoms in particular may be very confusing. Sensory alteration in carpal tunnel syndrome does not always follow a classical median nerve distribution. There are no receptors within the nerve and therefore it has little ability to convey localising information. Provocative clinical tests of nerve compression may reproduce sensory symptoms. Accurate motor testing of the upper limb is required, as is a knowledge of the normal anatomy and the possible variations.

Electrical testing can accurately locate the site of the lesion and as the ulnar nerve may be compressed at multiple sites, errors may be made without such confirmatory evidence. Electrical testing may also be used as an accurate indication of the rate of return of function. The aim of electrical testing is to determine whether there is a localised reduction in the functional capability of the nerve and, if so, to identify the site.

## MANAGEMENT

In patients where sensory symptoms are intermittent, conservative management may be attempted, particularly if the cause is thought to be postural or temporary, for example carpal tunnel syndrome in pregnancy. Rest, splintage and the avoidance of aggravating postures may produce some relief of symptoms. However, where symptoms have persisted for 3 months and spontaneous resolution is not occurring, surgical decompression may be undertaken. Surgical treatment must be instituted immediately if sensory symptoms become continuous or if there is any sign of motor weakness or muscle wasting.

## FUNCTIONAL RECOVERY

The degree of functional recovery after decompression is dependent upon the underlying pathology. The duration of motor symptoms is of crucial importance in determining the likely outcome. Complete paralysis in excess of 15 months is unlikely to respond to surgical decompression. If there is dissociated loss of either motor or sensory function, the prognosis is more favourable as this may indicate either a mild compression of the nerve, sparing central elements, or a localised compression of one or two fascicles which will respond to surgical release. In general, relief of sensory symptoms following surgical release may be expected even many years after the onset of symptoms. In the elderly, however, prolonged sensory symptoms may not respond to surgical decompression.

## MEDIAN NERVE COMPRESSION SYNDROMES (Fig. 18.3)

### Carpal tunnel syndrome

This is the commonest compression syndrome affecting the median nerve. In its earliest phase, it is typified by noctural tingling, waking the patient from sleep, and requiring a variety of postural manouevres to relieve the symptoms. These may include shaking the hand and elevation or dependency of the arm. Any history of upper limb discomfort which wakes the patient at night or is most marked on rising in the morning may indicate carpal tunnel compression. The paraesthesia may involve the classical median nerve distribution affecting the radial three and a half digits, but more often it is less specific. Most commonly only one or two digits within the median nerve territory are involved, usually the middle and ring. As compression progresses, the patient begins to notice clumsiness. The clumsiness is due to a combination of impaired sensibility of the radial side of the hand and a reduction in motor control of the thumb. Moving light touch appreciation and proprioception are affected and the function of the thumb abductor and opponens muscles as well as the radial lumbricals may be impaired. If untreated, compression may progress with muscle wasting and an inability to abduct the thumb; intermittent paraesthesia changes to permanent numbness.

Carpal tunnel syndrome may arise in pregnancy or thyrotoxicosis and is thought to be related to fluid retention as a result of the altered metabolic state. In other patients, anatomical abnormalities within the carpal tunnel may reproduce symptoms. Numerous structures may compress the median nerve, such as lipomas, abnormal muscles (palmaris profundus) or a median artery. Rheumatoid arthritis produces significant synovial proliferation and carpal tunnel syndrome is frequent. Synovitis has been suggested as a frequent cause of idiopathic carpal tunnel syndrome. However, such findings are more likely to represent a non-specific reaction to compression or may indicate an episode of previous oedema associated with trauma. The median nerve may be enlarged in neurofibromatosis. In many patients, there is no obvious cause of external compression; the carpal tunnel appears normal but computerised axial tomography suggests that there may be an absolute reduction in the cross-sectional area of the tunnel. Carpal tunnel syndrome may be associated with Dupuytren's disease either as a presenting symptom or as a later problem 2–3 months following contracture release.

Phalen's test and the reversed Phalen's test are provocative tests which may reproduce the patient's symptoms (Figs. 18.4, 18.5).

Electrical confirmation of the diagnosis is optional in patients with classical nocturnal symptoms associated with positive responses to provocative testing. When symptoms are atypical, nerve conduction studies are most useful. Constant sensory or any motor changes make the diagnosis obvious and early treatment essential.

Nocturnal splintage or steroid injections at the entrance to the carpal canal may help to diminish symptoms in pregnancy. In the third trimester of pregnancy, conservative management is satisfactory as symptoms usually ressolve after delivery. When other metabolic abnormalities (e.g. thyrotoxicosis) precipitate carpal tunnel syndrome,

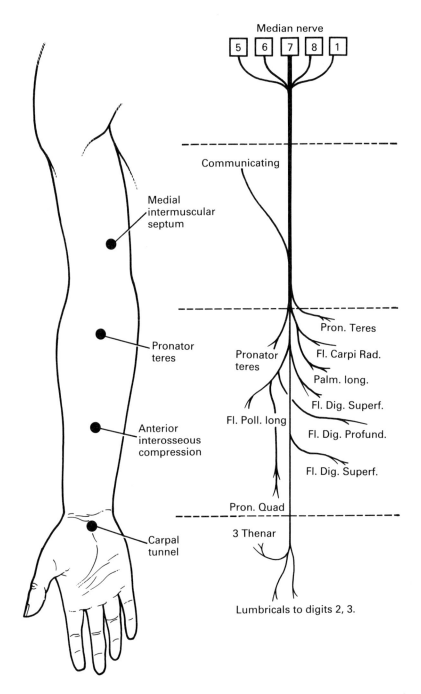

**Fig. 18.3**   Sites of median nerve compression in the upper limb

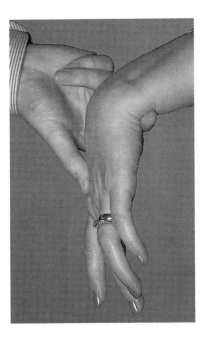

Fig. 18.4 Phalen's test for carpal tunnel syndrome

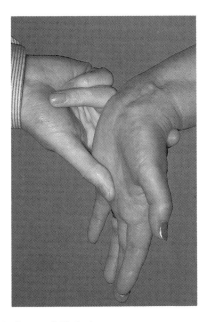

Fig. 18.5 Reversed Phalen's test

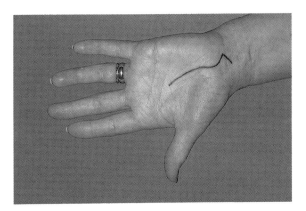

Fig. 18.6 Incision for carpal tunnel decompression

progressive symptoms in excess of 3 months require surgical decompression.

When planning the surgical incision, care should be taken to avoid the palmar cutaneous branch of the median nerve, or troublesome neuromas may result with impairment of sensation in the palmar triangle (Fig. 18.6). The volar carpal ligament should be released and the median nerve should be visualised from the ligament's proximal margin to the superficial palmar arch (Fig. 18.7).

The nerve is inspected after decompression to see if it remains flattened. The tourniquet is released and the rate of revascularisation of the nerve is noted. Should a persistent area of pallor remain, it has been suggested that an external neurolysis involving release of the epineurium be undertaken. A simple longitudinal split is made in the epineurium. It is not our practice to undertake a more extensive internal neurolysis of the nerve as we feel that this is likely to produce further damage, promote fibrosis, and perhaps exacerbate any tendency towards dystrophy.

Dissociated symptoms with more motor than sensory involvement may alert the physician to the possibility of differential compression of the motor branch. In such circumstances, the motor branch to the thenar muscles should be traced as it passes through the carpal tunnel as it may penetrate through a separate tunnel in the roof of the carpal canal and require individual decompression. This is a delicate and technically demanding procedure.

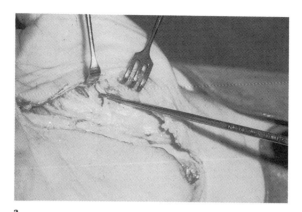

a

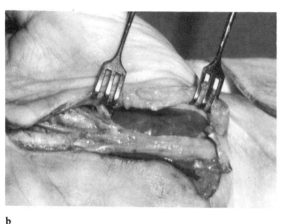

b

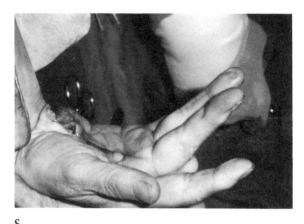

c

**Fig. 18.7  a** Incision showing the median nerve with the thenar branch going through the roof of the carpal tunnel. There was a separate hole through which this branch went, and in this patient motor symptoms outweighed sensory. **b** Release of the tourniquet, showing the prompt return of colour to the median nerve. If the nerve remains white, it may be necessary to incise the epineurium, but no further surgical intervention should be undertaken other than this. **c** Flexion of the wrist after release of the carpal tunnel produces prolapse of the median nerve. It can become adherent to the cutaneous scar producing a permanent pain syndrome. This is easily avoided by placing the wrist in dorsiflexion and keeping it there with a plaster for 2 weeks

The variations in the origin of both the motor branch and the palmar cutaneous branch of the median nerve make blind decompression of the carpal tunnel a dangerous procedure which should not be performed under any circumstances.

Postoperative immobilisation of the wrist in a position of slight extension, using a volar slab, rests the healing wound, prevents median nerve prolapse or adherence to the skin and is more comfortable for the patient. It is important to warn patients that full power and mobility of the wrist will not return for approximately 8 weeks following the operation.

## Prognosis

The prognosis in carpal tunnel syndrome is mainly dependent upon the age of the patient and the duration of symptoms. Rapid recovery may be expected in the young patient, but in the elderly full sensory recovery may not occur. This is particularly true if symptoms have been present for some considerable time. In general, surgical release of the carpal tunnel effectively terminates troublesome nocturnal paraesthesia. Its effect on established numbness is, however, less predictable. In the older patient with prolonged compression and muscle wasting, motor recovery is so uncertain that many surgeons undertake tendon transfers to restore abduction at the time of surgical decompression.

### Acute carpal tunnel syndrome

This extremely important syndrome is often overlooked but it can occur in any situation in which the hand becomes rapidly swollen. Carpal injuries such as volar dislocation of the lunate or Colles' fractures may produce direct compression of the median nerve. The oedema resulting from crush injuries is particularly likely to produce this syndrome. It may also occur following elective surgical treatment, particularly carpal procedures. If symptoms do not show signs of rapid resolution, urgent decompression of the median nerve is required.

### Pronator syndrome

This rare syndrome may be detected in a patient who is suspected of having carpal tunnel syndrome but who presents with paresthesia in the median nerve distribution in association with a negative Phalen's test. There may be sensory changes in the palmar triangle, indicating that the lesion lies proximal to the carpal tunnel. Discomfort may be noted in the forearm. The syndrome is due to compression of the median nerve as it passes through the pronator teres, by the muscle itself, the lacertus fibrosis or the sublimis arch. In association with this, there may be pain in the forearm on resisted pronation, and a 'Tinel' may be present at the point where the median nerve penetrates the two heads of pronator teres. Electrical testing is essential to localise the level of compression prior to surgical decompression.

### Anterior interosseous syndrome

The condition is often heralded by the abrupt development of pain in the forearm which lasts for several hours. As the discomfort subsides it is followed by weakness which may lead to a full paralysis of flexor digitorum profundus to the index finger, flexor pollicis longus, and pronator quadratus. It is a condition in which there are no sensory symptoms or signs. The patient is unable to make the 'O' sign and pinches in a characteristic fashion between thumb and index finger (Fig. 18.8); there is excessive index proximal interphalangeal joint flexion and hyperextension of the distal interphalangeal joint but without pulp-to-pulp opposition. The index pulp is placed against the ulnar border of the thumb. Variations in this pattern do occur. On occasion the index finger

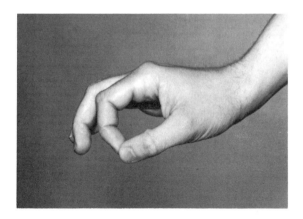
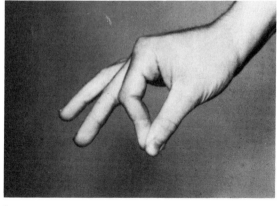

a                    b

**Fig. 18.8**  a The O sign, showing function of flexor pollicis longus and flexor digitorum profundus to the index, indicating an intact and functioning anterior interosseous nerve. **b** The posture adopted when the nerve fails

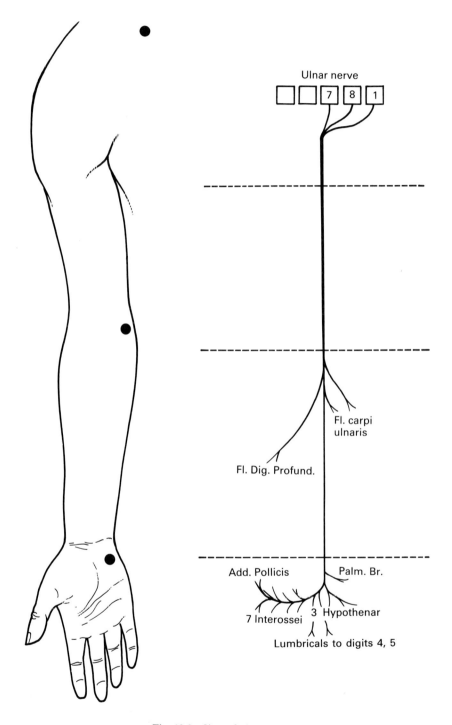

**Fig. 18.9**  Sites of ulnar nerve compression

profundus or flexor pollicis longus may be affected in isolation. Patients presenting with forearm pain and inability to flex the tip of the thumb should not be assumed to have a tendon rupture.

In many cases, the tenodesis test (see Ch. 20) or firm pressure of the flexor pollicis longus tendon proximal to the wrist will demonstrate the continuity of the musculo-tendinous unit and indicate a need for confirmatory electromyography.

Many patients will have a satisfactory return of function without surgical intervention. However, if spontaneous recovery, both clinically and electromyographically, is not commencing within 12 weeks, exploration should be undertaken. Exploration may reveal compression arising from a bicipital bursa, abnormal muscle bellies such as Gantzer's muscle (an accessory head of flexor pollicis longus), or a fibrous arch related to pronator teres or sublimis. The ulnar collateral vessels may also produce compression. On occasion no obvious cause of compression can be found.

## ULNAR NERVE COMPRESSION SYNDROMES (Fig. 18.9)

The ulnar nerve is unusual in that simultaneous 'compression' may occur at several sites from the thoracic outlet to Guyon's canal at the wrist. It supplies few structures proximal to the wrist but is the principal motor supply to the intrinsic muscles of the hand. Excellent intrinsic co-ordination is required to perform fine manipulative skills. These features make localisation of the site of compression particularly important. The benefits of surgical release are slow to appear and are unpredictable.

### Thoracic outlet syndrome

The roots of the brachial plexus accompanied by the subclavian vessels emerge from the neck between the scalene muscles, crossing on the first rib. Compression within this area is called thoracic outlet syndrome. It may be caused by cervical ribs (or more commonly their fibrous bands) or, rarely, fractures of the clavicle. The prolonged abnormal postures required in certain working environments may contribute to symptoms.

Discomfort is present in the upper arm and is often of an aching nature. Tingling or numbness may be present in the ulnar distribution of the hand and forearm, and the small muscles of the hand may become wasted. Diminished sensation on the inner aspect of the arm and forearm are suggestive as is a positive Tinel sign in the neck. Flexion of the neck towards the normal side, or compression at the suspected site may provoke the patient's symptoms. The pulse, colour and temperature of the affected limb may differ from the normal side and occasionally a thrill or bruit may be detected over the subclavian artery, indicating associated vascular compression.

Clinical signs are unreliable in this syndrome and electrical testing is necessary to establish the diagnosis. Arteriography is indicated if vascular signs are present (Fig. 18.10).

Conservative treatment by postural exercises helps many patients. Persistent disabling symptoms may rarely require anterior scalenotomy, cervical rib resection or fibrous band removal. Recurrence of symptoms following such surgical treatment has been treated by resection of the first rib. The efficacy of this treatment is the subject of much debate.

### Cubital tunnel

The ulnar nerve may be affected at this site by compression, longitudinal stretching and friction. Compression may be caused by the Anconeus muscle or the roof of Osborne's canal (the two heads of flexor carpi ulnaris). Stretching and friction occur during normal movement, when the nerve may elongate by half a centimetre and slip anteriorly by three-quarters of a centimetre. Conservative management may be effective. Many of these patients sleep in the prone position with their shoulders abducted and their elbows flexed producing direct pressure on the ulnar nerve. The use of night splints, holding the elbow semi-extended, and altered sleeping habits may relieve symptoms. Surgical decompression should be performed only after the most careful consideration. The condition may be treated by anterior transposition of the nerve but care must be taken that the nerve is freed for a sufficient distance both above and below the epicondyle to permit

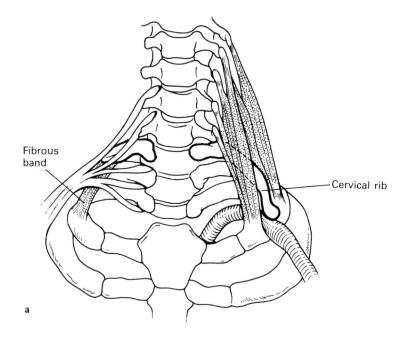

Fibrous band

Cervical rib

a

NERVE CONDUCTION STUDY REPORT

Conductance (Sympathetic Activity)

Some lack of conductance over the Ulnar side of the Ring finger the Radial side of the Middle finger and the Radial side of the Thumb.

Electrical Sensory Threshold

Lack of sensation over the Median Nerve Territory and the Radial side of the Ring Finger.

R.N.G. Results

| Median Nerve | | Ulnar Nerve | |
|---|---|---|---|
| Amplitude. | 1300 $\mu$V | 494 $\mu$V | |
| Distal Latency. | 3.8 ms | 2.4 ms | |

Nerve conduction Velocity

| Elbow to Wrist. | 59 M/s | 63 M/s |
|---|---|---|
| Upper arm to Elbow | 107 M/s | 127 M/s |
| Axilla to Upper arm | 60 M/s | |

The delayed Conduction Velocity across the Brachial Plexus confirms your suspicion that this lady has thoracic outlet syndrome.

b

Fig. 18.10   a Diagram of thoracic outlet syndrome. On the right side of the neck a fibrous band is seen compressing the lower roots of the brachial plexus. On the left side, vascular symptoms have occurred. There is compression of the subclavian artery by a cervical rib and evidence of poststenotic dilatation. This patient presented with vague symptoms of nerve compression, but clinical signs indicating thoracic outlet syndrome. X-rays did not reveal any gross abnormality. b Nerve conduction studies confirmed thoracic outlet syndrome

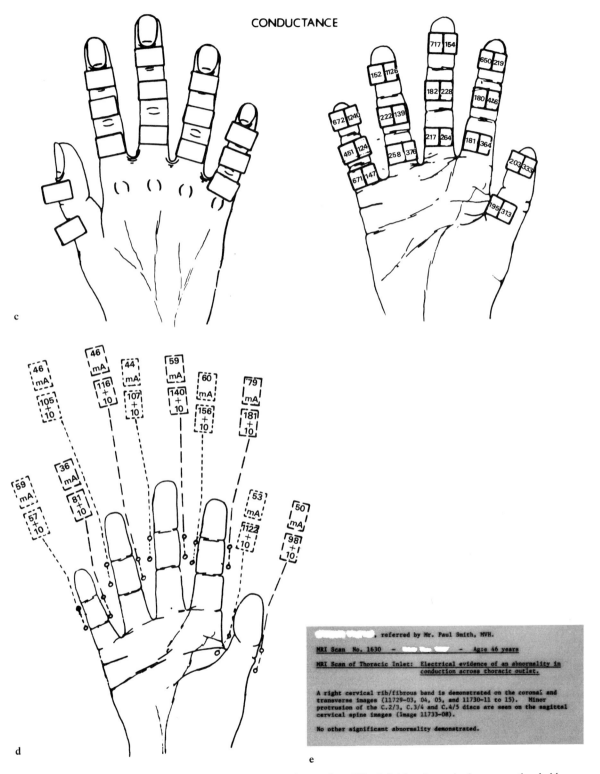

**Fig. 18.10  c** Conductance measurements, showing no gross abnormality. **d** No definitive change in the sensory threshold measurements. **e** Report of the MRI scan

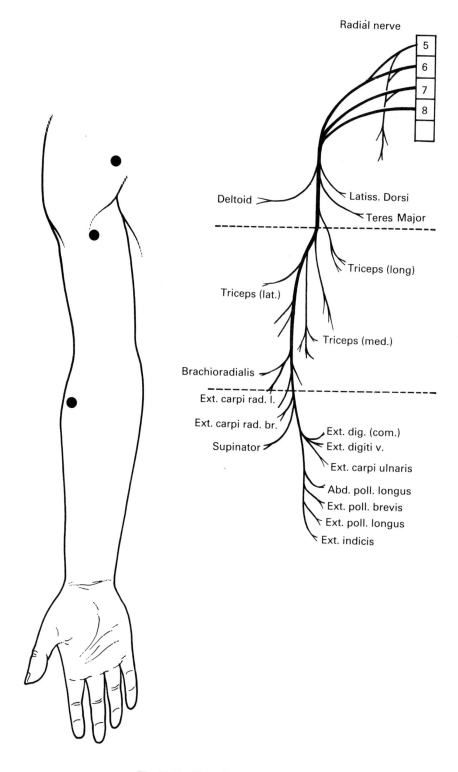

**Fig. 18.11** Sites of radial nerve compression

adequate transposition or a 'migrating compression syndrome' may be provoked by tethering the nerve. Proximally, after anterior translocation, the nerve may be compressed by the lower border of the medial intermuscular septum. Distally the nerve should be released from the cubital tunnel. Learmonth advised placing the nerve deep to the flexor/pronator muscle mass, but there is a risk that subsequent fibrosis may produce secondary compression. If surgical treatment is required the nerve should be handled with great gentleness. Poor surgical technique can add direct injury to a nerve whose function is already impaired. The response to surgical treatment is slow and often incomplete with maximal improvement taking up to 18 months to occur. The outcome is so uncertain that splintage has become the mainstay in the treatment of this condition in some centres in preference to surgery. Steroid infiltration is contraindicated as the benefits are minimal and the hazards of nerve injury too great.

## Guyon's canal

Compression of the ulnar nerve within Guyon's canal is much less common than carpal tunnel syndrome. Ulnar nerve compression within Guyon's canal may be suspected when the patient complains of sensory abnormalities in the ulnar nerve distribution in the hand. This may involve associated motor loss, although sensation on the dorsum of the hand is normal. This sparing of the dorsal branch clearly indicates compression within Guyon's canal. When the lesion lies proximally within the canal, motor and sensory fibres are involved. Distal lesions may produce dissociated motor or sensory loss. Like carpal tunnel syndrome with which it is often associated, there is usually no anatomical abnormality detected on surgical exploration. If a mechanical cause of compression is found it is most frequently a ganglion associated with degenerative changes in the adjacent intercarpal joints. Abnormalities of palmaris longus, the hypothenar or palmaris brevis muscles, ligamentous or Dupuytren's bands, and fractures of the hook of the hamate may also be responsible. This condition appears to respond well to surgical decompression and is usually associated with rapid resolution of symptoms, provided that their duration has not been excessive.

## Radial nerve (Fig. 18.11)

Radial nerve palsies may be caused by fractures of the humeral shaft with compression of the nerve in the spiral groove. They usually resolve spontaneously, provided that the fracture is adequately reduced. However, if no clinical or electromyographic evidence of recovery is apparent within 8 weeks of reduction, exploration is indicated to exclude nerve disruption.

'Saturday night palsies' are caused by compression of the radial nerve due to abnormal postures adopted during prolonged periods of unconsciousness (alcohol or drug overdoses).

'Spontaneous' paralysis of the posterior interosseous nerve may occur. The finger and thumb extensors are paralysed but brachioradialis and extensor carpiradialis longus (which are innervated by the radial nerve above the elbow) retain their function. Hence the patient is capable of dorsiflexion at the wrist, but with deviation in a radial direction. Finger extension is possible because of intrinsic action producing interphalangeal joint extension. However, the metacarpophalangeal joints cannot be actively extended by the patient (Fig. 18.12). The arcade of Frohse (a thickening of the proximal edge of the superficial head of supinator) may compress the posterior interosseous nerve. Compression may also be caused by local ganglia, bursa, lipomas, radial head fractures, degenerative changes in the elbow or the radial recurrent artery.

In 'spontaneous' paralysis, the duration of the total paralysis is the key factor in determining its management. If present for 15 months, recovery is unlikely and tendon transfer should be undertaken. The shorter the period of paralysis, the more likely that surgery will produce complete recovery and surgical decompresion should therefore be attempted. Surgical decompression of a *partial* nerve palsy can be surprisingly effective despite prolonged compression. In the recovery phase, pain on compression of the muscles indicates reinnervation and may be regarded as a

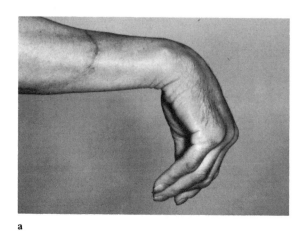

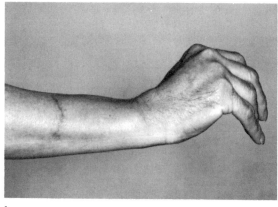

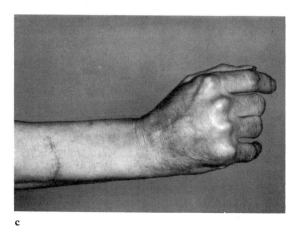

**Fig. 18.12   a** Laceration of the dorsal forearm. **b** Wrist extension is possible, but with radial deviation. Finger extension is not possible, nor is extension of the thumb. **c** Showing the radial deviation of the wrist and lack of finger extension typical of a posterior interosseous palsy

positive 'Muscle Tinel.' Tendon transfer is undertaken if surgical decompression fails to produce recovery (see Ch. 10).

## THE ROLE OF ELECTRICAL STUDIES

Numerous electrical tests are available in the study of peripheral nerve injury and compression. The three common tests that are used in clinical practice are direct nerve stimulation, electromyography and nerve conduction velocity measurement. Nerve action potential studies may be used but require highly sophisticated equipment to amplify very small voltages of less than 80 microvolts.

Electrical studies play a subservient role to clinical examination. They are used to confirm a diagnosis for the assessment of the rate and completeness of recovery following treatment and for research purposes. The clinician should have a clear idea of what he specifically wishes to know and should convey his request clearly to the neurophysiologist.

The effects of direct *nerve stimulation* are observed. Nerves may be depolarised transcutaneously (without any insertional requirement). In compression syndromes, if the nerve is stimulated proximally, the localisation sign may develop; the patient feels discomfort at the site of the nerve compression. Nerve stimulation proximal to a suspected site of compression may fail to evoke distal motor function. Stimulation distal to the site of compression will normally produce function, hence localising the problem area.

The condition of a motor unit can be determined by an *insertional electromyograph*. During the process of insertion, some information may be obtained about the consistency of the muscle and in particular the presence of fibrosis may be determined. A knowledge of the detailed anatomy is essential as the accuracy of insertion is of paramount importance in formulating a diagnosis. The careful insertion of the needle electrode into the muscle in question is checked by asking the patient to perform the movement appropriate for that muscle. Electrical activity can then be detected confirming accurate placement of the needle. As the needle is inserted, typical electrical patterns develop. Normal resting muscle is electrically silent. Denervated muscle, however, does not remain polarised in the fashion that normal excitable tissues do; spontaneous electrical depolarisation occurs, with discharges or fibrillations appearing as positive sharp waves on the oscilloscope. Their presence is significant if a clinical picture leads one to suspect muscle denervation. Insertional electromyographic changes persist for at least 6–8 months after clinical recovery has occurred.

*Nerve conduction velocity measurements* require the presence of an amplifier, oscilloscope and timer. A stimulating electrode is placed well proximal to the site of the suspected compression and recordings are taken proximodistally. The distal recording is normally taken from muscle so that the initial insertional pattern can be obtained and electromyographic evidence provided by this means. By noting the distance between the two recording electrodes, the rate of conduction may be determined. It is normally of the order of 55 m/s in motor nerves. This technique can be applied to sensory nerves which may be stimulated in an orthodromic or an antidromic fashion. Nerve conduction velocity measurements are influenced greatly by temperature (markedly slower when cold) and the age of the patient. The intensity of the stimulus, which needs to be higher where regenerating fibres are present, is another variable. Conduction velocity measurements are particularly useful in nerve compression syndromes, but it should be realised that the presence of only a few normally conducting axons may give rise to normal results. Conduction studies should not be undertaken in limbs which are grossly swollen, because in such circumstances the results are unreliable.

Electrical testing is particularly useful when the presenting features are unusual. However, if no electrophysiological changes are detectable, repeat studies in 6 or 12 weeks' time may reveal an abnormality. Nonetheless in carpal tunnel syndrome there remains a small group of patients who consistently show no electrical abnormality and yet demonstrate a convincing clinical picture and who respond to surgical decompression. Even with the most sophisticated electrophysiological testing, false-negative results will occur. In the diagnosis of the pronator syndrome, electromyographic evidence is more useful than nerve conduction velocity measurements. Anomalous innervation such as the Martin Gruber anastomosis (a median to ulnar motor contribution in the forearm) may be detected using these tests.

Electrical testing is used to confirm a clinical diagnosis, in particular to localise the level of a suspected lesion. It may be used to detect suspected anomalous innervation. Primary muscle pathology or neuropathy may be excluded. Intraoperatively, fascicular recordings and stimulation can be used in the assessment of a neuroma in continuity.

Where symptoms are classical and provocative signs confirmatory electrical testing is optional. If the nature of the diagnosis or the site of the lesion is in question, such testing is of great benefit. When the ulnar nerve is involved the sites of compression may be multiple and electrical testing is always desirable.

# 19. Tumours, lumps and ulcers

*Principal authors: F. D. Burke, D. A. McGrouther*

The term 'tumour' is ambiguous both to the patient and the surgeon. We have restricted its usage to neoplastic conditions. There exists also a large number of non-neoplastic conditions of the hand which may present as a lump or ulceration. A knowledge of all these conditions is of considerable clinical value. Although the majority of such lesions is benign, and delay in diagnosis inconsequential, a minority is of sinister significance where delay in referral will inevitably affect the prognosis.

Most neoplasms of the hand present as either a lump or ulceration. Many non-neoplastic conditions also present in this way. To an experienced surgeon the appearance of the lesion and its site provide strong clues to diagnosis. For this reason we have chosen to discuss together all swellings in the hand. Histological confirmation is always necessary if a neoplasm is suspected. The value of the pathologist's report is undermined if it is based on inadequate information. Sufficient clinical detail should always be supplied and, if ambiguity persists, a case conference is often of benefit.

Tumours and non-neoplastic lumps and ulcers in the hand may be classified as arising from:

Skin and subcutaneous tissues
Bone
Joints
Tendons and tendon sheaths
Nerve tissue

## TUMOURS ARISING FROM SKIN AND SUBCUTANEOUS TISSUES

Differential diagnosis:

Benign lesions
  chronic ulceration
  foreign body
  pyogenic granuloma
  viral wart
  sebaceous cyst
  dermoid cyst
  lipoma
  haemangioma
  lymphangioma
  fibromata
Malignant lesions
  squamous carcinoma
  variants    squamous cell carcinoma-in-situ
              Bowen's disease
              keratoacanthoma
  malignant melanoma
  basal cell carcinoma
  miscellaneous

### Benign skin lesions of the hand

*Chronic inflammatory conditions* of the skin of the hand occur more frequently than neoplasms and can simulate their appearance, presenting as either an ulcer or a lump. An example of such an ulcerated lesion is the fissure which may occur in a skin crease, particularly in the thick-skinned hand in cold weather. A simple traumatic wound may be accompanied by delayed healing giving rise to prolonged ulceration. This is most frequently seen in association with chronic mechanical irritation, exposure to chemicals or chronic immersion in water. A more sinister pathology, however, must be excluded histologically if extension of the lesion occurs. Where there is no clear history of trauma, or the wound fails to heal despite appropriate treatment, a diagnosis of dermatitis artefacta (self-inflicted injury) should be considered.

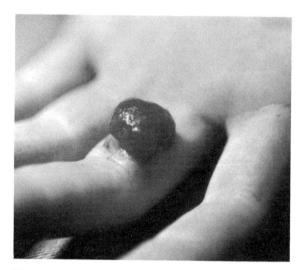

**Fig. 19.1** Pyogenic granuloma

A *foreign body granuloma* may present as an intracutaneous or subcutaneous lump. This represents the inflammatory reaction which surrounds retained foreign material. Organic material, such as wood, is particularly prone to form a vigorous reaction. *Pyogenic granuloma* may develop at a laceration site and presents as a rapidly growing mushroom-like papillomatous outgrowth (Fig. 19.1). The differential diagnosis between pyogenic granuloma and malignant melanoma is not always easy. Early histological confirmation should be sought in all such cases, particularly those close to the nail-bed. Excision biopsy is curative in pyogenic granuloma.

The *viral wart* (synonym verruca vulgaris) (Fig. 19.2a) is perhaps the most frequent tumour-like condition occurring on the skin of the hand and is particularly prevalent in children. These lesions are not ulcerated unless secondarily infected. Slow-growing lesions tend to be flat, whereas rapidly growing lesions are papillary. Treatment by cryotherapy, using topical liquid nitrogen, is generally effective. Three treatments at weekly intervals will be adequate in the majority of cases. If the history or appearance of the lesion leave doubt about the diagnosis, an excision biopsy is indicated, particularly in adult patients. The wart must be excised with an adequate margin of clearance to include the epithelial shoulder, or recurrence in the scar is likely. Large warts may be too extensive to allow excision and closure.

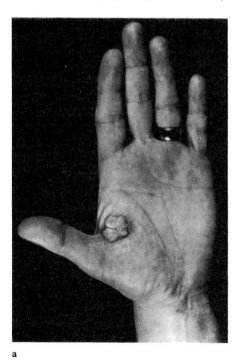
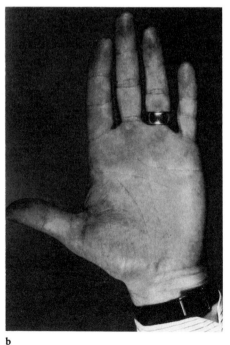

a        b

**Fig. 19.2** **a** A viral wart. **b** After treatment by diathermy, curettage and further diathermy of the base

Diathermy and curettage is possible; after initial diathermy the soft warty tissue is removed by curettage and the wound bed diathermised a second time to kill intracellular virus (Fig. 19.2b). Experience is necessary to judge the correct depth of treatment. Diagnostic difficulties may be encountered if a patient presents with a partly treated viral wart, which is ulcerated and infected. The lesion should be excised and the specimen sent for histological examination. The infection is controlled by frequent antiseptic dressings and the wound managed by secondary skin suture or graft.

*Sebaceous cysts* are rare in the hand and occur on the dorsal surface. *Epidermoid cysts*, by comparison, are common and occur on the palmar surfaces (Fig. 19.3), usually on the digital pulps. They are thought to arise from traumatically implanted epidermis following pin-prick or laceration and sometimes an adjacent or overlying scar is seen. These generally arise in the subcutaneous pulp but are firmly attached to overlying dermis. In longstanding cases indentation of the adjacent phalanx may be apparent on radiographs. The cyst wall and contents are excised intact in a bloodless field, taking care to avoid the neurovascular bundles which may have been displaced by the soft tissue mass.

*Lipomas* may arise at any site in the hand. Smaller lesions may be mistaken for other more common swellings, but larger lipomas of long duration are also seen and these have the typical clinical appearances of a soft, almost fluctuant, swelling. Lipomas in the thumb web may reach a considerable size before presentation. Care is required in their removal to avoid damage to neurovascular bundles.

*Haemangiomas* may present as swellings which vary in size from time to time. These are generally of the *cavernous type* and are occasionally sufficiently localised to permit total and local excision (Fig. 19.4). More frequently they are diffuse and the vessels may extend through many tissue layers including muscle, fascia and skin. Such lesions are often incompletely removed. A small number of patients become difficult therapeutic problems. Recurrences may be associated with pain. Surgery by debulking is often performed for cosmetic reasons, but, particularly in childhood, consideration should be given to leaving the lesion undisturbed. Angiography assists in outlining the extent of the lesion, but rarely succeeds in identifying the source of feeding vessels or predicting the ease of excision. Vascular embolisation therapy is potentially hazardous in the upper limbs. *Capillary* haemangiomata tend to produce areas of skin discoloration of the port-wine variety and these are rarely seen in the hand.

'*Strawberry*' *naevi* are occasionally seen in the hand. These rapidly growing lesions have a dramatic appearance. They have a characteristic history of appearing for the first time 1–2 weeks after birth and growing rapidly thereafter. They may bleed if they· become infected. They are, however, self-limiting and should be allowed to regress spontaneously. *Lymphangiomata* are rare and difficult to treat (usually at 7–10 years of age).

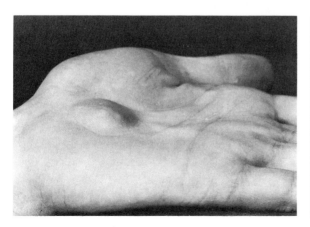

**Fig. 19.3**  Epidermoid cyst arising in a palmar scar

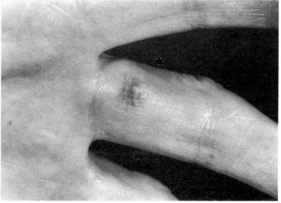

**Fig. 19.4**  Cavernous haemangioma of a digit

They may present as a swelling or as skin blisters. Excision and suture or skin grafting may be necessary.

A *dermatofibroma* presents as a small firm dome-shaped intracutaneous nodule. Such nodules are slow growing and resemble in appearance a small hypertrophic scar. Curiously the operative scar often becomes hypertrophic. The patient must be warned about this before surgery. The lesion can be confused with amelanotic malignant melanoma.

*Fibromas* presenting as nodules on the digits of children may look very aggressive histologically, but have been reported to be self-limiting. These should not be treated aggressively if their biological course appears benign.

Other benign tumours are rare in the hand and an exhaustive list would be superfluous for the diagnosis is only obtained after histological examination. In cases of doubt, the surgeon may chose to seek the advice of a dermatological or plastic surgical colleague whose experience in skin pathology may spare the patient unnecessarily aggressive treatment at one end of the spectrum or inadequate excision at the other. Excision

biopsy and prompt histological examination will suffice in the majority of cases.

## Malignant skin tumours

### Squamous cell carcinoma

The clinical diagnosis of squamous carcinoma is immediately suggested by the classical appearance of an area of ulceration with overlying crust and a rolled edge (Fig. 19.5). This is, however, an advanced stage of the lesion and at earlier stages it may present as an area of hyperkeratosis, later followed by ulceration, with little initial evidence of a surrounding rolled edge.

The prognosis of malignant tumours of the skin depends upon whether they arise on normal skin or skin damaged by some physical or chemical agent. Tumours arising in normal undamaged skin have a much poorer prognosis in general. Such patients are generally younger. Ultraviolet radiation in sunlight, ingestion of arsenic, or oil contamination may damage the dermis. Actinic ultraviolet damage is by far the commonest cause of injury to the dermis and is ubiquitous in fair-

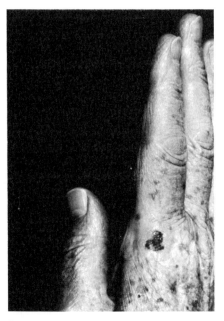
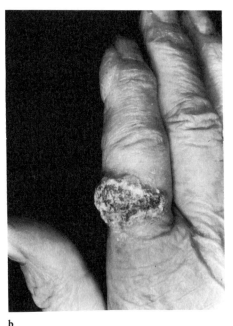

a          b

**Fig. 19.5** Different appearances of squamous carcinoma. **a** Ulceration. **b** Rolled edge

skinned Northern European stock exposed to sunlight. In tropical and subtropical regions, such as Northern Australia, skin cancer is very common and occurs at an earlier age than in temperate climates.

The clinical appearance of actinic skin damage is of areas of hyperkeratosis (Fig. 19.6a) on a background of dry wrinkled skin. Most actinic keratoses have. not progressed to malignancy. *Squamous carcinoma-in-situ* is the next histological stage of severity followed by invasion of deeper layers. *Bowen's disease* is a distinct clinical and histological variety of squamous carcinoma-in-situ with a clinically well-defined margin and an

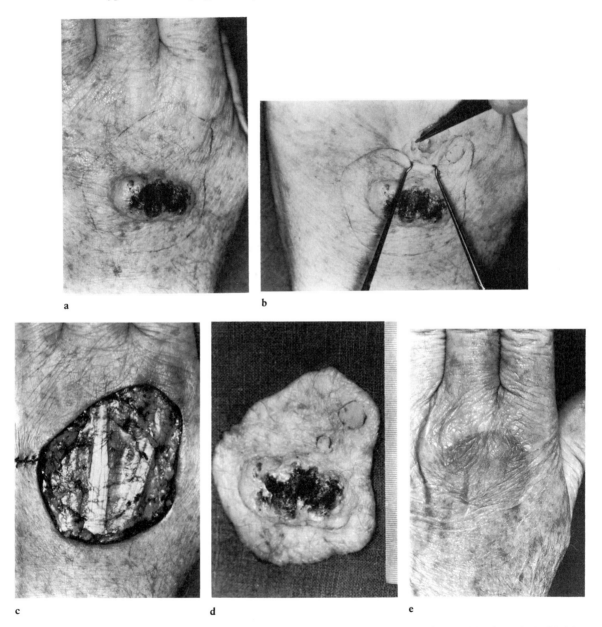

**Fig. 19.6** **a** Squamous carcinoma. Adjacent actinic keratoses are noted. **b** The periphery of the excision is marked with ink. **c** The lesion is excised down to the paratenon over the extensor apparatus and a split skin graft applied. **d** The excision specimen. **e** The late appearance

appearance of crusting. Actinically damaged skin may show all gradations of the above changes and, in addition, irregularity of pigmentation (melanocytic dysplasia). Damage of this type is most marked on the dorsal surface of the hands and other commonly affected sites are the face and lower legs.

Squamous cell carcinoma is the commonest skin tumour of the hand. Other malignant tumours in this site are relatively rare and the treatment of squamous carcinoma illustrates general principles which are widely applicable. Some tumours are neglected by the patient for a considerable time, but, regrettably, many are misdiagnosed by the physician or mistreated by the surgeon. Perhaps the most important principle is to encourage all surgeons to maintain a high index of suspicion when a 'wound' remains unhealed or a 'wart' becomes ulcerated. Almost always a history of previous trauma will be offered by the patient in an attempt to allay his fears of more sinister causes. Delay in treatment is a major factor in influencing prognosis.

The treatment of choice for squamous carcinoma is adequate excision and reconstruction (Fig. 19.6a). This is curative in the vast majority of patients. Biopsy may be indicated in rare cases of doubt or in advanced neglected cases, but complete excision is the preferred form of biopsy. This management principle leaves little place for radiotherapy as a sole treatment modality, it should be reserved for rare tumours which are particularly radiosensitive (e.g. lymphomata). It is not good practice to employ radiotherapy where surgical excision has been inadequate. A combined surgical and radiotherapy treatment programme is indicated if a squamous carcinoma has penetrated deeply. Adequate surgical excision, immediate flap cover (by free tissue transfer or radial flap cover) followed by radiotherapy, offers the best chance of local disease control without hand amputation (see below).

*Technique of excision.* The margins of the tumour should be clearly indentified by marking the visual peripheral margin with dots of Bonney's blue dye. The surgeon should then decide on the margin of clearance, 1.5 cm being generally satisfactory for a squamous carcinoma. This again should be marked with a line of Bonney's blue dye

(Fig. 19.6b). This marking discipline should be adhered to as only in this way can the prescribed clearance be assured once the operation has commenced. The dye leaves no need for further consideration of the peripheral clearance during the raising of the skin specimen and allows the surgeon to concentrate on the adequacy of the depth clearance. There is a plane of loose connective tissue on the dorsum of the hand, and it is possible to excise the skin specimen down to this plane (Fig. 19.6c). The operation must be performed under tourniquet to allow adequate inspection of the planes of clearance. It is good practice to mark the excised specimen (Fig. 19.6d) with a black silk suture at the twelve o'clock position (in the anatomical position), thereby allowing the pathologist the possibility of orientating the specimen and identifying areas where the histological clearance may not be quite adequate. Bipolar haemostasis should be performed, as necessary, throughout the operation and larger veins ligated with catgut. Wound closure may be possible by direct suture, if a small lesion has been removed, but, in general, split skin grafting will be necessary. Flap reconstruction is unnecessary for superficial tumours and it is easier to watch for recurrence under a split skin graft. The latter has a satisfactory cosmetic appearance (Fig. 19.6e). A useful indicator of prognosis in squamous carcinoma is the histological depth of the lesion. Clark has described a classification, by levels of invasion of the dermis, for malignant melanoma (see below), which may also be applied to squamous carcinoma.

Clark levels 1–4 (see Table 19.1) are usually adequately treated by wide local excision, whereas deeper lesions (Clark level 5, i.e. invading through dermis into fat) are likely to metastasise to the regional lymph nodes. Deep tumour extension

**Table 19.1**   Classification of levels of invasion

| | |
|---|---|
| 1 | Intra-epidermal |
| 2 | Papillary–dermal |
| 3 | Papillary–reticular dermal interface |
| 4 | Reticular–dermal |
| 5 | Subcutaneous fat |
| 5+ | Bone, joint or tendon |

with further spread along tendon planes may occur in advanced cases (Clark level 5+). Such deep tumours are likely to metastasise and the surgeon should not mistakenly believe that more radical local surgery will ensure a good outcome for the patient. Compartment amputation is rarely considered in squamous carcinoma as the patients are usually elderly. A combined policy of management is possible for deep tumours with wide local excision and immediate skin cover using a radial forearm flap (Fig. 19.7). The excellent vascularity of this flap allows radiotherapy to be given through the flap to the wound bed. Extensive skin tumours most frequently require a transverse amputation which should be sufficiently proximal to clear the necessary compartment. Amputation above the elbow joint may be indicated for advanced tumours of the hand and wrist.

Metastasis to lymph nodes requires block dissection. Curiously, tumour generally develops in the axillary lymph nodes without deposition in intermediate lymphatics. If the tumour is found to have spread through the capsule of the axillary lymph nodes, radiotherapy would be clearly indicated at this site.

### Keratoacanthoma

The keratoacanthoma is a tumour which has an appearance identical to squamous carcinoma. It tends to grow rapidly and be self-limiting. It should not, however, be treated expectantly, but should be excised for histological examination in the usual way, as certain differentiation from squamous carcinoma is impossible.

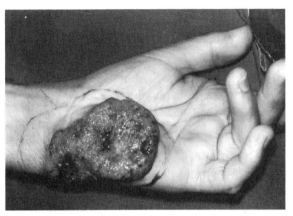

a

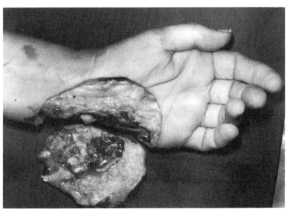

b

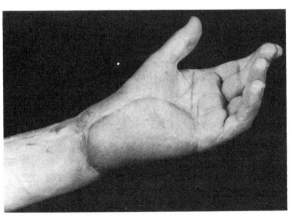

c

**Fig. 19.7 a** Extensive squamous carcinoma of the palm. **b** The lesion widely excised. **c** The defect has been reconstructed with a radial forearm flap. The wound bed was irradiated through the flap

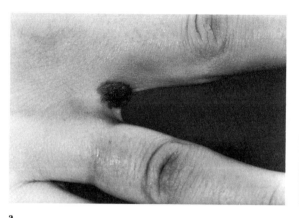

a

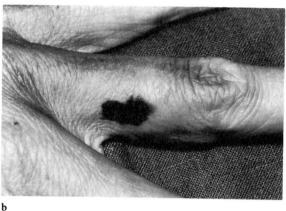

b

**Fig. 19.8** Pigmented skin lesion. **a** Simple compound naevus. This lesion had not changed for many years. **b** Superficial spreading malignant melanoma slowly growing in the digital web. This was treated by excision and skin grafting with no recurrence

### Malignant melanoma of the hand

Malignant melanoma, arising in the hand, is sufficiently uncommon for many surgeons to see only a few cases in a lifetime, but as the prognosis is determined by early adequate excision, it is necessary for every hand surgeon to have a working knowledge of the salient features. Every medical student knows that a naevus which undergoes change and ulcerates or bleeds should be excised immediately. Such lesions are advanced and probably widely disseminated, and excision of an ulcerated or nodular lesion is 'closing the stable door after the horse has bolted'. This attitude shows a significant defect in medical training, for ideally such lesions should be excised earlier with the likelihood of a much better prognosis.

Malignant melanoma presents in a number of different ways. Lentigo maligna presents as a flat enlarging freckle, often with irregular pigmentation. The lesion is not palpable and usually arises in actinically damaged skin. Superficial spreading malignant melanoma (Fig. 19.8b) (see Table 19.1) is the next grade of development, with a relatively good prognosis. The clinical appearance is like lentigo maligna and the distinction can only be made histologically. Nodular malignant melanoma (Fig. 19.8c) may develop from a lentigo maligna or superficial spreading melanoma or de novo. The lesion is palpable and the prognosis is much worse. The usual prognostic indicators of Clark (level of depth of incision, see Table 19.1) or Breslow (histological depth as measured by a micrometer; <0.76 mm prognosis good, >0.76 mm poor) are of limited value in the hand, because of the specialised nature of the skin. Any enlarging freckle or flat pigmented area (lentigo) should therefore be excised. It is generally advised that all freckles, whether enlarging or not, should be excised when they occur in the palm of the hand. The true incidence of malignant melanoma arising in such lesions is unknown, but palmar melanoma is rare. Certainly the author has seen many patients and colleagues with such freckles. It seems wise, however, to advise excision. Malignant melanomas, arising on the palm or digit, frequently have no pigment (acral lentiginous malignant melanoma). They generally do not present until the stage of ulceration or fleshy granulomatous outgrowth, mimicking the appearance of a pyogenic granuloma. The diagnosis is not immediately apparent. Subungual melanoma is extremely rare and is often mistakenly treated as a chronic 'paronychia'.

The treatment of superficial spreading melanoma is by *wide* excision and skin grafting. Nodular melanoma is also treated in this way, although perhaps with a wider margin (Figs 19.8c, d,e). The current advice is that limb lesions should be cleared by a margin of 5 cm. This is rarely practicable in the hand and experience is

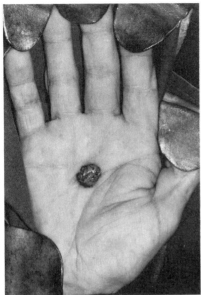

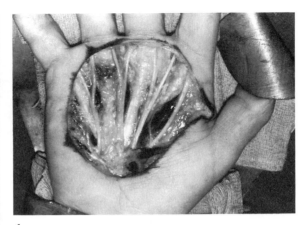

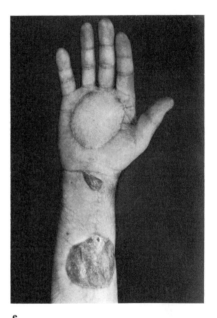

**Fig. 19.8** **c** Nodular malignant melanoma of palm. **d** After histological confirmation, this lesion was widely excised, including the palmar fascia. **e** The area was reconstructed by a radial forearm flap

required in achieving a balance between adequacy of clearance and excessive ablation of function. The overriding principle is adequate ablation rather than functional conservation. If the likelihood of metastasis is high, the patient must be kept under frequent review, checking for enlargement of axillary lymph nodes. Block dissection of the axillary lymph nodes may be necessary at a later stage. Subungual melanoma requires amputation of the digit. In the digits, ray amputation is normally advised and, in the thumb, at the level of the metacarpophalangeal joint. The patient should have the benefit of current advice on the additive therapeutic role of chemotherapy, but the mainstay of curative treatment remains early surgical intervention.

*Basal cell carcinoma* (Fig. 19.9)

By contrast with the high incidence of basal cell carcinoma in the head and neck region, this tumour is rare on the hands. It may, however, occur on the dorsal surface with the typical appearance of an area of ulceration having a raised pearly edge.

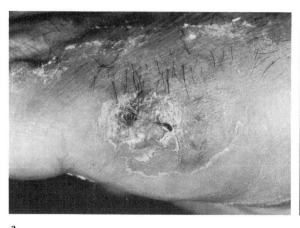

a

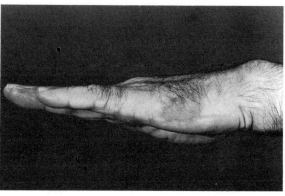

b

**Fig. 19.9** **a** Basal cell carcinoma **b** After treatment by excision and split skin grafting.

*Miscellaneous*

Other malignant primary and secondary skin tumours may occur in the upper limbs. The histological diagnosis will indicate the appropriate treatment.

## TUMOURS ARISING IN BONE

Differential diagnosis:
    Simple cyst
    Enchondroma
    Osteoid osteoma
    Giant cell tumour
    Aneurysmal bone cyst
    Myeloma
    Ewing's tumour
    Osteosarcoma
    Secondary tumour

Tumours arising in bone are not readily diagnosed by clinical examination alone. A firm, usually smooth enlargement of the bone is apparent. Nevertheless, much information can be obtained from the *history* before resorting to a radiograph. *Pain* may be absent and the diagnosis made as an incidental finding during unrelated investigations. Absence of pain suggests the lesion is benign (e.g. enchondroma or simple cyst). Increasing discomfort of gradual onset indicates a more active process. The osteoid osteoma characteristically presents with discomfort in the limb of several months' or years' duration. An abrupt onset of pain suggests that the weakened bone has fractured spontaneously. *Enlargement* over many months or years suggests the lesion is benign, usually an enchondroma. Rapid expansion is characteristic of an aneurysmal bone cyst, or giant cell tumour. Secondary tumours rarely cause massive enlargement of the bone and such expansion as occurs is usually of short duration and associated with relentlessly increasing discomfort. The age of the patient is also an aid to diagnosis. Simple bone cysts and enchondromas may present at any age. Osteoid osteomas, giant cell tumours, aneurysmal bone cysts and Ewing's tumours usually present before the fortieth year. Myeloma and secondary tumours present in middle or advanced age.

A wealth of information can be gleaned from the *radiograph*. The *site of a lytic lesion* in the bone may give important clues as to the diagnosis, especially in the long bones. Both giant cell tumours (Fig. 19.10) and aneurysmal bone cysts (Fig. 19.11) tend to occur at the end of long bones, eccentrically placed. The giant cell tumour may extend up to the articular surface, while the aneurysmal bone cyst remains behind the growth plate. However, in the hand, the bones are so small, that diagnosis on a basis of site of lesion is infrequent.

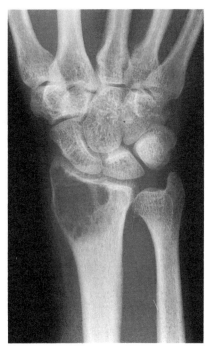

Fig. 19.10  Giant cell tumour of radius

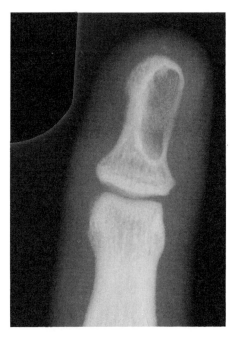

Fig. 19.12  Simple cyst of distal phalanx

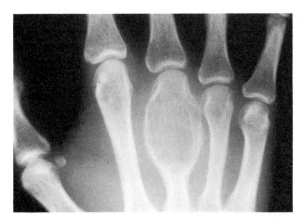

Fig. 19.11  Aneurysmal bone cyst

Simple cysts (Fig. 19.12) may present in any of the upper limb bones, but enchondromas (Fig. 19.13) are usually found in the phalanges or metacarpals. Osteoid osteomas (Fig. 19.14) may present in any long bone, but most frequently in the phalanges.

The radiographic *appearance* of the lesion will aid diagnosis. A clear cavity without calcification is probably a simple cyst. Stippled calcification suggests an enchondroma. The osteoid osteoma classically presents with a central calcified nidus in a surrounding radiolucent area. This in turn is surrounded by an area of bone sclerosis. The giant cell tumour may be totally radiolucent, but commonly there is a 'foamy' calcification present. Trabeculated calcification is the usual feature of the aneurysmal bone cyst. Secondary tumours are generally osteolytic in their action, the bone appearing poorly calcified rather than completely absent.

The *appearance of the interface* between the tumour and the bone is of considerable significance. A well-demarcated line between normal bone and the lesion indicates a slow-growing benign process. Simple cysts are well demarcated, with little or no expansion of the bone. The enchondroma has a distinct margin at the interface, but moderate expansion of the bone does occur, with thinning of the cortex. If fracture of the cortical bone occurs, healing callus may give the lesion a more sinister appearance. The general appearance of the enchondroma, however, is of a bone adapting to a benign lesion, which is slowly increasing in size.

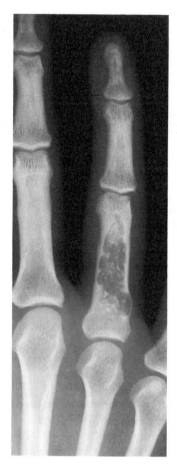

**Fig. 19.13**   Enchondroma

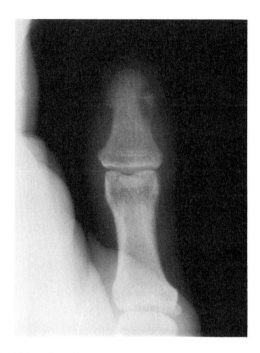

**Fig. 19.14**   Osteoid osteoma

The laminated appearance of the osteoid osteoma has been described already. Mild expansion of the bone may occur, but the lesion rarely becomes larger than 1 cm in diameter. Some swelling of the surrounding soft tissues commonly occurs. The aneurysmal bone cyst may produce rapid and massive expansion of the bone. The cortex may be so expanded and thin that the bone takes on the appearance of a distended periosteal sac. The interface with normal bone is usually fairly distinct, but less so in the more active type.

Giant cell tumours often present with expansion of the bone and thinning of the cortex; the margin with normal bone is generally distinct. The appearance of secondary tumours of bone (Fig. 19.15) is quite different. The tumour appears to infiltrate the normal bone; there is no abrupt

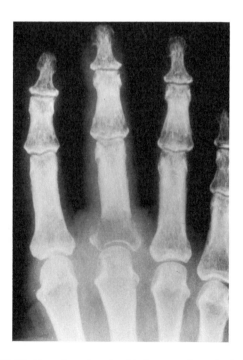

**Fig. 19.15**   Secondary deposit with fracture of proximal phalanx

interface, simply a hazy edge to the lesion. Expansion of the bone is uncommon, the cortex and medulla being replaced by tumour tissue.

In the upper limb, enchondromas only rarely undergo sarcomatous change. Giant cell tumours have a broad range of activity, the majority being benign, but the most active being malignant. Any alteration in the rate of growth of either of these tumours, or radiological evidence of an indistinct tumour margin, suggests malignant change may have supervened.

## Myelomatosis

Myelomatosis is a neoplastic condition arising from plasma cells of the bone marrow. The condition is uncommon under the age of 55 years and frequently presents with bone pain and pathological fracture. Upper limb involvement is uncommon, particularly in the distal parts. Radiographs reveal a lytic lesion of the bone with diffuse tumour bone interface. Skeletal survey frequently reveals multiple lytic areas, particularly in marrow sites (pelvis, vertebrae, ribs and skull).

## Ewing's tumour

Ewing's tumour is an uncommon, but highly malignant neoplasm, which arises in the long bones of children. They may present with pyrexia, leucocytosis and bone pain, misdirecting the clinician towards a diagnosis of osteomyelitis. The radiological appearance may lend support to this diagnosis, with extensive involvement of the long bone shaft. On occasion, a characteristic laminated 'onion skin' appearance to the bone makes diagnosis of Ewing's tumour more obvious. Early metastasis to lungs or other skeletal sites is frequent. Extensive infiltration of the bone makes en bloc excision rarely practicable.

## Osteosarcoma

This rarely presents in the upper limb. The majority occurs between the ages of 10 and 30 years with a further group presenting in the 60s and 70s as malignant change in Pagetoid bone. Osteosarcoma is more common in the lower limb, generally near the end of long bones. The bone is involved from within and the lesion may be lytic in nature, sclerotic, or a combination of the two. The interface with normal bone is indistinct. Radiographs may reveal that the expanding tumour has raised the periosteum from adjacent normal bone (Codman's triangle). Lines of calcification may be present outside the bone, perpendicular to the long axis (sunray spicules). Neither Codman's triangle nor sunray spicules are specific to osteosarcoma and both may, for instance, occur in the case of long bone osteomyelitis. Spread is local and via the bloodstream to the lungs. Chest radiographs may reveal secondary deposits.

## The role of biospy in tumours arising in bone

A detailed history, examination and radiographic assessment will often permit definitive surgery to be performed at the time of biopsy. If, however, the diagnosis remains in doubt, or if ablative surgery is under consideration, a preliminary biopsy is required. A cortical bone flap is raised, a portion of the tumour removed, and the cortical lid replaced. This reduces the risk of local spread of tumour. Pre-operative discussion of the differential diagnosis with a pathologist may indicate that frozen section examination will be of value. Many bone tumours require decalcification prior to staining, but differentiation of giant cell tumour from an aneurysmal bone cyst is feasible on frozen section. If preliminary biopsy is performed, every effort should be made to contain the tumour within the bone and definitive surgery should follow swiftly. On re-exploration, excision of the biopsy incision margins would seem prudent.

## The management of bone tumours

**Bone cysts.** Many of these present as incidental findings on radiographs. No active treatment is required for the majority. If the structure of the bone is weakened, it is prudent to curette and bone-graft the lesion. A lid is fashioned in cortical bone overlying the cyst. This may be done most easily by using a fine power drill, making a series of holes in the shape of a rectangle. The lid is lifted, the cyst curetted and cancellous bone packed into the cavity and the lid closed. If the cyst is in a metacarpal or phalanx, the dorsolateral approach gives good access with retraction of the extensor tendon. Replacing the cortical lid reduces the risk of subsequent extensor tendon adhesion. Early mobilisation is advised, unless there is skeletal instability.

**Enchondroma.** This tumour continues to grow slowly and many tend to be situated close to the articular surface, particularly at the base of the phalanges. Management depends on their site and size, the patient's age and general health. Curettage and bone graft is preferred in most cases. The tumour is soft, grey-white in colour with gritty calcified particles. If fracture of the cortex has occurred, management becomes more complex. Providing the alignment of the fingers remains satisfactory (particularly in rotation), it may be preferable to allow the fracture to heal spontaneously and then perform a curettage and bone graft at a later date. This delay is not in the expectation of the enchondroma disappearing spontaneously (a situation which occasionally happens with cysts, but rarely with enchondromas). If no significant shift of the fracture has occurred, early curettage of the cyst will turn a fairly stable fracture into an unstable one and may increase the chance of rotatory malalignment. If, however, significant malalignment of the phalanx has already occurred, or the fracture shows no signs of uniting with conservative management, then open reduction of the fracture, curettage and bone grafting, must be performed. If the tumour lies close to the joint, problems may be experienced in stabilising the fracture while the graft consolidates.

**Giant cell tumours.** These tumours also tend to lie close to the articular surfaces. A minority (approximately 15%) of these tumours is malignant with local soft tissue invasion and spread via the bloodstream to the lungs. Chest X-ray should be performed and lung tomography, or scan, may be required. A close study of the interface between the tumour and adjacent bone may reveal the degree of local invasion. The tumour is soft, often lobulated and friable. Recent or old haemorrhage into the tumour is frequently seen, its colour being red or brown. Regrettably, the proximity to articular surface often means that en bloc resection is possible only if one attempts to arthrodese the involved joint at the same time. In these circumstances, surgeons frequently opt to curette the cavity and pack with bone graft, thus preserving the adjacent joint. A review of the literature suggests that local recurrence of tumour following curettage is approximately 40%. Therefore, if this treatment is used, the curettage must be radical to minimise this risk. The grafted cavity will require monitoring with serial X-rays to identify possible recurrence. Should this happen, it may respond to further curettage, or en block resection. If the lesion is in a finger, amputation of the digit may be appropriate. Recurrent metacarpal tumours, with possible soft tissue extension, require a ray excision, with resection of the finger metacarpal and adjacent intrinsic muscles. Radiotherapy is not advised for giant cell tumours of the bone. It increases the risk of the tumour becoming malignant.

**Aneurysmal bone cyst.** On occasion these tumours are more dramatic in their presentation than giant cell tumours, but they are less likely to recur following curettage and bone grafting. The cavity is filled with serous, often blood-stained fluid and thrombus. Failure to control the tumour with curettage and bone graft may lead to en bloc resection. The tumour is not malignant, but on occasion is very aggressive locally. Problems are best avoided by prompt treatment following diagnosis. If the grafted cavity shows signs of recurrence, swiftly move to en bloc resection.

**Osteoid osteoma.** These lesions respond well to localised resection. This may take the form of excision of a block of tissue, including the nidus, or cutting a window in the adjacent cortex and clearing the area of the tumour. The nidus is small and indistinguishable clinically from the surrounding bone. It is prudent in these circumstances to use radiological control in theatre in the planning of resection and to check that excision is complete before the wound is closed. If the nidus is missed, recurrent symptoms may occur. If the osteoma is present in a phalanx, we prefer the 'open window' technique. The majority of the cortex can be left intact and the cavity packed with cancellous bone graft.

Isolated myelomas, involving the long bones of the upper limb, may be treated by en bloc resection, bone graft and stabilisation with intramedullary rods or plates. If the tumour is multifocal, curettage, bone graft and intramedullary rod fixation will relieve pain and maintain skeletal stability. Survival rates for osteosarcoma and Ewing's tumour remain low. Both are, to a degree, radiosensitive. If lung and body scans indicate no secondary spread, amputation may be considered in combination with both radio- and chemotherapy. Combined chemotherapy has improved survival rates for osteosarcoma in recent years.

**Secondary tumours.** Management of these cases depends on the source of the primary. Tumours commonly metastasising to bone are breast, lung, prostate, kidney and thyroid. Breast and prostate metastases may respond to hormonal therapy. Radiotherapy and chemotherapy are used as indicated by the nature of the primary tumour. The predominant symptom in a bone metastasis involving the wrist or hand is pain. This is often severe, even if a fracture has not occurred. The symptom is best managed by removing a cortical window over the secondary deposit, curetting out the involved bone and packing the area with bone graft. Frequently the involvement of the bone is so extensive that skeletal stability will be lost. If this seems likely, the cavity is best filled with acrylic bone cement. This supports the remaining shell of bone and maintains stability. Tumour secondaries in the larger long bones of the upper limb may be treated in the same manner, but it is necessary to supplement acrylic cement with an intramedullary rod.

If fracture occurs through a secondary deposit in the bone, stabilisation of the fracture is required. This is particularly important in larger long bones of the upper limb. If the fracture causes significant pain, the tumour should be curetted, an intramedullary nail inserted, and the bone cavity packed with cement. This remains the treatment of choice, even if the patients are in poor general health and close to death. The temptation to treat with external splintage should be avoided, unless it is felt the patient has only a very short time to live. Stabilisation of the fracture

greatly eases the pain and permits the use of the upper limb.

### The choice of bone for grafting

Bone grafting has been advocated in the management of several bone tumours. In the majority of cases cancellous bone alone is required, although larger block resections in humerus or radius and ulna require corticocancellous blocks. The most plentiful source of good-quality cancellous bone is the iliac crest. The disadvantages to iliac crest graft lie in the disturbance of the cutaneous nerves overlying the hip and discomfort around the scar. To an extent, this can be reduced by careful surgical technique, lifting the cortical rim of the iliac crest, hinged on the periosteum at its inner edge. If necessary, large amounts of cancellous bone may then be removed, using curved gouges. The lid is then sutured back and the tissue closed in layers. Smaller amounts of good quality graft may be obtained from the lower radius. Care must be taken not to disturb the sensory branches of the radial nerve. The upper end of the ulna produces a small amount of poor-quality cancellous bone. Its use as a source of bone graft is less satisfactory.

## TUMOURS ARISING FROM JOINTS

Differential diagnosis:
    Heberden's nodes
    Mucous cyst
    Ganglia (dorsal or volar)
    Pigmented villonodular synovitis
    Rheumatoid synovitis
    Synovial sarcoma

### Heberden's nodes

Osteoarthritis of the distal interphalangeal and, occasionally, the proximal interphalangeal joints produces exostoses and nodularity adjacent to the articular surface (see Fig. 16.21). The condition is commonly seen in the elderly, producing cosmetic deformity, mild to moderate discomfort, and some stiffness in the involved joints. It rarely causes significant functional problems. Management involves reassurance of the patients that the function of the hand will remain satisfactory, although some discomfort may be experienced. Rarely instability of the joint merits arthrodesis.

## Mucous cyst (Fig. 19.16)

The cyst is a ganglion which usually arises from the distal interphalangeal joint. Herniation of the capsular tissues occurs on the dorsal aspect. Characteristically the cyst lies very close to the skin, which is considerably thinned. Pressure may occur to the germinal matrix producing deformation of the nail. The attenuated skin over the cyst renders it liable to rupture by trivial injuries, with the risk of sepsis travelling retrogradely into the distal interphalangeal joint. Surgery is advocated for this reason. The thin skin overlying the cyst makes closure following excision difficult. Excision of the cyst is performed with the overlying attenuated skin. A local skin flap is raised and swung to cover the defect in the distal interphalangeal joint. A small triangular skin graft may be required to cover the defect more proximally.

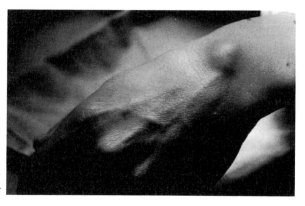

Fig. 19.17   Ganglion of wrist

## Ganglia of the wrist (Fig. 19.17)

**Dorsal.** The majority arise from the wrist joint, while others appear in sites where tendons cross (e.g. extensor pollicis longus crossing ECRL and ECRB). The cysts are filled with clear mucinous material which appears to arise from the adjacent joint. The area around the scapholunate ligament on the dorsal aspect of the wrist is the principal site from which the ganglia develop. Initially, the discomfort may be considerable, with no mass evident on clinical examination. As the ganglion grows, the discomfort may get less marked. If surgery is felt to be required, it is best done through a transverse incision under tourniquet and local anaesthesia. Care is taken to preserve the terminal sensory branches of the radial nerve. The ganglion is excised down to the wrist capsule. Oversewing of the neck of the cyst is not necessary and may increase, rather than diminish the recurrence rate. The skin is sutured and a light, but firm, dressing is applied. Early movement of the fingers and wrist is encouraged.

**Volar.** Volar wrist ganglia intimately relate to the radial artery and arise between flexor carpi radialis and abductor pollicis longus in either the radiocarpal or trapezioscaphoid joints. Exploration of these cysts is best performed through an oblique incision, curved towards the carpal tunnel. Local anaesthesia is less satisfactory for this type of ganglion, and a Biers block, in particular, is to be avoided. Great care must be taken to avoid injury to the radial artery or its

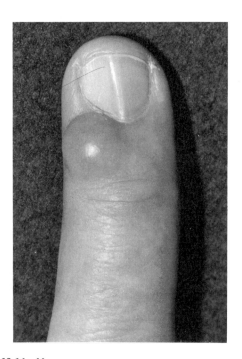

Fig. 19.16   Mucous cyst

branches during the dissection. Frequently it is valuable to let down the tourniquet before closure to ensure that no damage to the artery has occurred. The Biers block does not permit the release of the tourniquet at this stage. During surgery, it is important to preserve the palmar cutaneous nerve, which lies close to the incision. It is worthwhile performing a separate closure of the deep fascia, reducing the chance of adjacent tendons adhering to the overlying skin.

### Pigmented villonodular synovitis (giant cell tumour) of the joint (Fig. 19.18)

It is unclear whether this condition represents true neoplasia or simply a reactive condition. Malignant change does not occur. The characteristic appearance is of a firm lobulated intra-articular swelling. If the condition has been present for several years, damage to the articular surface of the joint may occur, but this is uncommon. A radiograph of the joint usually reveals soft tissue swelling only, without calcification. Exploration reveals a firm, lobulated, red-brown pigmented tumour, which dissects free from surrounding tissue without undue difficulty. All age-groups may be affected and this tumour is quite commonly found in metacarpophalangeal and interphalangeal joints. Recurrence following excision is uncommon and suggests a lobule of tissue has been left behind at previous surgery.

### Rheumatoid synovitis

The rheumatoid process may involve any joint in the upper limb, but only rarely affects the distal interphalangeal joints. The joint is often warmer than surrounding tissue, and the swelling relatively soft. Examination of the synovium is best performed by pressing on both sides of the joint, while ballotting the dorsal aspect with a third examining finger. The synovium feels thick and fluid is present within the joint. There may be other stigmas suggestive of rheumatoid arthritis. The patient may have rheumatoid nodules on the subcutaneous border of the forearm. Ulnar drift or swan-necked deformity may be present. Synovitis of the proximal interphalangeal joint may produce attenuation of the central slip (see Fig. 16.8a,b) and a boutonnière deformity. Management of rheumatoid synovitis is considered in Chapter 16.

### Synovial sarcoma

This is an uncommon but highly malignant tumour principally involving young adults. The synovium is markedly thickened and in subcutaneous joints may appear warm. An effusion may be present, or spontaneous haemorrhage into the joint. Radiographs may reveal erosion of the articular cartilage and flecks of calcification are commonly seen within the tumour mass. Tumour circulation may be apparent on an arteriogram. Amputation is usually indicated.

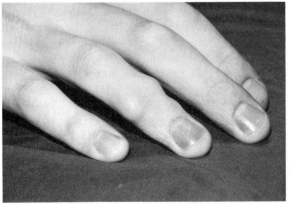
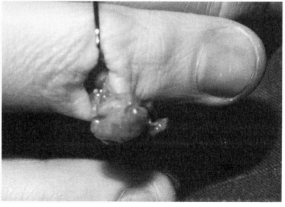

a                                    b

**Fig. 19.18  a, b** Giant cell tumour of the distal phalanx

## TUMOURS ARISING FROM TENDONS AND TENDON SHEATHS

Differential diagnosis:

Pigmented villonodular synovitis of flexor tendon sheath

Trigger finger

De Quervain's syndrome

Seed ganglion

Rheumatoid synovitis of flexor or extensor tendons

### Pigmented villonodular synovitis of the flexor tendon sheath

This presents as a nodular swelling over the volar aspect of the finger. The sheath is distended on palpation and flexion may be limited by the bulk of the tumour. Triggering or crepitus may be apparent on flexing the finger. It may prove difficult by examination alone to differentiate villonodular synovitis from rheumatoid synovitis of the flexor tendon sheath. The former tends to be firmer and lobulated. Clinical appearance and management is similar to that described for villonodular synovitis of the joint.

### Trigger finger

The site of triggering, where the tendon nodule catches against the sheath, is almost invariably at the metacarpophalangeal joint. Uncommonly, the lateral bands may trigger over an exostosis on the dorsal aspect of the metacarpal head. Triggering is usually associated with nodularity of the tendon rather than stenosis of the flexor tendon sheath. The condition is most frequently seen in middle-aged females, but can occur at any age and in either sex. Several fingers may be involved and there is an association between trigger finger, de Quervain's (stenosing tenovaginitis) and carpal tunnel syndrome. The precise cause of the swelling on the tendon is unclear. It may well relate to a disturbance to the blood supply of the tendon, or perhaps damage to the tendon lymphatics. A minority of cases is due to rheumatoid synovitis around the flexor tendons. The congenital trigger thumb presents in infancy and the child is found to be unable to fully extend the

interphalangeal joint of the thumb. True triggering of the thumb in these cases is uncommon. A nodule in the flexor tendon is palpable at the level of the metacarpophalangeal joint.

Management of triggering may be conservative if the symptoms are mild. A small amount of steroid may be infiltrated around the mouth of the A1 pulley in the palm. However, this treatment is inadequate for any significant disproportion between tendon and sheath. In most cases surgical release of the more proximal part of the A1 pulley is required. This is performed under direct vision with local infiltration anaesthesia. Early mobilisation of the fingers is preferred to ensure that no adhesion develops between tendon and sheath. Care must also be taken to identify and preserve the digital nerves adjacent to the A1 pulley. Particular care must be taken when releasing a trigger thumb. The digital nerves lie very lose to the skin and may be divided as the skin is incised. Congenital trigger thumbs noted at birth may with safety be observed in the first instance, as one-third of the involved thumbs will be released spontaneously within the first months. If surgical release is required, loupe magnification is helpful to identify and protect the digital nerves.

### De Quervain's syndrome (stenosing tenovaginitis)

This condition presents as pain and often swelling at the base of the thumb overlying the radial styloid (Fig. 19.19). There may be fullness over the first dorsal compartment containing extensor pollicis brevis and abductor pollicis longus. Finkelstein's test is positive (ulnar deviation of the wrist with the thumb held in flexion reproduces the pain). Occasionally crepitus may be present on movement of the thumb. A radiograph of the wrist will reveal if there is any significant first carpometacarpal arthritis, non-union of the scaphoid, or scaphotrapezial arthritis. These are all conditions which may produce discomfort around the radial styloid.

De Quervain's syndrome frequently arises because of an episode of unaccustomed vigorous activity. In such cases it is reasonable to rest the wrist and thumb on a splint. Non-steroidal anti-inflammatory agents may also be of benefit. However, if symptoms do not settle within 3

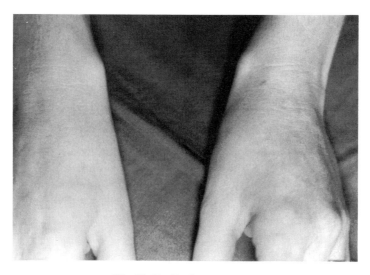

**Fig. 19.19** De Quervain's syndrome

weeks, alternative treatment is indicated. A steroid infiltration around the mouth of the first dorsal compartment will frequently relieve the discomfort. This technique is not without problems. If the commonly used depot-type steroid injections are given subcutaneously, local fat atrophy and depigmentation of the skin may occur. Significant blemishes to the skin may be produced and women with thin wrists are better treated with the shorter-acting hydrocortisone acetate, which seems to cause these problems infrequently.

Surgical decompression of the first dorsal compartment is indicated if more conservative measures do not control the symptoms. Extensor tendon anatomical variations are so common that the classical textbook appearance is the exception rather than the rule. At exploration a full decompression of all local extensor tendons must be performed. On occasion a duplication of extensor pollicis brevis is found, both tendons travelling in separate fibro-osseous tunnels. More frequently, the abductor pollicis longus is found to be composed of several slips and one of these may travel in a separate compartment. All must be fully released. Great care must be taken to preserve all the sensory branches of the radial nerve which lie close to the incision. A tender scar, due to inadequate protection of the radial

nerve branches, remains the most common complication of surgical decompression.

*The seed ganglion* (Fig. 19.20)

The history and presentation of this lesion is quite characteristic, and no difficulty should be experienced in diagnosis. The patient presents with a lump at the base of the finger on the volar aspect. The lump overlies the proximal phalanx near its base and is eccentrically placed, rarely in the midline. The pea-like nodule is firm, smooth and small. It usually causes discomfort when grasping narrow objects like a bucket-handle or car steering wheel. The nodule does not move with the flexor tendons and there is no triggering of the finger. Injection of the ganglion may rupture it, but recurrence is not uncommon. Exploration and excision of the ganglion with a small segment of tendon sheath resolves the problem and recurrence is rare. The defect in the flexor tendon sheath is left open. Care must be taken to protect the adjacent digital nerve and vessels. Early mobilisation reduces the likelihood of adhesions developing between the tendon and sheath.

*Rheumatoid synovitis involving the tendons*

**Extensor tendon synovitis** (see Fig. 16.2b). On occasion difficulty may be experienced in

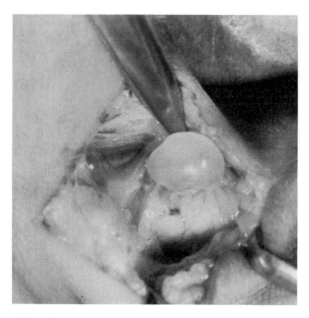

Fig. 19.20    Seed ganglion of flexor tendon

differentiating between a soft multiloculated ganglion on the dorsal aspect of the wrist and rheumatoid synovitis. Transillumination is often a useful test in these circumstances and will reveal which of the swellings are ganglia. The presence of an extensor tendon rupture strongly suggests a rheumatoid process at work. The management of the condition is described in Chapter 16.

**Flexor tendon synovitis.** This is a frequent manifestation of rheumatoid disease, but often overlooked clinically (see Fig. 16.3). Flexor tendon rupture is probably somewhat less common than the extensor variety, but even in the absence of rupture the condition reduces the function of the hand considerably. Synovitis may extend from the forearm to the palm, producing a compound palmar ganglion. There is fullness in the forearm which may be squeezed through the carpal tunnel into the palm by gentle forearm pressure. Thickening of the synovium in the carpal tunnel may give rise to median nerve compression (see Fig. 16.4). In the fingers, the thickened synovium erodes and distends the flexor tendon sheath. Examination will reveal reduced flexion of the fingers, a distended flexor tendon

sheath, and perhaps crepitus over the tendons on attempted flexion. Profundus or superficialis tendon ruptures may be present (see Ch. 16).

## TUMOURS ARISING FROM NERVE TISSUE

Differential diagnosis:
    Neurofibroma
    Neurilemmoma
    Glomus tumour
    Cutaneous neuroma

### Neurofibroma

Solitary lesions are extremely rare, the usual presentation being multiple tumours in von Recklinghausen's disease (multiple neurofibromatosis, *café au lait* spots and skin nodules). The neurofibromas are usually small and firm. They appear more mobile in the transverse than the longitudinal plane in the upper limb and percussion over them commonly causes tingling distally. Elongated plexiform tumours may on occasion be found to extend over several centimetres. The tumour tissue is not readily dissected from the nerve bundles and it is fortunate that surgery is rarely required. If excision of a neurofibroma is performed, some loss of nerve function may be anticipated. Increasing pain or enlargement of the tumour may indicate sarcomatous degeneration. Malignant change is uncommon.

### Neurilemmoma (a tumour of Schwann cell) (Fig. 19.21)

This is a more common variety of nerve tumour. Neurilemmomas are usually solitary and may appear in any part of the body, particularly the upper limb. The tumour may lie on the route of a major nerve. Percussion over the mass may produce tingling distally, but this feature is frequently absent. Exploration reveals a soft yellow tumour, commonly related to a nerve. The nerve fascicles are splayed out by the neoplasm but retain their integrity, and excision can be performed without major loss of nerve fibres. Recurrence is rare.

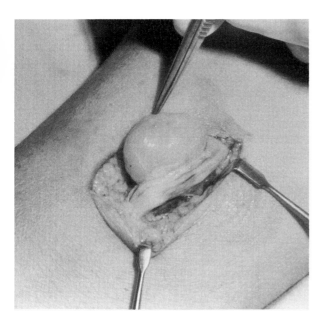

**Fig. 19.21** Neurilemmoma

*Glomus tumours*

These arise from the perivascular tissues which control the blood flow to the skin. The arteriolar flow mechanism is under neurological control. The lesion contains many nerve elements and pain is a prominent symptom from an early stage.

Glomus tumours are usually seen in the hands and feet, commonly distally placed; the nail bed may be involved. Shooting spontaneous pain, or a discrete trigger spot in the fingertip would suggest the diagnosis, even if no mass is palpable. Exploration under magnification and excision of the small tumour is required. Inadequate excision results in continuing discomfort. The less painful glomus tumours may present with a long history of discomfort in the fingertip and a more obvious mass. The tumour may be up to 1 cm in diameter. Palpation causes discomfort. On exploration a soft yellow well-encapsulated tumour is readily dissected from surrounding tissue.

*Cutaneous neuromas*

These are fortunately uncommon. The patient gives a history of a laceration, usually overlying the route of a digital nerve of the finger. There is an exquisitely tender nodule in the scar which the patient attempts to protect from any form of contact. The finger is commonly held flexed for this reason. At the time of injury the nerve has been divided and the proximal stump permitted to lie adjacent to the healing skin edges. Management involves exploration and either nerve repair or burying the nerve stump in a more protected area.

# 20. Patient assessment

*Principal author: P. J. Smith*

The comprehensive evaluation of hand disorders requires experience in a number of areas. The examiner must have a profound knowledge of the normal anatomy and physiology. In addition, the disturbance in hand function will depend not only upon the pathological process but also upon the patient's physiological and psychological responses.

**The immediate examination of the hand following trauma** requires an expeditious approach. It differs in extent and technique from the examination of a patient with a longstanding condition, seeking elective surgery. In the acute situation the patient is apprehensive and may be in pain. Gentleness in examination, early reassurance and the relief of pain is essential.

In assessing such injuries, certain questions must be answered:

*1. Does this patient require exploration in theatre?*

All but the most superficial skin lacerations should be treated in a theatre with good illumination, tourniquet control and fine instruments. In particular, penetrating glass wounds must always be explored in this way.

*2. Is the hand or injured digit viable?*

This can be rapidly assessed by observing the colour, capillary refill and response to pulp compression.

*Colour.* The normal colour of the human hand defies description and artistic ingenuity. Total ischaemia renders the hand pale or white in appearance when compared to normal areas of skin, although this may be difficult to assess in dark-skinned patients. Venous obstruction initially renders the hand more livid in appearance with a bluish, purplish hue and, if prolonged, a marked degree of mottling of the skin results. It can be difficult to assess circulation on the basis of colour alone. In the presence of an open wound associated with a devascularised digit, bleeding may obscure the colour of the skin, making interpretation of this sign difficult.

*The capillary refill.* When part of a nail-bed or the skin is firmly compressed and then released, there is a relaxed and gentle return of colour to the pale area. This capillary refill tends to be quicker in the nail-bed than it does in the surrounding skin. A sluggish return indicates poor arterial in-flow. Venous engorgement may lead to a more rapid capillary refill associated with a slight bluish hue to the finger. In early venous congestion, the change in colour may not be obvious, but capillary refill will be rapid. This is a valuable sign following replantation.

*Pulp compression test.* Tissue with a normal circulation has a characteristic turgor; firm compression of a finger-pulp for 10 or 20 seconds will produce an indentation which expands and refills. The return of tissue turgor is an invaluable method of monitoring circulation following replantation (Fig. 20.1). In an ischaemic digit, pulp compression will leave an indented and pale area which does not re-expand.

*3. Is the skeleton stable?*

Good radiographs taken in two planes are essential to determine the nature of any skeletal injury. It is possible to miss a fracture if a single view is relied upon.

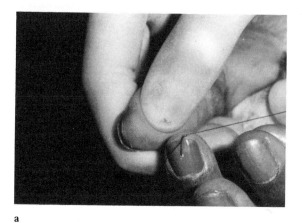
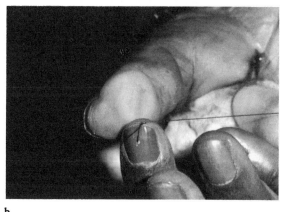

a                                                                                    b

**Fig. 20.1** **a** The pulp compression test. Used to assess whether there is adequate arterial input in the finger. The pulp is firmly compressed and then the compression is released, as in **b**. An immediate return of tissue turgor indicates adequate arterial in-flow. Poor arterial in-flow is indicated by the presence of a continuing pale tip which does not refill, as illustrated in **b**

### 4. Is there any evidence of tendon injury?

The tenodesis test assesses the integrity of the flexor and extensor tendons by comparing their relative movement on flexion and extension of the wrist. Flexing the wrist increases the tension on the extensor tendons thus extending the fingers. Extension of the wrist does the reverse, the fingers falling into a more flexed position. The thumb is similarly affected. Any alteration in the normal digital cascade is immediately apparent, particularly if a single digit is injured and both tendons are divided, giving rise to a classical pointing sign.

### 5. Is there any evidence of nerve injury?

The plastic pen (tactile adherence) test will detect immediate cessation of sweating in denervated areas. This test is easy to perform and is tolerated well by the youngest of children. It requires no patient co-operation and can be performed on an unconscious patient (Fig. 20.2).

### 6. Is there evidence of actual or impending skin loss?

This can be difficult to assess clinically and should be undertaken in the operating theatre. Actual loss is obvious once débridement has been undertaken,

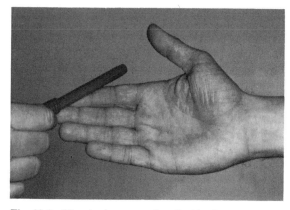

**Fig. 20.2** The plastic pen test described by Stewart Harrison. In this test a plastic pen is drawn over a suspected area of denervation. Such areas do not sweat and are dry and the pen does not adhere to the finger. Tactile adherence in uninjured areas is normal

however, impending skin loss in a degloved area is more difficult to assess. An extensively undermined area may proceed to skin necrosis. The likelihood of this can be assessed by inspecting the edge of the skin flap to see if there is capillary bleeding from the dermis. The capillary refill of the flap itself may also give an indication of the likelihood of survival. The skin may be obviously bruised and crushed with a large underlying haematoma. The edge of the wound should be

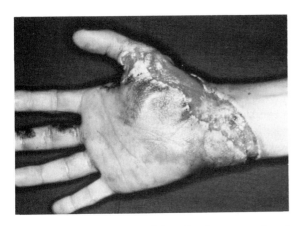

**Fig. 20.3** Degloving injury of the palm. Some contusion of the palmar skin can be seen. Serial trimming of the wound edge until dermal bleeding is present will return the skin margins to viability. This patient was treated by immediate free flap cover

gradually débrided by serial excision until dermal bleeding is obtained; delayed closure without tension of grafting may avert skin loss (Fig. 20.3). The use of intravenous fluorescein may be invaluable in such circumstances.

A patient with an injured hand should be examined once preferably or at the most twice if a more experienced opinion is sought. It is therefore important that the initial dressing should allow easy pain-free removal. A polythene bag may prove useful. Any dressing required to provide rest or compression may then be applied and the hand elevated to control oozing. Subsequent examination may be performed without patient discomfort. Once a treatment plan has been established analgesic blocks may be administered, particularly if there is to be a delay before exploration.

**The assessment of a patient with a non-urgent problem** in the outpatient department is different. A more detailed examination is required pertinent to the particular problems raised in the history. The examination commences as the patient walks through the consulting room door. Much information can be gained both from the patient's entry and that of any companions. The unaccompanied 14-year-old, the 21-year-old with parents and the opinionated spouse all give cause for concern. The

patient's approach to the surgeon is important. Failure to engage in direct conversation and addressing comments to nursing staff may indicate a patient with whom rapport may be difficult. Excessive vocalisation about minimal symptoms indicates the patient's symptom threshold and an assessment must be made as to whether the symptoms are proportional to the pathology involved.

The surgeon's approach to the patient is equally important and establishing rapid physical contact is valuable in this regard. It is wise to sit the patient so that the examining surgeon can manipulate and examine the hands with ease. The presence of a desk between the patient and the doctor inhibits this. A general examination of texture, turgor and mobility of the hand can be obtained as the history unfolds. Early contact of this type will usually put the patient at ease. The patient's response to this manoeuvre tells the surgeon much about how he responds to his own hand. Some patients constantly look at their hand while others never look at it. A normal patient looks at the involved hand occasionally, but shifts attention to the surgeon and others as the conversation dictates. Indifference or fixation are poor prognostic signs. The general appearance of the hand can, of course, convey hints about possible systemic disease. Numerous volumes have been written on this subject alone. It is important that the hand surgeon does not lose sight of the fact that beyond the shirt cuff there lies a complete patient.

There are two groups of elective patients; those who have sustained a previous injury and who return for consideration of reconstructive procedures, and those who present with primary pathology. In the post-traumatic patient, a detailed history of the injury and previous treatment is necessary. In all cases, the surgeon should ascertain the symptoms and the degree to which they limit function. Factors which aggravate or relieve symptoms may offer valuable diagnostic clues. These features must be put in the context of the patient's age, occupation, interests and hand dominance. The medical history must include details of previous injury, treatment, and any relevant general medical information. *Examination is undertaken to confirm or refute a presumptive diagnosis, to grade the severity of the underlying pathological processes, to monitor a response to treatment and to assess reconstructive possibilities.* The surgeon must determine the answers to certain specific questions:

1. Is the hand soft and supple?
2. Are there contractures present?
3. Does deformity exist?
4. What is the specific functional impairment?

*The suppleness and softness of the hand* is determined by observation and palpation of the skin and the underlying tissues. In the patient undergoing rehabilitation, both induration and swelling must be assessed. The mobility of the skin upon underlying structures and the presence of scars must be determined. If further incisions are proposed, the maturity and direction of an existing scar may determine the location of subsequent incisions. The presence of excessive sweating or increased hair growth may indicate a reflex sympathetic dystrophy and treatment of this should be completed prior to undertaking reconstructive surgery. In certain elective conditions such as Dupuytren's, scleroderma and Still's disease, the hands may be indurated and stiff.

*An examination for the presence of contractures* must be made. If present, the surgeon must determine whether joint, tendon or skin is primarily responsible. In certain injuries such as severe burns all three structures may be involved. The presence of skin contractures can generally be diagnosed on visual inspection when a flexion or extension deformity exists related to a scar, graft or flap. A linear scar crossing a flexion crease at right angles, a sheet of burn scar tissue or contracted graft may all produce such deformities. In the digits it is possible to measure the distance between the flexion or extension creases and compare them with the other hand. This indicates the presence of absolute shortening of skin. It should be possible to differentiate between a skin contracture and the involvement of underlying structures. In a flexion deformity due to skin shortage, the tenodesis effect will not influence the position. It may be possible to demonstrate a full range of joint movement by appropriate manipulation of other interlinked joints. Tendon shortening may be ascertained by the tenodesis test; the wrist is put through its normal range of flexion and extension and the posture of adjacent fingers in the normal digital arcade is observed. A discrepancy may arise suggesting either shortening of a tendon or tethering. The presence of a joint contracture may be determined by testing whether the joint in question can be fully extended when all other interlinked joints are flexed (or vice versa for an extension deformity). However, inability to passively correct a contracture by this means does not always indicate that the joint is responsible.

However, if *deformity* is present it is important to ascertain whether it is postural and thus passively correctable (postural) or fixed (structural) requiring corrective surgery. Passively correctable deformity is associated with nerve paralysis. Alternatively, the development of such deformity may indicate reinnervation of previously paralysed muscle groups, leading to imbalance. For example, in high ulnar nerve injuries clawing may appear for the first time during the recovery phase and indicates profundus reinnervation. In such circumstances its development is a good prognostic sign.

Structural deformity may require surgical correction to improve function. Objective measurements of the range of motion allows progress to be assessed at each visit. *A detailed examination should now be undertaken to determine any specific impairment of function*, with each system being examined in turn.

## EXAMINATION OF THE SYSTEMS

### VASCULAR

*Allens test* assesses the patency of larger vessels. The radial and ulnar arteries are firmly compressed at the wrist and residual pooled blood is pumped out of the hand by the patient rapidly opening and closing his fist. The radial artery is released while maintaining compression on the ulnar artery. Rapid capillary refill should occur and the time taken documented. The same procedure should be repeated and the patency of the ulnar artery assessed. Compression should be maintained for

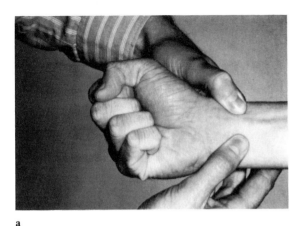
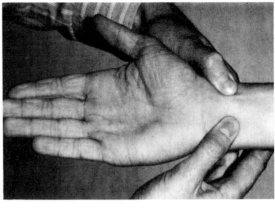

a

b

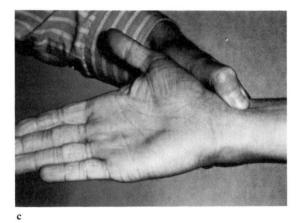

c

**Fig. 20.4 a, b, c** Allen's test. The patient's radial and ulnar arteries are compressed, and at the same time the patient is asked to make a fist and open his fingers several times. This has the effect of pumping blood out of the hand and rendering the hand relatively ischaemic. The patient is then asked to extend the fingers as in **b** and compression to both arteries is continued for a further 10 seconds. In this way the presence of an abberant median artery can be detected. The finger is then removed from the artery in question to assess whether or not it is patent. In the illustration, pressure has been removed from the ulnar artery and the whole hand has become pink, indicating the patency of the ulnar artery

at least 10 seconds prior to release to exclude the presence of a median artery. (This particularly applies in cases of carpal tunnel syndrome.) (Fig. 20.4). *Digital Allen's test*—in this test the radial and ulnar digital arteries of a finger are compressed in the same way as previously described and released in turn to assess their patency.

The Doppler flow meter may prove useful in assessing circulatory status, detecting abnormalities in the direction and type of flow. Arteriography may be required for accurate assessment of vessel anatomy.

## NEURAL

### Motor testing

An evaluation of muscle power is required. It is particularly important in the assessment of peripheral nerve injuries to be aware of trick movements.

### *Median nerve*

**Thumb abduction.** The thumb is placed in the abducted position and the patient is asked to maintain it there while the examiner tests for active contraction of the belly of abductor pollicis

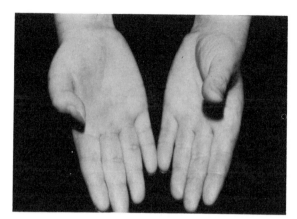

**Fig. 20.5**   Patient showing a median nerve palsy on the right hand where there is inability to abduct the thumb, as shown on the left hand

brevis. If the patient abducts both thumbs against each other, early weakness may be detected (Fig. 20.5).

*Thumb opposition.* Opposition of the thumb occurs when the thumb is abducted and then flexed across the palm. In pure abduction the metacarpal pronates. This can be seen by looking at the thumb nail. When adducted against the side of the index finger the thumb nail lies at right angles to the index finger nail. In palmar abduction a considerable amount of pronation has

occurred (approximately 65–70°) and thus when the metacarpal is flexed across the palm, pulp-to-pulp opposition is possible. Opposition will not occur without this automatic metacarpal rotation on abduction of the thumb (Fig. 20.6).

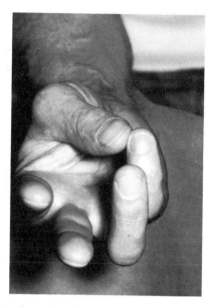

**Fig. 20.6**   Opposition of the thumb, as viewed from the distal end of the hand. One can see quite clearly that the nail of the thumb has pronated through some 60° from its normal position lying at the side of the hand and at 90° to the plane of the palm of the hand. Opposition involves metacarpal rotation

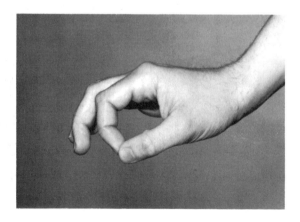

a

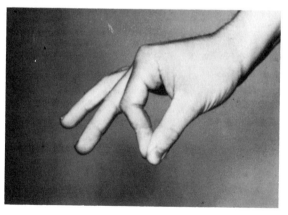

b

**Fig. 20.7**   a The normal hand is capable of forming an 'O' between the thumb and the index finger. To do this, the action of flexor pollicis longus and flexor digitorum profundus to the index is required. In anterior interosseous palsy, both of these muscles are paralysed and hyperextension occurs at both the interphalangeal joint of the thumb and the distal interphalangeal joint of the index finger as shown in **b**

*Anterior interosseous*

The anterior interosseous nerve can be tested by asking the patient to make the 'O' sign between the index and thumb. In order to do this contraction of the index profundus and flexor pollicis longus is necessary. Both of these muscles are innervated by the anterior interosseous nerve, Inability to flex either the tip of the thumb or the tip of the index finger may indicate an anterior interosseous nerve palsy (Fig. 20.7).

*Ulnar nerve*

In general the ulnar nerve supplies the small muscles of the hand with the exception of some thenar muscles. The palmar interossei are responsible for adduction of the fingers and each of these can be tested in turn. The dorsal interossei are responsible for abduction. When testing for interosseous function it is important that the whole of the forearm is placed on the examining table with the wrist in neutral and the digits unable to flex or extend from the table. Attempted digital extension can be prevented by the examiner exerting a slight degree of compression on the proximal interphalangeal joint. Abduction and adduction trick movements are common and the interossei must be tested with care. Abductor digiti minimi

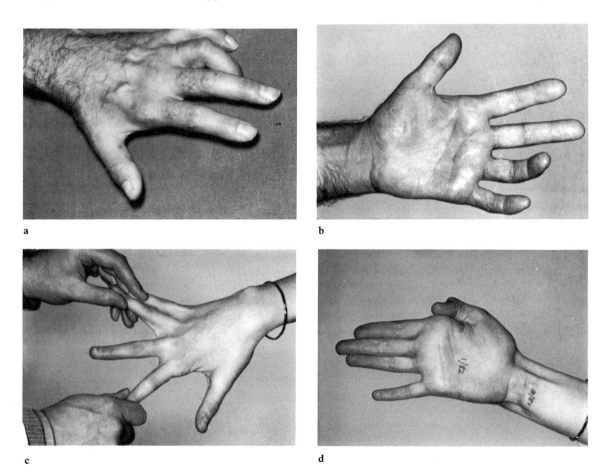

a        b

c        d

**Fig. 20.8** Ulnar nerve palsy. **a** Wasting of the first dorsal interosseous and the remaining interossei can be seen, as well as clawing in a low ulnar nerve palsy. **b** The palmar view of the same hand, displaying clawing, and flattening in the palm of the hand due to interosseous palsy. **c** The patient is unable to move the middle finger from side to side. Each digit is tested in turn to assess dorsal and palmar interosseous function. **d** A patient recovering from an ulnar nerve lesion, in whom the Tinel has just reached the proximal palmar crease. Wartenburg's sign is still positive, due to paralysis of the fourth palmar interosseous, preventing adduction of the little finger

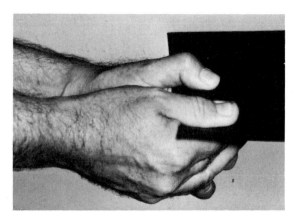

**Fig. 20.9** Froment's test. Due to paralysis of the adductor of the thumb, key pinch can only be maintained by the use of flexor pollicis longus, as seen in the left hand which suffers from an ulnar nerve palsy

can apparently tense and abduct the finger (despite being paralysed), due to powerful wrist flexion and metacarpophalangeal joint hyperextension (Fig. 20.8).

*Froment's test.* The patient is asked to grasp a firm object between the thumb and the side of the index finger in the key grip position. If the adductor is paralysed the patient will use flexor pollicis longus. Pronounced flexion occurs at the interphalangeal joint of the thumb. However it should be noted that this is the mechanism of key grip in some patients and that they may therefore exhibit this sign despite normal ulnar nerve function (Fig. 20.9).

*Radial nerve*

Testing brachioradialis, extensor carpi radialis longus and brevis will demonstrate function in the radial nerve above the elbow. All the other extensors are supplied by the posterior interosseous nerve distal to the elbow. Thus an injury to the posterior interosseous nerve will affect thumb and finger extension. Wrist extension still occurs but the hand is radially deviated. Extensor carpi ulnaris is paralysed but extensor carpi radialis longus functions (Fig. 20.10).

Objective assessment of the active and passive range of movement on each outpatient visit will determine where progress is being made. Muscle

power may be objectively determined using dynamometers (Fig. 20.10).

**Sensory testing**

*The acutely injured nerve*

**The plastic pen test.** The plastic pen test is the most useful test in acute nerve injuries. A plastic pen is stroked across the area under investigation. Resistance to the movement of the pen is greater in normally innervated skin which sweats; in denervated areas the pen slides freely over the dry skin (Fig. 20.2).

*The repaired nerve*

Some patients will describe an immediate improvement in sensation following repair. Such comments are normally received with scepticism by attending medical staff. This symptom disappears 2 or 3 days later with the onset of Wallerian degeneration, but conduction of impulses across recently repaired nerves has been demonstrated in research animals and in man.

*Tinel sign.* The Tinel sign only becomes apparent several weeks after nerve repair. It is believed to be related to the advancing margin of regenerating axon sprouts. These cross the nerve interface approximately 1 month after injury. On average, subsequent advancement is at a rate of only 1 mm a day. An advancing Tinel's sign is not usually detected until 6 weeks after repair at the earliest. Percussion of the nerve is initiated distally, moving proximally towards the site of injury. The distance from the site of injury, at which percussion gives rise to tingling within the distal distribution of the nerve, is noted at each visit. The rate of advance may be thus determined. A comparison should be made between the relative strengths of the advancing Tinel and the static Tinel at the nerve repair site. If the advancing Tinel is more pronounced it implies good axonal regeneration. If the static Tinel exceeds the advancing Tinel it indicates axonal entrapment in scar tissue at the repair site. The prognosis is less favourable. With the passage of time a point is reached when the advancing Tinel sign comes to the fingertips and disappears.

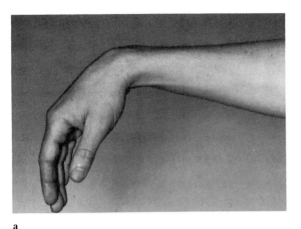

a

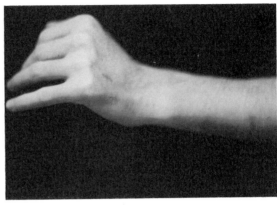

b

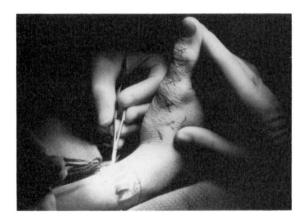

c

**Fig. 20.10**  **a** The position adopted in a radial nerve palsy. The patient is unable to extend both the wrist and the fingers and thumb. **b** Posterior interosseous palsy due to laceration over the extensor muscle mass. The patient is able to extend the wrist but it is deviated in a radial direction, due to the unopposed action of extensor carpi radialis longus. However, digital and thumb extension are not possible. A tenodesis test is necessary in patients who are unable to extend their fingers to exclude the possibility of tendon damage. **c** A more distal radial nerve injury involving the terminal branch of the radial nerve and leading to loss of sensation over the dorsal aspect of the thumb and first web space

Sensory improvement can then be expected at the fingertips. A margin of advancing sensation creeps distally with the Tinel sign. The patient is hyperaesthetic at this margin and his response to moving light touch is exaggerated. The hyperaesthetic margin advances to the fingertip and is immediately followed by the development of spontaneous tingling within the areas it has vacated. This settles, leaving paraesthesia in response to moving light touch stimulation. Later, moving light touch is interpreted as touch, but it feels distant. It is as though the patient is being touched through a glove, or through thickened skin. Protective sensation then develops, with the patient able to withdraw from noxious stimuli such as pain and extremes of temperature. Interpretation of pin prick may be delayed and altered in quality, as is interpretation of heat. Appreciation of warmth is initially delayed but slowly improves and is followed by a return of discriminating sensation. The patient can distinguish between textures. It is only at this stage that tests of discriminating function are appropriate (Fig. 20.11).

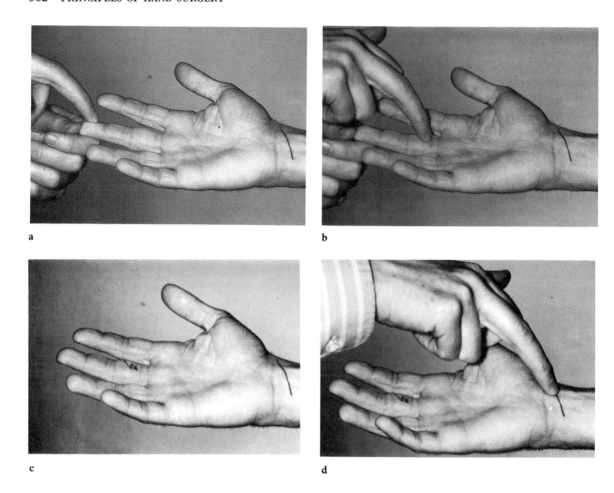

a       b

c       d

**Fig. 20.11** The Tinel test. **a** Percussion is commenced distally at the fingertip, in one of the involved fingertips of the median nerve. The patient has a laceration of the wrist (marked in ink) and loss of sensation in median nerve territory. Percussion is continued proximally until a point is reached as in **b**, in which the patient experiences a sensation like an electric shock. This point is then noted as in **c** and a distance from the scar site is measured on serial visits. In this way the Tinel sign can be seen to advance. The advancing Tinel sign is then compared with a Tinel sign which is elicited over the scar site in **d**

*Two-point discrimination.* Dellon's moving two-point discrimination test can be used prior to re-establishment of static two-point discrimination (Fig. 20.12).

A paper clip or two-point discriminator is gently applied to the distal pulp and drawn proximally over the skin, producing virtually no indentation. The gap between the stimulating blunt ends is increased if no response is obtained and the area retested after an interval of at least 3 seconds. In the static test the clip is applied gently without producing indentation and a measurement is taken when the patient first indicates that he can distinguish two points.

*Ridging.* The use of the ridging device gives a further indication of sensory function (Fig. 20.13). It should be noted that two-point discrimination and ridging tests are difficult to perform, difficult to interpret, and difficult to replicate. These tests only partially quantify sensory recovery; their interpretation is difficult and their significance indeterminate.

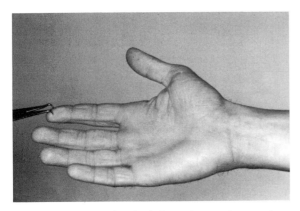

**Fig. 20.12** A two-point discriminator is moved across the pulp to determine the smallest distance between the two points at which they can be appreciated.

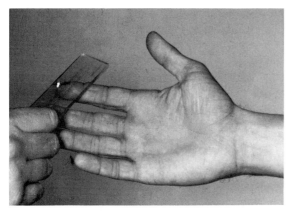

**Fig. 20.13** The ridging device being used to assess sensation. It is drawn across the digits in an oscillating manner and the point at which the patient first notices the ridge is determined and compared with other areas

## MUSCLE TESTING

An assessment of *passive joint mobility* is an essential preliminary to muscle testing ensuring that there are no skin or joint contractures. *Muscle wasting* may be noted in advanced nerve lesions and *postural deformities* such as clawing or wrist drop may be observed. The presence of *muscle contractures* should be excluded. The first web space and the interossei should be carefully examined and accessible muscle bellies should be palpated for induration. The long flexors should be fully

stretched by simultaneous dorsiflexion of the wrist and extension of the fingers to exclude the presence of muscle shortening or adhesions. The long extensors should be tested by simultaneously flexing the wrist and digits. The interossei should also be tested (Fig. 20.14). *The principle of testing for a muscle contracture is to put the hand in the position in which the muscle concerned is maximally stretched.* Thus for the interossei muscles which flex the metacarpophalangeal joints and extend the interphalangeal joints, contractures are detected by inability to flex the interphalangeal joints fully and simultaneously extend the metacarpophalangeal joints.

*Voluntary power* in the muscles should then be assessed. The surgeon knows the main action of each muscle to be tested. He should, therefore, not waste time and risk misunderstanding, explaining to the patient the task he would like performed. Instead, he should perform the movement for the patient, and then instruct the patient to 'keep it in that position and don't let me move it'. Any attempt that the examiner then makes to move the part will call into action the muscles he wishes to test. The surgeon should be observing and palpating the muscle under test. A comparison should then be made with the contralateral limb. All the individual muscles below the elbow can be seen or felt contracting, with the exception of supinator, opponens pollicis, adductor pollicis, lumbricals, the palmar interossei, pronator quadratus and opponens digiti minimi. It is important to be aware of *trick movements*. These are performed by other active muscles giving the impression of activity in a paralysed muscle. *Common trick movements are:*

1. Apparent active flexion of the interphalangeal joints of the thumb caused by the tenodesis effect acting on the flexor pollicis longus tendon associated with dorsiflexion of the wrist.
2. Active extension of the interphalangeal joints of the thumb by the action of abductor pollicis brevis, often in association with wrist flexion.
3. Apparent active abduction of the fingers occurring as a normal accompaniment to active extension of the metacarpophalangeal joints by the long extensors rather than the interossei.
4. Apparent activity of abductor digiti minimi

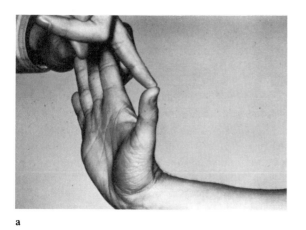

a

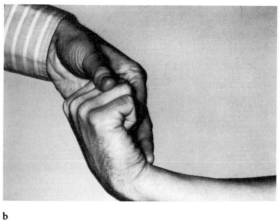

b

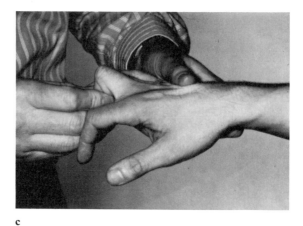

c

**Fig. 20.14**    **a** Extension of the wrist and digits to detect the presence of any flexion contractures. **b** Flexion of the wrist and fingers to test for the presence of any extensor contractures. **c** Extension of the metacarpal joint of the digit plus flexion of the proximal interphalangeal joint to test for the presence of intrinsic contracture. A refinement of this is then to deviate the digit both to the radial and the ulnar direction. Patients with rheumatoid arthritis may have tightness limited to the ulnar intrinsics

due to powerful wrist flexion and metacarpophalangeal joint extension. Flexor carpi ulnaris pulls on the pisiform, tensing the abductor digiti minimi, thus giving the impression of active contraction.

If the muscle bellies are normal, attention should be directed towards the tendons and their surrounding synovial tissue. Inflammation of this lining membrane gives rise to tenosynovitis in which a painful creaking is noticed on active movement of the tendon. This is particularly important in the assessment of patients with rheumatoid arthritis. The swelling of dorsal synovitis

is usually obvious but more minor synovial thickening can be detected by resting the examiner's hand on the dorsum of the wrist and asking the patient to move his fingers. Palpation of the flexor tendons in the fingers and palm may also reveal crepitus. Examination of the digital theca area for synovitis is usually accomplished by Saville's test. Normally it is possible to tent the skin away from the underlying tendon sheath when palpating the sides of the digit between finger and thumb. If there is synovitis, Saville's test reveals a doughy consistency and the normal yielding to pressure is absent.

Finklestein described a test for the diagnosis of De Quervain's tenosynovitis of the thumb, in which gentle ulnar deviation of the carpus with the thumb joints flexed, provokes discomfort over the radial styloid area. The test may cause some discomfort in a normal wrist and a comparison between the two sides is informative.

## SKELETAL EXAMINATION

Palpation of the skeleton should be undertaken, and areas of localised pain noted. Fractures are diagnosed from radiographs and the demonstration of crepitus is both painful and unnecessary. The stability of all relevant joints should be assessed and the active and passive ranges of motion noted. X-rays, bone scans, computerised axial tomography and nuclear magnetic imaging all have roles to play.

## SUMMARY

The assessment of the hand must always be pertinent. Examination of the acutely traumatised hand differs from the examination of the same hand 3 months later, when secondary surgery is being considered. The initial examination requires assessment of viability, skeletal stability, integrity of the skin and gross tendon and nerve function, to determine whether surgical intervention is necessary. In the immediate postoperative phase the examination is concerned with skin viability and wound healing. The presence of infection, swelling, or signs of reflex sympathetic dystrophy, are relevant, as they may delay rehabilitation. When the wound is healed and the hand is soft and supple, the examiner turns his attention towards signs of functional recovery. Is sensory recovery adequate? Can the patient make a flat hand? Is key grip possible? Is power grip or precision grip effective? The effect of such disabilities on the patient's occupation, hobbies and interests should be noted. In the presence of functional impairment, reconstructive procedures may be considered. A detailed assessment is then required to analyse the individual function of all the remaining parts. Thus, examination of the hand should not be performed as a monotonous routine but should be pertinent to the clinical situation.

# Index